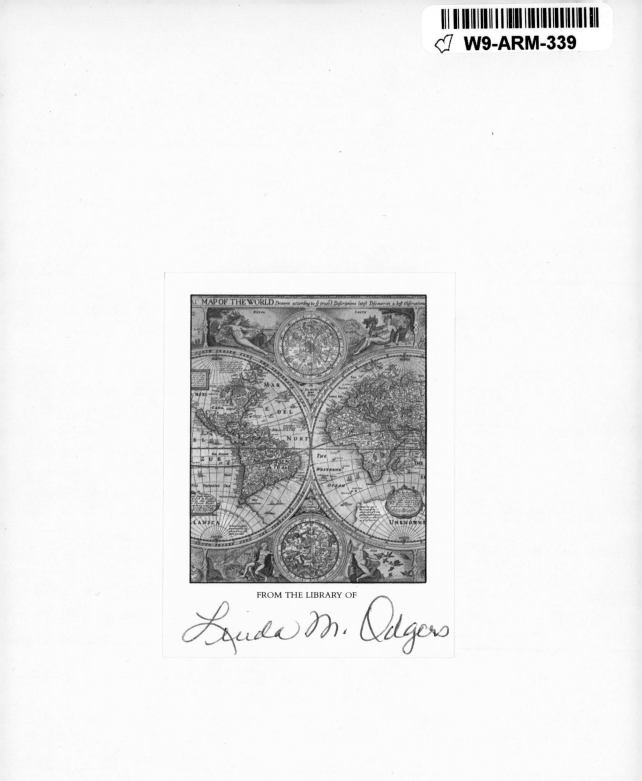

FROM THE LIBRARY OF

Linda M. Odgers

NURSING ADMINISTRATION
in the hospital health
care system

NURSING ADMINISTRATION
in the hospital health care system

EDYTHE L. ALEXANDER, R.N., M.A.

Nursing Consultant,
Hospital Patient Care Systems,
New York, New York;
formerly Assistant Executive Director,
Allegheny General Hospital,
Pittsburgh, Pennsylvania

SECOND EDITION

with 43 illustrations

THE C. V. MOSBY COMPANY

Saint Louis   1978

SECOND EDITION

Copyright © 1978 by The C. V. Mosby Company

All rights reserved. No part of this book may be reproduced in any manner without written permission of the publisher.

Previous edition copyrighted 1972

Printed in the United States of America

The C. V. Mosby Company
11830 Westline Industrial Drive, St. Louis, Missouri 63141

Library of Congress Cataloging in Publication Data

Alexander, Edythe Louise.
  Nursing administration in the hospital health
care system.

  Bibliography: p.
  Includes index.
  1. Nursing service administration.   2. Hospital
care.   I. Title. [DNLM: 1. Organization and
administration.   2. Hospital nursing service.
3. Nursing, Supervisory. WY105 A375n]
RT89.A43 1978   658'.91'61073   77-18114
ISBN 0-8016-0110-X

TS/CB/B   9   8   7   6   5   4   3   2   1

PREFACE

The second edition of *Nursing Administration in the Hospital Health Care System* has been revised completely in order to update the contents of this book in relation to recent events and concepts that are influencing the clinical and management roles of nurses in a hospital environment.

This book is designed for nurses who are preparing themselves for a managerial role at any level in a nursing service organization, for self-study, and as resource material for those in workshops or seminars on the management (administration) of nursing services in patient care. Although the material focuses on the programs and actions within a hospital, many of the concepts are applicable to nurses' roles in other health institutions.

The purpose of the book is to assist the reader in gaining more awareness of the factors affecting problems of how to manage, plan, organize, coordinate, communicate, and control the behavioral actions of people, as well as the material and financial resources of organizations. With the application of scientific technology and medical sophistication in patient care services, the nurse-manager at any level needs the knowledge and capabilities to relate current role concepts to achieve desired outcomes in quality patient care and must understand the meaning of leadership in resolving problems with others.

Current literature and periodicals have presented many suggestions by individuals and professional health organizations concerning the role of nursing and the improvement of nursing services. This book is designed to contribute to their efforts. The references at the end of each chapter indicate the valuable contributions of others.

This book is not intended to be a panacea for all nursing care and service problems. It is not intended to serve as a strictly "how-to-do-it" book. It is an attempt to present information in an operational way by relating concepts and methodology to the management of nursing service input for the achievement of desired outcomes. This book does not present theoretical and educational content of staff development and nursing research programs. The literature offers valuable guidelines.

Chapters 1 through 5 provide a frame of reference concerning the concepts of administration from the past to the present time in our society. These chapters present factors influencing nursing service programs and actions, such as actions by legislative and controlling bodies, standards of the practice of nursing and services, introduction of many categories of workers, and collective bargaining by nurses.

Chapters 6 through 8 focus on administrative theories and principles and the need to define goals and objectives, as well as to plan and make appropriate decisions concerning the behavioral actions of personnel. The process of organizing nursing service resources within a viable dynamic structure is discussed to achieve both organizational and personal goals of staff members.

Because an effective communication system is crucial to achieve objectives and establish a collegial approach to decision making, Chapters 11 and 12 emphasize the mechanisms and methodologies to coordinate, direct, and control activities related to nursing problems, assignment and staffing, budgeting, quality assurance, and performance evaluation.

I am aware that there is no one best structure, method, or leadership style in the management of people and things. However, I hope that this book will assist professional nurses in developing their managerial roles for the achievement of the goal of nursing: providing good individualized care for patients at a reasonable price.

I wish to express my appreciation to the many nurses, physicians, and administrators who provided ideas and criticisms that helped me in writing this book, as well as professional organizations, authors, and their publishers for permission to use their material to illustrate a management concept. A very special thanks to Hadley Smith who gave of herself so graciously in the preparation of this manuscript.

Edythe L. Alexander

CONTENTS

1 | Emergence of nursing in the hospital system

In affluent nations the costly, complex, and technological approach to the delivery of medical and hospital services is an expansion of the road that has been traveled in the history of health care. The famous trilogy of theology, law, and medicine has been replaced by many specialites in various professions.

The advances and setbacks of medicine, nursing, and hospitals have been and continue to be closely associated with the cultural, political, and socioeconomic forces in each society. In addition, values, ethics, intellectual thought, and education have influenced nursing, medical status, and the role of hospitals in each society.

History indicates that many new concepts and procedures are sophistications of those of the past. Understanding the forces that have shaped our present medical and nursing professions and the hospital care system will help to explain their existing strengths and weaknesses and provide direction for the future.[1,26]

THE BEGINNING OF NURSING STANDARDS

The first breakthrough in medical isolation in Europe came with the translation of writings from the Brahmanic and Arabic. The fundamental Indian medical text is that of Susruta, declared as ancient in A.D. 400. The book of Charaka, written around A.D. 100, defines a nurse's ethical standards and responsibilities:

The Physician, Drugs, Nurse, and Patient, constitute an aggregate of four . . . . Knowledge of the manner in which drugs should be prepared or compounded for administration, cleverness, devotedness to the patient waited upon and purity (of both mind and body) are the four qualifications of the Attending Nurse.*

In discussing the type of building necessary, he further states:

This should be secured a body of attendants (nurses) of good behavior distinguished for purity or cleanliness of habits, . . . possessed of cleverness and skill, endued with kindness, skilled in every kind of service that a patient may require, competent to cook food and curries, clever in bathing and washing a patient, well-conversant in rubbing or pressing the limbs; or raising the patient, or assisting him in walking or moving about, well-skilled in making or cleaning beds, competent to pound drugs, or ready patients, and skillful in waiting upon one that is ailing, and never unwilling to do any act that they may be commanded (by the physician or the patient) to do.*

In ancient times, Susruta pointed out that "A qualified physician is alone capable of relieving the pain of many a suffering patient, just as only a helmsman is capable of taking his boat across a river without the help and cooperation of a single oarsman."* In most situations today the physician may be thought of as the patient's skipper. Caring for patients is accomplished through the efforts of many professionals and other members of the team. Each professional must be able to function effectively in his or her discipline. All members coordinate their in-

---

*From Charaka-Samhita, translated by Kaviray Avinash Chandra Kaviratna, vols. 1-4, Calcutta, 1890-1925, published by the translator. (Austin, A. L.: History of nursing source book: a compilation of selections from original documents, New York, 1957, G. P. Putnam's Sons, pp. 26-28.)

dependent responsibilities with other members of the team to provide quality care for their patients.

Susruta also stated his ideas about the qualifications of the so-called nurse: "that person alone is fit to nurse or to attend the bedside of a patient, who is cool-headed and pleasant in his demeanor, does not speak ill of anybody, is strong and attentive to the requirements of the sick, and strictly and indefatigably follows the instructions of the physician."* Susruta's writings do indicate the existence of a hospital hierarchy and a division of labor—some were delegated to give direct care, some to do the cleaning, and others to prepare the food. It is interesting to compare Susruta's ideas with the present management of nursing care concepts and the professional code formulated by the American Nurses' Association.[3] The code states:

1. The nurse provides services with respect for human dignity and the uniqueness of the client unrestricted by considerations of social or economic status, personal attributes, or the nature of health problems.

2. The nurse safeguards the client's right to privacy by judiciously protecting information of a confidential nature.

3. The nurse acts to safeguard the client and the public when health care and safety are affected by the incompetent, unethical, or illegal practice of any person.

4. The nurse assumes responsibility and accountability for individual nursing judgments and actions.

5. The nurse maintains competence in nursing.

6. The nurse exercises informed judgment and uses individual competence and qualifications as criteria in seeking consultation, accepting responsibilities, and delegating nursing activities to others.

7. The nurse participates in activities that contribute to the ongoing development of the profession's body of knowledge.

8. The nurse participates in the profession's efforts to implement and improve standards of nursing.

9. The nurse participates in the profession's efforts to establish and maintain conditions of employment conducive to high quality nursing care.

10. The nurse participates in the profession's effort to protect the public from misinformation and misrepresentation and to maintain the integrity of nursing.

11. The nurse collaborates with members of the health professions and other citizens in promoting community and national efforts to meet the health needs of the public.*

State nurses associations and districts should form committees to establish policies and procedures for the investigation of code violations. A code for nurses focuses on areas of accountability that nurses choose to accept because of personal integrity to clients and to the community.

PATIENT CARE IN THE EARLY CHRISTIAN ERA

The patient care concept was a synthesis of Greek medicine and Christian ideals. The parable of the Good Samaritan was applied in caring for each patient, and the attitude of *ministering* to a patient developed. The most unpleasant activity was ennobled by a sense of dedication to the individual in need of care. The emphasis on personalized service was based on the ascetic belief that caring for the poor, blind, or crippled was a way of atoning for one's sins.

In the early Middle Ages, medical care existed outside of the body. The medicine man carefully guarded the little knowledge he had and concealed his ignorance behind his superior judgment and authority. The lay healers and practitioners used the herbs they believed appropriate for their patients, and clung to their old superstitions. The monks carried out minor surgery and blood letting.

---

*From Charaka-Samhita, translated by Kaviray Avinash Chandra Kaviratna, vols. 1-4, Calcutta, 1890-1925, published by the translator. (Austin, A. L.: History of nursing source book: a compilation of selections from original documents, New York, 1957, G. P. Putnam's Sons, p. 28.)

*From American Nurses' Committee on Ethical, Legal, and Professional Standards: The 1976 revised code for nurses with interpretive statements, pub. no. G-56R25M, Kansas City, Mo., 1976. The Association. Reprinted with the permission of the American Nurses' Association.

Design and management of monastery infirmaries

Monasteries' infirmaries were designed with separate buildings for the acutely ill, the lepers, the mentally ill, those with chronic ailments, and the ambulatory patients. This was the beginning of separation of patients in relation to their severity of illness and type of health problems.

The St. Benedict Order of management was established in most infirmaries.[1,5] The abbesses came to be respected for their ability as administrators. The sisters and lay sisters cared for the patients; the latter bathing patients, making beds, changing bed linens, and housekeeping. The hierarchical pattern of delegation of duties promoted the traditional organizational structure that has been adapted by hospitals for centuries.

Design and management of the knights hospitalers

The authoritarian system of hospitals stems from the Knights Hospitalers established during the eleventh and twelfth centuries. These hospitals were built primarily to care for military casualties of the Crusades. Statutes, sanitary regulations, engineering innovations, and the organizational structure contributed to improved care. Lavatories were built outside the hospital. A pure water supply was brought to the hospital by an aqueduct system. Drainage canals were constructed for water overflow.

In Rhodes, Greece, the Knights set up a health commission to prevent the spread of epidemics. The regulations included a 40-day quarantine period for those who had come in contact with a victim. This practice began epidemiology as a branch of medicine.

The overall management of the Knights Hospitalers was delegated to a commander. He was responsible for caring for sick cheerfully without grumbling and complaining. Sergeants were assigned to each ward, and their duties posted. One of their duties was to wash the feet of a patient upon admission, for religious and symbolic, rather than sanitary, reasons. In general, the sergeants cared for the sick. The convalescent patients were given considerable freedom as long as they did not disturb the sick patients or the staff.

The physicians were a part of the staff. They were required to examine urine, diagnose disease, administer the appropriate medications, and visit patients at least twice a day. On rounds, the physician was accompanied by a brother (secretary). An interesting innovation was the placement of a board at the head of each bed. The brother wrote the physician's orders on it as dictated by the physician. This management plan contributed to the beginning role of the army nurse and the nurse in civilian hospitals.

PATIENT CARE IN THE MIDDLE AGES

With the rapid spread of sickness and increased religious fervor, many church and some secular orders were established to care for the poor, elderly, and disabled. The affluent were cared for in their homes.

Under the influence of early Christianity, hospitals proliferated as refuges for travelers and victims of disaster. In 542 the Hôtel-Dieu was founded in Lyons, France. Many hospitals were established along the Crusade routes (1091-1291). In London the St. Bartholomew (1137), St. Thomas (1200), and St. Mary of Bethlehem (1247) Hospitals were established.

In the fourteenth century when the Black Death spread across Europe, hospitals began to concentrate their efforts on the treatment of the sick and injured rather than the aged, orphaned, and poor. The main objectives of the hospitals shifted to focus on the protection of healthy individuals by admitting those infected with a known dangerous disease.

The public, in general, knew little of what took place in the hospitals. Patients were cut off from communication with the outside either because they were friendless or because there were restrictions on visitors. Officers and staff disliked the intrusion of outsiders, who were prejudiced against hospitals because of the neglect, poor treatment, and high incidence of death, primarily due to infection, that occurred.

The Reformation resulted in further stagnation of European medicine and a resurgence of priestly medicine, especially in England, where the Reformation was more closely connected to the conflict of church and state than was the Reformation on the continent. The conflict of King Henry VIII with Rome led to the Act of Supremacy in 1534.[6] This act resulted in a firm rejection of papal control. Most of the monasteries' infirmaries and charitable institutions were closed and secular and state hospitals were opened.

They were miserable, damp, dark, dirty places overrun by pests. Hospital care sank to its lowest ebb. Frequently three or more persons shared one bed without regard to type of disease, degree of illness, age, or sex. Medical practice was no better than the administration of the institution.

Women of little education and social background were hired to work in these hospitals. These women received little or no training by their peers or physicians. Due to tremendous public criticism the St. Bartholomew and St. Thomas hospitals in London were reopened to treat the sick and injured.[28,30]

The Renaissance, the rebirth of classical thought and creativity, had an everlasting impact on hospital patient care. Many intellectuals began to explore the sciences, and from their enlightened attitude and benevolence, philanthropy emerged. Inspired intellectuals and the wealthy groups directed their energies, ideas, efforts, and money toward improvement of hospital patient care.

Emergence of medical training programs

Beginning in the 1420s, there occurred a great revolution in medical training based on medical theory and practice. The number of medical schools increased throughout Europe and laws were passed to prevent lay healers and practitioners from practicing medicine. Restrictions also were placed on healers and monks who used surgical tools. The lay practitioners and healers of the 14th century did not understand the relationship between medical theory and practice.[28]

In many European countries, physicians

and surgeons formed two groups of healers. Physicians were concerned with internal medical problems and thought it undignified to use their hands as surgeons did. In England, surgery was delegated to university-trained surgeons and barber-surgeons who previously had been monks' assistants. The Union of Surgeons and Barbers existed until 1800, when the present Royal College of Surgeons was founded.[14]

PATIENT CARE IN EARLY AMERICAN HOSPITALS

Beginning about 1700, a significant characteristic trend of the early voluntary hospital was the care of the acutely ill. The so called charity hospitals were organized, controlled, and supported by influential and wealthy people in the cities. The objectives and concepts of patient care initiated in most American hospitals were those of the European settlers of the 16th and 17th centuries, who instituted their own traditions and concepts of patient care. Some hospitals were church controlled; others were state supported or secular voluntary hospitals. In seaport towns such as Boston, Philadelphia, or New York, hospitals or places of refuge were first established for the care of shipboard victims of contagious diseases, indigents, the insane, and criminals. Conditions in these first American hospitals were not much better than those in European medieval times.[11]

INFLUENCE OF THE INDUSTRIAL REVOLUTION ON HOSPITAL SERVICES

From the middle of the 18th century to the middle of the 19th century the Industrial Revolution contributed to dramatic socioeconomic changes through inventions and technological innovations. The factory system was created.

Hospitals were influenced by the forces of industrialism, capitalism, and enlightened despotism and other political and social currents, as well as private initiative and cooperative action of some individuals. Medical practices also paralleled the growth of hospitals.

The scientific and technological advances,

along with the socioeconomic forces of society, began to change methods of medical treatment, as well as the environment of the hospital. In 1842, Dr. Crawford Long of Georgia demonstrated the use of anesthesia in surgery. The application and development of Pasteur's discoveries, Joseph Lister's aseptic principles, Edison's invention of the incandescent light, Roentgen's discovery of the x-ray—all these inventions and other scientific advances produced a great need for better hospital management and better controls of medical and surgical patient care services.

In Great Britain the laboring population, formerly employed predominantly in agriculture, gathered increasingly in cities. Capitalism began on a large scale, and a new type of commercial entrepreneur developed from the old class of merchant adventurers. An expanding middle class and a wealthier population demanded better hospitals.

Emergence of the not-for-profit hospital

The "charity" (voluntary) hospital became important in the cities as a place where people who were sick would be cared for and treated. To many physicians it was an important place to gain new medical knowledge and skills and an opportunity to use the skills of others in an apprenticeship system of training. For the trained, qualified physicians the hospital was a place where they could win honors or renown that would open the way to professional success.

It was also believed that the hospital, unlike a business enterprise, could be managed by a lay person who had little understanding of business matters, physical sciences, or human relations.

In these hospitals the nursing personnel worked long hours and carried out many oppressive duties. They were motivated by a feeling of dedication stemming from the ascetic concepts of the medieval period. Exploitation of student nurses resulted in a new set of circumstances. The concern of physicians of the time for competent nurses is revealed in many historical writings.[25] Fuller,[5] a Scottish physician, discussed the qualifications of the nurse as follows:

Of a Middle Age, fit and able to go through with the necessary Fatigue of her Undertaking.

Healthy, especially free from Vapours, and Cough.

A good Watcher, that can hold fitting up the whole Course of the Sickness.

Quick in Hearing, and always ready at the first call.

Quiet and Still, so as to talk low, and but little, and tread softly.

Of good Sight, to observe the Pocks and their Colour, Manner, and Growth and all Alterations that may happen.

Handy to do everything the best way, without Blundering and Noise.

Nimble and Quick agoing, coming, and doing everything.

Cleanly, to make all she dresseth acceptable.

Well-tempered to humour, and please the Sick as much as she can.

Cheerful and Pleasant; to make the best of Everything, without being at any time Cross, Melancholy, or Timorous.

Constantly Careful, and diligent by Night and by Day.

Sober and Temperate, not given to Gluttony, Drinking, or Smoaking.

Observant to follow the Physician's orders duly; and not be so conceited of her own Skill, as to give her own Medicines privately.

To have no Children, or others to come much after her.*

In the eighteenth and nineteenth centuries many of Dr. Fuller's qualifications for nurses were accepted by hospital staff, physicians and patients.

NURSING, A PART OF THE HOSPITAL SYSTEM

With the expansion of medical care for patients, the need for nursing assistance became an urgent reality. Beginning in 1873, hospitals established schools to train women in the care of the sick. The students were expected to give nursing care and other services to patients to the extent that their

---

*From Fuller, T.: Exanthematologia; or a rational account of eruptive fevers, London, 1930, Charles Revington, pp. 209-210 (Austin, A. L.: History of nursing source book, New York, 1957, G. P. Putnam's Sons, p. 118.)

service hours interfered with their training classes and personal self-development. Nursing involved the dichotomous goals of training prospective nurses and meeting existing nursing care needs of patients. Nursing education became closely identified with and controlled by the hospital.

The charity hospital became important to society for several reasons:

1. The cure and care of patients with low incomes
2. The education and training of physicians
3. Continued medical training

At the International Hospital Congress in 1961, Giordina,[16] speaking on the role of nursing in hospital care said:

If Napoleon had emphasized the military importance of nurses, as he did doctors, if the Crimean War had been fought 20 years earlier, if Florence Nightingale had started her work in a civilian organization instead of in the Army, scientific nursing would probably have been firmly established in the hospital long before the physician made it his workshop for teaching and research . . . instead of being the servant girl to medicine, nursing would in that case have entered into an equal partnership with medical practice, both serving the patient from different sources of knowledge and skill as Florence Nightingale originally hoped to achieve.*

The introduction of trained nurses and students created conflicts between the physicians, older experienced nurses, and the hospital administrators. In the beginning of the 19th century the hospital behavioral environment was such that the director of nursing, known as the matron, had to establish her own power system to accomplish what she considered to be her duties in the care of patients. Working in an autocratic, paternalistic environment, the matron centralized the administration of nursing services and took over many medical and hospital management responsibilities. This centralization of authority lowered the status and responsibility of other nurses.[30]

*From Giordina, Camillo: Role of nursing in hospital care. In Proceedings of the 12th International Hospital Congress: The changing role of the hospital in a changing world, London, 1961, International Hospital Federation, Hospital Center.

The authoritarian and paternalistic approaches were used and reinforced by the directors in nursing. With medical advances in hospitals, industrialism, and demands for socioeconomic improvements by laboring groups, the hospital became more dedicated to the treatment of disease. The physician enjoyed a highly autonomous role in the hospital organization with power to direct its course. Medical power rested on two interrelated complexes of factors: (1) the nature of the organizational structure and (2) the independent professional ideal that focuses on vocational freedom, responsibility to the client, and intellectual and technical capacities and skills unique to the profession.

In this situational environment, socialization conflicts began to confront the nurse, physician, and hospital administrator. The nursing department began to function as an independent department in which the director had a position of authority between the medical staff and the lay administrator, even though the organization primarily was physician directed.

Early nursing schools

During the first period of nursing development (1870-1900) the creativity and independent thinking of the nurse was, to say the least, stifled because of the public concept of a nurse, the social background of the majority of nurses, the inadequate training courses, and the authoritarian system of hospitals. The many demands of caring for patients and many hospital duties during a long workday did not motivate the nurse to study and devise new methods to meet the demands more effectively.

According to Nightingale,[25] the training school of St. Thomas in London was established in 1860 with the primary objective "to produce nurses capable of training others." In describing her achievements she said, "In thirty years I have helped raise nursing from the sink." A review of the St. Thomas nursing curriculum indicates that it was based on the philosophy that education of a nurse involved two distinct qualities—character and knowledge.

During the early years of the 1900s there seemed to be little awareness of the need to develop nursing programs within a university along with other recognized professions. Because of Florence Nightingale's success, by 1897 nursing itself was becoming independent, so much so that a group of nurses proposed the creation of an independent body of examiners, separate from all the training schools, to examine nurses. Any nurse passing the test of the examining board would be entitled to have her name placed on a registry for nurses and be called a registered nurse.

After much opposition, including that of Florence Nightingale, in 1893 the Royal British Nurses' Association was given the only right to the maintenance of a list of persons who applied to have their names entered as nurses. This was the beginning of the establishment of uniform standards for nurses.

Miss Nightingale fought against the restrictions placed on women's activities and the socioeconomic conventions that placed them in subordinate positions. However, the nursing schools were based on her ideas, which were primarily maternalistic. She did not demand a very liberalizing, creative, educational program for nursing students. The St. Thomas School was secular and independent. The administration, the curriculum, and the daily regimen of the students were greatly influenced by Miss Nightingale's own past experience in an apprenticeship nursing program and military nursing in the Crimean War. Unfortunately, the financial independence of the school was not considered an important or essential factor, even though Miss Nightingale and others believed that the education of nurses required financial support as much as other educational programs for the preparation of teachers, physicians, and lawyers.

Until the 1930s most hospital schools of nursing operated merely a so-called in-service training program under the direction and control of the hospital.

EMERGENCE OF CONFLICT BETWEEN MEDICINE AND NURSING

During the development of medical programs for the preparations of physicians, nurses were almost as well educated as the physicians themselves. During the first part of the 20th century, physicians believed that the trained nurse would become discontented with nursing and want to become a physician; therefore, although the physicians realized the great need for more and better nursing care, the majority of them did not support the establishment of training schools. Many of them feared that the trained nurse might supplant them.

In the early 1900s in the United States attempts by nurses to establish the minimum requirement of a high school diploma as a qualification for training were bitterly opposed by most of the medical profession as well as by the hospitals themselves. The wide differences in medical and nursing attitudes and skills created problems in the evaluation of nursing care and promotion of nursing education. They also created professional problems between the well-prepared nurse and the less well-prepared physician with whom she worked.

In the early decades of this century the Ethical code of Nursing was loyalty to the physician at all times in all situations. Aware of the attitude of physicians toward the goals of nursing, nurses in general accepted a status subservient to the physician, such as always standing when a physician entered a room or opening a door for a physician.[6]

EMERGENCE OF MEDICAL ASSOCIATION AND EDUCATION PROGRAMS

In 1870 few of the medical schools required as much as a high school diploma for admission, and none required a bachelor's degree. Most medical programs were not more than 2 years in length, whereas the training program for nursing was soon established as a 3-year program.

The American Medical Association, which was founded in 1847 and reorganized in 1901, established its Council on Medical Education and Hospitals in 1905. The purpose of the council was to establish standards and initiate an ongoing plan for medical schools.

The Flexner Report (1910)[15] on medical education had a most beneficial effect in establishing a cooperative relationship between universities and medical schools in our country. The hospital became a major element in the medical educational process. Thus the emergence of the sciences and medicine began. Many people viewed medicines as more of an art than a science. Few medical students had actual hospital training until the twentieth century. Medical schools in the late 1920s ranged from excellent teaching institutions to commercial diploma enterprizes.

As a result of the Flexner Report, several hundred so-called medical schools were closed, and standards for medical programs were formulated.

The modern voluntary teaching hospitals, along with university-connected medical centers, have continued as focal elements in the formal and informal medical educational process. Under the direction of the Council on Medical Education of the American Medical Association the internship and residency programs have continued to improve in keeping with socioeconomic and medical advances.

The Council's publications, *Essentials of an Approved Internship* and *Essentials of Approved Residencies*, continue to provide current information about qualifications, requirements, and responsibilities of the medical staff and hospital administration.

DEVELOPMENT OF HOSPITAL PATIENT CARE STANDARDS

In 1918 the American College of Surgeons initiated a hospital standards program to help improve American surgery and the conditions affecting the care of patients. By 1951 the one-page sheet of 1918 had become a 147-page manual. The program outgrew the capabilities and financial resources of one organization. The American College of Surgeons realized that such a program required a broad base.[14]

Formation of the Joint Commission on Accreditation of Hospitals

In keeping with the concepts of the American College of Surgeons, the American Medical Association, and the American Hospital Association, the Joint Commission on Accreditation of Hospitals was formed in 1952.[14] The JCAH is an independent, voluntary, nonprofit corporation organized to render public service that aims to assist the hospital and its staff in improving quality of care through education and training and offers suggestions in the application of basic standards in the delivery of patient care. On January 1, 1959, the Canadian Council on Hospital Accreditation assumed full responsibility for accrediting hospitals in Canada. From 1959 on, the JCAH has included representatives from the following health associations: American Medical Association, American College of Surgeons, American College of Physicians, American Hospital Association, American Association of Homes for the Aging, and American Nursing Home Association.

The latter two associations were included in January, 1966, at which time the commission inaugurated a program for extended care facilities. JCAH recommends that hospital policies and regulations should be realistic and in keeping with existing circumstances, yet adhere to established recommended criteria. Its actions are not subject to ratification by the parent bodies. A hospital that desires to be accredited by JCAH must meet a long list of minimum essential standards in relation to facilities, services, and organizations and pay a small fee. A copy of the current standards for hospital accreditation should be in every nursing library.

The quality of nursing service care is influenced by and closely associated with the quality of hospital and medical care. Many nursing leaders and the American Nurses' Association have recommended that nursing services be reviewed in accordance with specific criteria by the JCAH. This is now a reality; however, ANA does not have representatives on the commission. See Chapter 5 for recent JCAH Standards for Nursing Services.

Emergence of the American Hospital Association

The American Hospital Association was formed in 1906 to improve the management of hospitals. It was an outgrowth of the Association of Hospital Superintendents, which was organized in 1898. The AHA has provided leadership in the field of hospital administration. It has directed much of its efforts toward establishing standards of hospital equipment, management training of personnel, development of better rapport with the board of trustees, medical staff, and administrators in hospitals, for financing, construction or remodeling of hospital facilities, and joint planning with federal, state, and local governmental agencies and the public.

The American College of Hospital Administrators is a supplemental branch of the AHA. Its efforts are directed toward upgrading the standard practices of hospital management and promoting hospital administration as a profession through collegiate administration programs in health care, scientific hospital management, and research. In 1934 the University of Chicago offered the first program in hospital administration.

The New York Academy of Medicine Survey

In 1922 the New York Academy of Medicine published a prelminary report of its nursing section's survey of New York hospitals and 52 schools of nursing in Greater New York.[23] This was the first recorded time study of institutional nursing. The Pfefferkorn and Rovetta analysis[27] indicated that hospitalized patients' requirements far exceeded the nursing man-hours available to perform the nursing care activities for each patient. This study also showed the failures of the directors of nursing services and hospital administrators to inform boards of trustees of the poor nursing care rendered and the poor morale of the graduate and student nurses. The study emphasized that such conditions lowered nursing educational standards as well as nursing services, since most of the care was given by students.[29]

At the time of this study not one of the 52 nursing schools in the survey could give cost expenditures showing whether the school was an economic asset or a liability to the hospital that operated it. It has been difficult, some 50 years hence, to secure separate input and output financial figures for the nursing school and nursing service in some hospitals.

NURSING EDUCATION AND STANDARDS
Nursing associations

To protect the public, establish a uniform standard of education, and favor well-trained nurses over poorly trained women in hospitals, the superintendents of nurses realized that unity of nurses was necessary to initiate reforms. At the Congresses held in Chicago during the World's Fair in 1893, one was included for trained nurses, as a subsection of the hospital section of the Congress of the Associated Charities. This first meeting of nurses resulted in the founding of the American Society of Superintendents of Training Schools for Nurses. The aim and objective of this organization was to develop realistic and uniform educational standards and to support the best interests of the nursing profession.[4,22]

Through the efforts of many nurse groups on a state and local level, steps were taken to form a national association. The first meeting of the Associated Alumnae of the United States and Canada was held in April, 1898. This Association represented nurses in patient care services, and the American Society of Superintendents represented the teachers and leaders. To meet the goals of members on state and local levels and provide greater unification within nursing, the Nurses' Associated Alumnae of the United States was changed to the American Nurses' Assocation in May, 1911. Moreover, when the American Society of Superintendents was organized, its membership only included superintendents and assistant superintendents. When state and local sections were organized, its membership was expanded. At the 1972 convention it was agreed to adopt the name National League for Nursing Education. Together these two organizations (ANA and NLNE) worked for reform in nursing care, nurse licensure, educational nursing programs, and better working conditions for nurses.

The Goldmark Study

With advances in medicine, increase in the number of hospital patients, and the new aim of teaching health concepts to citizens in the community to prevent the spread of infectious diseases, many people began to ask questions regarding the need for more trained nurses. The demand for nurses for health teaching, for hospital nursing, and for teaching nursing students was voiced in all states.

In 1918, under the sponsorship of the Rockefeller Foundation, a Committee for the Study of Nursing Education, composed of physicians, nurses, and representatives of hospitals and health agencies, was organized. Mr. C. E. Winslow, head of the Department of Public Health at Yale University, was appointed chairman, and Josephine Goldmark, well-known social researcher, was secretary.[13] The group studied graduate nurses as they were working in the various fields: institutions, private duty, and public health. The Goldmark study, which was published in 1923, brought to light the fact that courses of instruction had received meager attention during the period of rapid expansion. Many nurses in responsible positions had little preparation. Senior students were generally used as head nurses or were kept on night duty for long periods. Students were also sent out on private cases, with the financial return made to the hospital.

The courses of instruction were based on patient's needs of the day, and lectures were frequently modified to comply with the nursing service demands. As a means of remedying deficiencies, some of the Committee's recommendations seem to be most significant, even today. They advocated that through state legislation the definition and licensure of subsidiary grade nursing service workers be determined and that nurses in administrative, supervisory, and teaching positions complete additional courses beyond their basic nursing program. The committee also urged that financial support be given to university schools of nursing. This classic study introduced a methodology for conducting future national studies.

To resolve immediately some of the problems brought to light by the Committee, two endowed university schools of nursing were developed on a college level, independent of hospitals. The Yale University School of Nursing, established in 1923, granted their first bachelor's degrees to two graduates of the school 3 years later. Vanderbilt University School of Nursing (1925) and Western Reserve University School of Nursing (1923) were also pioneers in many experiments in nursing education.[29] The aim of these programs was to develop an educational program to prepare nursing leaders who were scientifically and culturally prepared.

Committee on Grading of Nursing Schools

The second far-reaching 8-year study, initiated by a proposal of the National League for Nursing Education to the Rockefeller Foundation group, resulted in the appointment of a Committee on the Grading of Nursing Schools.[7] Its purpose was to do a cooperative study of nursing practice in all its aspects. Health organizations, all initially interested in the project, elected representatives. William Darrach of the American Medical Association was made chairman of the committee, and Mary Ayres Burgess,[7,8] statistician, became director of the investigation. This study reminds us that over 50 years ago health professionals and educators endeavored to find new ways to increase nursing manpower resources to meet the increasing demands for patients' nursing care requirements at reasonable costs.

The study encompassed three major projects: the first was directed at the supply and demand for graduate nurses, the second was a job analysis of what nurses did and how they might be taught, and the third graded nursing schools. The results of the first project were reported in 1928 in the well-known publication *Nurses, Patients and Pocketbooks.*[8] The findings are still meaningful today because although more nurses are in practice, there are still too few qualified nurses to meet the many demands—the numbers game does not necessarily close the quality gap.

The findings of the second project of the Committee on the Grading of Nursing Schools were reported in 1934 in the publication *An Activity Analysis of Nursing.*[27] The goal of a job analysis of nurses' activities was to discover all activities that constitute nursing. In this report the question of what is good nursing was raised. Opinions of patients, physicians, hospital administrators, and community laymen were studied. The findings showed that patients looked for skill combined with kindness and willingness to adjust to particular duties in any situation. Physicians expected skill, reliability in transfer of information, and personal loyalty. Hospital administrators expressed a need for nurses who would assume responsibility for smooth functioning of their floor or department and interpret the policies and spirit of the hospital.

The third and final report, *Nursing Schools Today and Tomorrow,*[9] was on the grading of nursing schools. A survey approach was used, in which 74% of the schools accredited by the state boards (1,500) participated in the first grading and 81% participated in the second. The findings appearing in *Nursing Schools Today and Tomorrow* showed that the care of patients was considered the chief purpose of the hospitals, with their nursing schools operated as paying service departments and student nurses regarded as employees.

The findings of the grading committee did not provide much new information on proposals other than those the nursing profession had stressed. However, it did furnish factual data that strengthened the arguments for reform. The committee identified four steps that would have to be accomplished to effect both improvement in nursing practices and the education of future nurses.[6,9,22] They recommended (1) reducing the number of students admitted to nursing schools in the United States and raising entrance requirements so that only properly qualified women would gain entrance to the nursing profession; (2) assigning qualified graduate nurses in each hospital unit and delegating to them the responsibility for the nursing care rendered, instead of student nurses; (3) placing schools of nursing under the direction of nurse educators instead of hospital administrators and seeking public funds for the education of nurses; and (4) assisting hospitals in improving the quality of graduate nursing.

Introduction of licensure law

Another immediate outcome of the two national surveys of nursing education by the Rockefeller Foundation and the Committee on the Grading of Nursing Schools was the revision of nurse practice acts. With the increasing number of practical nurses and aides and no set standards for the training of practical nurses, the existing laws did not provide adequate protection for the citizen, physician, or trained nurse.

In New York on 9 November 1899, Sophia F. Palmer of Rochester and Sylveen Nye of Buffalo took the first definite steps to establish state registration of graduate nurses. The first licensure laws enacted were not uniform nationwide, but some regulations were common to all states. In each state the laws provided for a period during which nurses with varying lengths of training could be registered, usually without examination. This protected valuable nurses who trained or practiced prior to the time of the legal enactment. By the early 1900s the nurse licensure laws included provision for the inspection and registration of training schools and gave only the licensee the title of registered nurse with the right to use the initials R.N.[2]

In 1938 the state of New York enacted a law requiring licensing of all who nursed for hire. The law established two groups, one entitled to practice as registered professional nurses, the other as licensed practical nurses. It became unlawful for any person not so licensed to be employed to care for the sick in any capacity in the state of New York. Other states followed with enactment of similar but often less inclusive legislation. With the demand for nurses in World War II, New York and other states temporarily suspended the practice law. Recent proposals to change professional practice acts are discussed in Chapter 4.

INFLUENCE OF WORLD WARS I AND II ON NURSING SERVICE

The government's positive attitude toward the importance of nursing was brought to light in World War I. A permanent Army Nurse Corps was established through congressional action in 1901, and a Navy Nurse Corps was founded in 1908.

World War I

United States entry into World War I resulted in an absence of trained nurses in civilian hospitals and private homes. Under the direction of Jane Delano, the establishment of classes for women in the home was advocated so that they could care for the sick at home and safeguard the health of their families.

The immediate postwar period presented the need for trained public health nurses. The federal government established hospitals requiring nurses to care for the injured and sick soldiers and their families. Expansion of the number of hospital beds and the indifference of young people toward a nursing career created a shortage of trained nurses. Hospitals wanted to train attendants, whereas nurses were trying to secure adequate state licensure and better education for nurses. The idea of training attendants in the same school as nurses was rejected by many nursing leaders. During the war the growing tendency toward less careful selection of young women for hospital schools reached its peak.

World War II

In July, 1940, Julia C. Stimson, president of the American Nurses' Assocation, called together representatives of the five national nursing organizations, the American Red Cross nursing service, and federal agencies closely concerned with the extension and use of nursing resources. From this group the Nursing Council of National Defense developed. The Council was a planning agency with some administrative responsibilities. Its functions were to determine the role of nurses and nursing in the program of national defense, unify all nursing activities, act as a clearing house regarding nursing and national defense, and cooperate with other agencies with related responsibilities.

Following the declaration of World War II, the Council's structure was broadened. The program of the U. S. Cadet Nurse Corps and the Procurement and Assignment Ser-

vice of the War Manpower Commission became additional work for the Council.

Emergence of aides for patient care

During the depression years when many nurses were unemployed, nursing aide training programs were unsuccessful. However, in 1938 the program was revised under the direction of Mary Beard, Director of Nursing Service for the Red Cross. The auxiliary workers were known as nurses' aides.

The revised program of 10 weeks was carried out in hospitals. The nurses served as instructors assisted by other medical and health officers. Many of the nurses' aides proved to be so efficient that the hospital wanted to keep them and pay them. In 1942 the Red Cross authorities agreed that aides could become paid hospital workers but ruled that they could no longer be members of the Volunteer Nurses' Aide Corps and must return their Red Cross insignia. Because there was so much controversy over this policy, in 1943 the Red Cross agreed to revise it and permitted aides both paid and unpaid to continue to wear the Red Cross and Office of Civilian Defense insignia, as well as the designated uniform.

Many of the trained aides became practical nurses by waiver when licensing for practical nurses was instituted.

Emergence of practical nursing programs

The first course in practical nursing was offered in 1890. In 1940 there were over 19,000 so-called practical nurses in the United States; however, only a small percentage had received any formal instruction. In 1941 the National Association for Practical Nurse Education (NAPNE) was organized.

The support given by the Ginzberg report and others helped develop the practical nursing programs and led to the utilization of the licensed practical nurse (LPN) or the licensed vocational nurse (LVN) as she was called in some states.

After World War II the Vocational Education Division of the U. S. Office of Education appointed a committee composed of nurses, hospital administrators, educators, and government representatives to conduct a job analysis of the practical nurse. The analysis was published in 1947. By 1950 the practical nursing curriculum and the accreditation program were introduced, and efforts were made to secure legal status for practical nurses in each state.

In the 1940s licensed practical nurses also organized their own association known as National Federation of Licensed Practical Nurses (NFLPN). By 1950 there were 30,000 licensed practical nurses and over a hundred approved practical nursing schools. Because of the legislative clause in licensure, many of the L.P.N.s were licensed by waiver, if they had worked as practical nurses, for a specified number of years before the licensure act was adopted.[29]

Emergence of nursing service standards

In 1936 the *Manual of Essentials of Good Hospital Service* was published under the sponsorship of the American Hospital Association and the National League for Nursing Education. It was the first time recognition of minimum standards of average nursing care required for patients classified by categories such as adult medical and surgical patients, mothers and newborn babies, and pediatric patients was given.

The purpose of the manual was to set up the principles by which nursing services could function without dependence on the students in the hospital school of nursing. This manual was revised in 1942 by representatives of the American Medical Association, American College of Surgeons, and American Nurses' Association. The third manual, entitled *Hospital Nursing Service Manual*, was published in 1950 under the guidance of the five organizations; however, the AHA and NLNE carried the major responsibility for this edition.[19]

When the United States entered World War II, the institutional staff nurse had taken a place in the center of the stage of professional nursing service.

ECONOMIC AND CULTURAL INFLUENCES ON NURSING AS A CAREER

A review of the editorial pages of the *American Journal of Nursing*, founded in 1900, tells us of the frustrations encountered and of actions taken by nursing leaders to improve education, raise standards, and increase the excellence of nursing to deliver better care to patients.

The status of nurses and their functions in hospitals stemmed from the Victorian concept of the woman's role in society. It was thought that because women possessed a loftier and finer nature than men they would gain personal satisfaction from performing drudging tasks of caring for the helpless and dependent and were therefore especially well-qualified by nature to minister to the sick. Even today the sex role continues to be an important factor in the pragmatic arena of hospital work.

As a cultural pattern, female occupations have not been given as much status or independence as the professions followed by males, and most women had little chance to select professional occupations. Between 1920 and 1930, there was a high potential recruitment market for women in nursing. The status quo in nursing was accepted by physicians, administrators, and nurses themselves. As long as a large reserve of potential student nurses was available, acceptance of and complacency toward existing nursing problems was fostered. Those individuals who attempted to disrupt the status quo were frequently accused of producing negativism.

One of the greatest difficulties nurses have had is their inability to establish acceptable minimum standards of hours and wages for the graduate nurse.[20] Prior to 1930 nurses were striving to establish themselves as professionals. Many of the nursing leaders of that time believed it to be "unprofessional" to limit working hours to a specific number of hours per week; they did not want to be classified with factory workers or domestic servants. Other dedicated nurses believed that nursing was a vocation to care for sick people. Also, the private duty nurses (in 1928 there were nearly 14,000) were afraid that increasing the pay of nurses or shortening the workday hours would decrease employment days.[29]

As a result of the depression in 1932, the

American Nurses' Association followed the recommendation of the National Recovery Administration plan, thus advocating cutting the working day to 8 hours so that 3 nurses could be employed instead of 2. Although the plan was not too effective because most nurses were in private duty, it did demonstrate that a nurse could do better work in 8 hours than in the longer 12-hour day (see Chapter 4 for recent labor relations law and ANA Economic General Welfare Program).

In 1940, basic information about the cost of nursing service and nursing education was published by Pfefferkorn and Rovetta.[27] The efficiency of industrial and business standards had an influence on nurses' attitudes.

During the 1920s, according to Burling, Lentz, and Wilson,[10] when wages were falling and the nurse saw herself exploited in many ways, the concept of the nurse as an angel of mercy came into disrepute among many nurses. They began to place value on higher education and technical competence. With more patients and equipment to care for in hospitals, nursing services became more rigid. Nurses were expected to follow a strict set pattern as outlined in the manual or as ordered by the physician. Frequently creativity and spontaneity were discouraged by the physician, director, hospital administrator, supervisor, and even the instructor. Along with the advances and expansion in medical care, more technical procedures had to be carried out, thus somewhat separating the technical tasks from those associated with the teaching and the humanistic aspects of nursing care.

In the 1930s, hospitals employed few graduate nurses, since more of the nursing care and supervision was done by instructors and student nurses. Many hospitals used student nurses almost as slave labor, which in turn permitted them to use graduate nurses to scrub floors, carry trays, clean equipment, repair linens and supplies, make bandages, and perform numerous other hospital tasks.[8,18]

By 1940 the hospitals were larger but fewer in number, as were the schools of nursing. Because of the expansion of facilities in the large hospitals, decrease in the number of available nursing students, and increase in nursing care demands, hospitals began to employ more graduate nurses.

HEALTH INSURANCE PLANS[27]

With public criticism of the scarcity of good medical care available during illness and demands for more and better medical services, the Committee on the Costs of Medical Care was established in 1927. Their study showed that medical and nursing services were unevenly divided among the different socioeconomic groups in each community. It was suggested that governmental bodies assume some responsibility for the health of citizens and medical services be provided by means of health insurance.

With the growing complexity of medicine came the growth of health insurance. With urbanization and increase in mobility a new importance was attached to hospitalization insurance, a service in many cases previously provided by friends, family, or neighbors. The movement for large-scale group insurance coincides with the 1929-1932 depression period. By 1934 over 100,000 subscribers and over 100 hospitals were participating in hospital insurance plans in American cities. In 1936 the American Hospital Association, with the support of a grant from the Julius Rosenwald Fund, established the Hospital Service Plan Commission. Its objective was to provide information and guidance to hospitals and others in the establishment of voluntary, nonprofit hospital care insurance plans and to act as an information clearing center for administrators of existing hospital service associations. The hospital insurance plans approved by this Commission became known as Blue Cross Plans. Its first listing of participating, nonprofit organizations was published in 1938.

For a hospital insurance plan to secure the Blue Cross approval, with a blue cross as its symbol, benefits had to be guaranteed to the subscribers through contractual arrangements with a group of member hospitals. During World War II, health insurance boomed because many industries were unable to increase wages above certain maximum levels in accordance with federal government regulations; therefore they gave health insurance as a so-called personnel fringe benefit. The private insurance companies that had not entered into this field of insurance began to offer health plans. After World War II, health insurance became an important socioeconomic issue in the formulation of industrial contracts negotiated by the large unions.

In New York the Health Insurance Plan known as HIP and in California the Kaiser Permanente Plan offered to Kaiser workers during the building of the Hoover Dam paid hospital and medical costs. Many physicians' and surgeons' organizations did not enter the insurance field. The California Physicians Service, composed of a large group of private physicians, offered a medical plan to their patients in 1939. As more medical societies throughout the United States entered the insurance field, the American Medical Association set up certain standards for approval; those plans found acceptable were permitted to display a blue shield as a symbol. Thus the Blue Shield policies became an integral part of Blue Cross group insurance practices. Recent health insurance plans are discussed in Chapter 4.

SUMMARY

History reminds us that scientific discoveries and development in the modern sense began their course hundreds of years ago. The health care system in hospitals continues to change in a society as the result of the forces active in that society. Changes affecting nursing care services and training of personnel within a hospital health care system involve a degree of similarity of socialization and agreement among the interested groups. And the only thing that is constant in life is change.

REFERENCES

1. Ackerknecht, E. H.: A short history of medicine, New York, 1955; The Ronald Press Co.
2. Aikens, C. A.: The registration movement: its past and its future; Trained Nurse and Hospital Review 44:1-11, January 1910.
3. American Nurses' Association: Code for nurses with interpretive statements, New York, 1970, The Association.
4. American Nurses' Association: Facts about nursing, New York, 1945, The Association, pp. 14, 41-45.
5. Austin, A. L.: History of nursing source book, New York, 1957, G. P. Putnam's Sons.
6. Bullough, V. L., and Bullough, B.: The emergence of modern nursing, 2nd ed., New York, 1969, The Macmillan Publishing Co.
7. Burgess, M. A.: A five-year program for the committee on the grading of nursing schools, New York, 1926, Committee on the Grading of Nursing Schools.
8. Burgess, M. A.: Nurses, patients and pocketbooks, New York, 1928, Committee on the Grading of Nursing Schools.
9. Burgess: M. A.: Nursing schools today and tomorrow, New York, 1934, Committee on the Grading of Nursing Schools.
10. Burling, T., Lentz, E., and Wilson, R.: The give and take in hospitals, New York, 1956, G. P. Putnam's Sons.
11. Burrow, J. G.: AMA—voice of American medicine, Baltimore, 1863, The Johns Hopkins Press, pp. 1-66, pp. 132-151.
12. Churchill, E. D.: The development of the hospital. In Faxon, H. W., editor: The hospital in contemporary life, Cambridge, 1949, The Harvard University Press.
13. Committee for the Study of Nursing Education: Nursing and nursing education in the United States, and a report of a survey by Josephine Goldmark, New York, 1923, The Macmillan Publishing Co.
14. Davis, L. E.: Fellowship of surgeons: a history of the American College of Surgeons, Springfield, Ill., 1960, Charles C. Thomas, Publisher.
15. Flexner, A.: Medical education in the United States and Canada, New York, 1910, Carnegie Foundation for the Advancement of Teaching.
16. Giordina, C.: Role of nursing in hospital care. In Proceedings of the 12th International Hospital Congress: The changing role of the hospital in a changing world, London, 1961, International Hospital Federation, Hospital Center.
17. Goodrich, A. W.: The contribution of the Army School of Nursing. In National League of Nursing Education, Annual Report, 1919, and Proceedings of 25th Convention; Baltimore, 1919, The Williams & Wilkins Co., pp. 146-156.
18. Health resources statistics; a report from the National Center for Health Statistics, Washington, D.C., 1968, U.S. Department of Health, Education, and Welfare, Public Health Services, pub. no. 1509.
19. National League of Nursing Education and American Hospital Association: Hospital nursing service manual, New York, 1950, The League and Association.
20. Jamme, A. C.: Department of Nursing Education, The California eight-hour law for women, American Journal of Nursing 19:525-530, 1919.
21. Johns, E., and Pfefferkorn, B.: An activity analysis

of nursing, New York, 1934, National League of Nursing Education.

22. Kalisch, B. J., and Kalisch, P. A.: Slaves, servants, or saints? (an analysis of the system of nursing training in the United States 1873-1948), Nursing Forum 14(3):222-263, 1975.

23. Lewinski-Corwin, E. H.: The hospital nursing situation, American Journal of Nursing **22:**603-606, 1922. (From the summary of the study of the hospital survey made by the Public Health Committee, presented at the New York Academy of Medicine, December 1, 1921.)

24. Majono, G.: The healing hand—man and wound in ancient world; Cambridge, Mass., 1975, Harvard University Press, pp. 266, 374-381.

25. Nightingale, F.: Nursing notes, London, 1859, reprinted 1946, Philadelphia, J. B. Lippincott Co.

26. Nutting, A., and Dock, L.: A history of nursing, New York, 1907, G. P. Putnam's Sons.

27. Pfefferkorn, B., and Rovetta, C. A.: Administrative cost analysis for nursing service and nursing education, New York, 1940, National League of Nursing Education.

28. Riesman, D.: The story of medicine in the middle ages, New York, 1936, Harper & Brothers.

29. Roberts, M. M.: American nursing—history and interpretation, New York, 1954, The Macmillan Publishing Co.

30. Woodham-Smith, C.: Florence Nightingale, New York, 1951, McGraw-Hill Book Co.

2 | Hospital nursing service in midcentury

By midcentury there were many different categories of paid workers and volunteers in hospitals. The physician took over the role of leader of the hospital team, composed of nurses, dietitians, social workers, and administrators. Specialization emerged as a new factor in the medical field.

SHORTAGE OF NURSES

Nurses, physicians, hospital administrators, and the public began to voice opinions on the shortage of nursing personnel. Nurses were in an ambiguous position in their role in the delivery of patient services. They were upset over the inadequacies of their professional and economic status and the demands for more and better nursing care. The gap between an expanding population requiring nursing care and the limited number of trained nurses with appropriate knowledge and skills to provide such care has been and still is a major problem.

POPULATION AND HOSPITAL BED INCREASES

During the 1940s the rising birthrate was reflected in a notable increase in the annual number of births, amounting to an increase of over 1 million births per year in the years 1946 to 1951.[33] During 1935 to 1950 the population increased 14.5% in the wartime decade, and the number of patients annually admitted to hospitals more than doubled.[4,33]

In 1951 the United States had over 1 million hospital beds exclusive of 190,000 in federal government hospitals.[14] The passage of the Hospital Survey and Construction Program (Hill-Burton Act) in 1946 helped hospitals increase their bed capacity and other facilities. From 1955 to 1965 the population increased 17%, the number of active physicians increased 22%, and the number of active professional nurses in practice increased 44%.

Since 1955 a substantial per capita rise in the availability and use of hospital facilities has taken place. The American Hospital Association annually conducts a survey of registered hospitals. The statistics for 1967 are based on 7,172 hospitals, a net increase of 12% over 1966.

Patient bed occupancy rate is the ratio of average daily census to beds. Between 1966 and 1967 almost all occupancy rates for hospitals in various types of service and control categories decreased, with the exception of the nongovernment, short-term general and other specialty hospitals.

HEALTH PAYMENTS AND EXPENDITURES

The health insurance plans of the 1940s were accelerated. The 10-year health program prepared by the federal Social Security Administration for President Truman aroused much controversy about compulsory versus voluntary insurance as a method of paying for medical care, which was rapidly becoming both more scientific and more costly to patient and hospital.[9] In 1948, 30 million people were enrolled in Blue Cross (hospital) insurance plans. By 1952, 90 million people had some type of prepayment insurance coverage.

The Social Security amendments of 1965 further established high quality, comprehensive health care as a human right and not a privilege to be enjoyed by relatively few Americans.

By midcentury, health professionals and potential consumers of health services began

17

to voice their opinions and demands concerning more and better nursing services. In 1969 Lewis[19] stated that "our future young investigators would classify the late 1960s as an era when things were not really as cool as they might have been because everyone was *hung-up* trying *to do his thing* or *uptight* trying to protect *his bag.*"

During the 1950s and 1960s the expenses for personal health services and sources of payments in the United States changed rapidly. In 1950, only 20% of all personal health care was paid by government sources. From private sources, about 66% was paid directly by patients and about 10% through insurance plans.[18] At the beginning of the 1970s direct payments by patients had decreased almost 36%, private insurance payments had increased over 50%, and government sources increased over 36% for all expenses. Of these payment funds, hospital payments continued to receive about 50% of the funds, and physicians about 25% of them.[4] Of these payment funds, the amount paid to hospitals and physicians increased. Between 1966 and 1971, expenditures for health care in the United States increased 87% and expenses for health care per person nearly doubled.[8]

NURSING SERVICE RESOURCES

By 1950, according to American Medical Association reports, hospitals had augmented their nursing services with well over 200,000 registered graduate nurses, approximately 100,000 student nurses, and 225,000 nursing assistants (practical nurses, nurses' aides, and male attendants).[4]

According to the Interagency Conference on Nursing Statistics (ICONS) for 1969, 680,000 registered nurses were employed part-time (25% of them) or full time.

Moxley,[22] in discussing the health manpower crisis, said, "the paradox has its roots in the fact that there are growing shortages in that component of medical care which can only be supplied by the physician-diagnosis. The individual consumer (patient) is demanding increasing amounts of care and is finding difficulty in entering the health care system."

Levine,[18] an expert on health manpower, predicted in 1969 that "the demand for nurses will continue upward. It is anticipated that by 1980 over 1 million registered nurses will be needed. . . . New roles for nurses will be established . . . which will enable the nurse to operate more independently and with greater initiative, including clinical specialists, patient care coordinators, and research nurses."

Although the average hospital stay was shortened by new therapies and earlier ambulation, resulting in more admissions, the number and complexity of diagnostic tests and surgical procedures required a longer hospitalization for some patients and above all a high degree of nursing skill.

NURSES' ECONOMIC STATUS

The United States Department of Labor's survey entitled The Economic Status of Registered Nurses 1946-47 showed that nurses worked longer hours, did more night and shift work, received less overtime pay, had fewer fringe benefits, and were paid lower salaries than most workers in industry or in comparable occupational groups. Nurses at the 1946 ANA biennial convention agreed that district state assocations would act as spokesmen and bargaining agents for their membership and negotiate with the nurses' employers concerning salaries, hours, and other working conditions and benefits.

The passage of the Labor-Management Act of 1947 (Taft-Hartley Act) complicated the ANA economic security and welfare programs. The act excluded nonprofit hospitals from the legal obligation of collective bargaining and tended to encourage hospital administrators and boards of trustees to refuse to engage in bargaining with their employees, including professional registered nurses.

After the passage of the Taft-Hartley Act, nurses in some states negotiated contracts. Prior to the late 1960s nursing organizations had not been very effective in improving the economic conditions of the profession for several reasons: the registered nurse's lack of interest and support of the organizations' economic and welfare programs, the nurse's ethical approach to the care of the sick, and the nursing organizations' lack of funds to promote such programs. (See Chapter 4, recent ANA collective bargaining program.)

At the 1969 convention of the National League for Nursing, Evelyn Hamil, in discussing the impact of the short workweek and daylight work hours of our society, hoped that nurses would accept their responsibility for around-the-clock coverage for patients, even though for the most part other professionals and technical personnel work daylight hours with weekends off.[12]

NURSING STUDIES BY NURSE EDUCATORS AND OTHERS

The functions, status, problems, and viewpoints of nurses, physicians, and the public were investigated from 1948 to 1960. From 1945 to 1955 almost every state nurses' association participated in one form or another in what came to be called surveys in nursing needs and resources. Basically most of the studies focused on solving nurse manpower shortages and utilizing personnel and human relations studies to discover nurses' satisfactions and dissatisfactions, as well as those of patients and the public.

The Brown Report

The national Nursing Council published its final report, *Nursing for the Future*, in 1948.[6] This report, commonly known as The Brown Report, was sponsored by the Carnegie Corporation and the Russell Sage Foundation.

The primary goal of the Brown study was to ensure society quality nursing care. The nursing council committee agreed and supported Dr. Brown's viewpoint that nursing service and nursing education should be viewed in terms of what is best for society, not what is best for the profession of nursing as a possibly vested interest. Much of the information presented in the report gave a vivid picture of how hospitals were predominantly operated. Most of them applied authoritarian principles rather than encouraging cooperative team relationships. Nursing service was caught between the authority exercised by medical directors on the one hand and by the hospital administration on the other.

The report indicated that nursing service administrative and supervisory staffs tended to be authoritarian and that the nurse had little freedom to make clinical nursing judgments in the care of patients and was given little initiative outside of specified duties, even within the service to which she belonged. It was found that the administrative orders were issued from the top hospital administrator, with little opportunity provided for nurses to participate in policy decision making. A similar approach was followed in the central nursing office by the director of nursing. No matter how simple the problem the nurses did not participate in the decision making. The staff nurses did not have a sense of being members of the health care team.[6]

The Brown Report pointed out the need for sound legislation regarding the training and functions of the practical nurse and other health workers. It also urged those hospitals engaged in complex forms of patient care to examine, analyze, and determine their clinical nursing service needs, interpersonal relationships, and hospital budgets and expenditures to initiate a better balance between the required technical and professional nursing manpower needs and the establishment of closer team relationships between the medical, nursing, and social work professionals. It stressed that the current system of nursing education could not produce the number of qualified graduate nurses needed for the care of patients. The report urged that professional and highly technical nursing education be undertaken by universities and colleges.

Classification and accreditation service

The committee for the Improvement of Nursing Services endeavored to implement some of the recommendations of The Brown Report. Their report, *Nursing Schools at the Mid-Century*, was published in 1949.[35] The report showed that only 55% of all nursing instructors had academic degrees, although this was a great improvement over 1929, when only 4% of all nursing instructors had 4 or more years of college education.

The report indicated that many patients thought their hospital experience was unsatisfactory. Nurses felt their work experience was unrewarding. The data also indicated that patients frequently preferred volunteer aides because they seemed less hurried and more interested in them than the nurses. A frequent comment voiced by the staff nurse was, "There are always too many patients, too few nurses, and too little time for the amenities of life."

An interim classification of schools of nursing was prepared that placed each school reviewed under one of the three defined classifications. This was a preparation for an accrediting service that was established in 1950 as the National Accrediting Service, under the direction of Dr. Helen Nahm of the NLN.

Study to determine nursing team organization and functions

A committee on the functions of nursing was formed through the efforts of Professor R. Louise McManus, then Head of the Division of Nursing Education, Teachers College, Columbia University.[7] The committee was composed of representatives of nursing and informed individuals in the fields of medicine and social science. Eli Ginzberg, a Barton Hepburn Professor of Economics at Columbia University, served as chairman. The committee reviewed the problems, focusing on the current and prospective shortages of nurses. Their deliberations and recommendations were published in 1948 in the book, *A Program for the Nursing Profession*. This committee endeavored to define the scope of nursing functions, emphasizing the clinical responsibilities of the trained nurse for patient care and her role as an associate of the physician.[7]

The committee's major recommendations may be summarized as follows:

1. Experimentation and research in the organization and functioning of nursing service should be initiated.
2. A nursing service organization that would effectively use 4-year professional nurses, 2-year registered nurses, and 1-year practical nurses should be developed, subdividing nursing functions among the professional and practical nurses.
3. Hospital nurses should utilize nursing assistants for duties that can be performed by less skilled individuals.
4. Hospitals should clarify and improve re-

lations between the nurse and other members of the health team.

Dr. Ginzberg, chairman of the committee, also urged hospital administrators, physicians, and nurses to apply an elementary principle of economics: *never use high-priced personnel for low-priced work*. In discussing the economic status of the nurse and the nurse manpower shortage, he recommended that the traditional economic incentives used to motivate nurses should be increased.[10]

Study on team nursing organization and functioning

In December, 1949, a research and experimental program on the organization and functioning of nursing teams was initiated by the Division of Nursing Education of Teachers College, Columbia University, in an effort to adopt some of the recommendations made by the Committee on Functions of Nursing. The experiment was aimed at establishing new standards for future nursing practice. The study was begun in a limited way under the direction of Amelia Leino. Later, with funds made available by the W. K. Kellogg Foundation, the research program was expanded under the direction of Eleanor C. Lambertsen, then Professor of the Department of Nursing, Teachers College, with the cooperation of the staff of the Department of Hospitals, New York City.[17] Working together, these two groups, faculty and nursing staff, were able to initiate a plan for the management of nursing care. The publication *Nursing Team Organization and Functioning*, by Lambertsen,[17] is a guide that sets forth the basic principles of team nursing and can be adapted to particular hospitals' needs.

The team is a synthesis of the case and the functional methods. The assignment plan aims to help meet heavy nursing care demands and provide a setting in which the knowledge and skills of the experienced professional nurse can be used more effectively. The team leader, a registered nurse, generally assigns specific duties to each member of the team at the beginning of the tour and plans and coordinates the care of each patient on the team. Team members may include R.N.s, L.P.N.s, and nursing aides. At the end of each tour another nursing team becomes responsible for the patients on that team. The head nurse or clinical coordinator, assisted by a secretary or clerk, is responsible for the overall management of nursing care for all the patients on the unit.

For the past 20 years many observers believed that team nursing could be an effective method if hospital management methods such as the establishment of the unit management system and on-going in-service training programs for nurses and team members were improved.

NATIONAL NURSING COMMITTEE ORGANIZED FOR ACTION

A national committee for the improvement of nursing services was appointed by the joint board of directors of the national health organizations to put into action the recommendations set forth in the various studies. This committee was composed of representatives from the fields of general education, hospital administration, and public health and the American Medical Association and nursing organizations.

After the restructuring of the national nursing organizations in June, 1952, the National Committee for the Improvement of Nursing Services became the advisory committee of the Nursing Service Division of the National League for Nursing. It jointly planned regional institutes on nursing service administration and in-service training.

A functional analysis of nursing service (1951)

The University of California School of Nursing and the California State Nurses' Assocation conducted several surveys and studies in the early 1950s.[16,31] The surveys indicated that precise and systematic information on *who does what in nursing when, why,* and *how* was most inadequate. It was agreed that much more information on nursing service activities seemed necessary to establish a factual basis on which to build better administration and examine nursing practices.

One study indicated the need to clarify the functions of the graduate nurse in various positions before an effective personnel utilization system could be initiated. The qualified graduate nurse was caught between the orders from above and personnel problems and duties on the floor; she frequently was obliged to assume many activities previously carried out by physicians. In turn, less qualified workers began to perform many tasks that had formerly been responsibilities of the professional nurse, some of which had come to symbolize nursing.

No one knew the appropriate distribution of the different categories of nursing personnel, what ratios might be considered stable and safe, and the range of differences in nursing needs of particular patients in various types of hospitals.

Study of nursing functions in twelve hospitals

A small pioneer study conducted in twelve hospitals in the state of New York[24] suggested methods to improve care through better administration. Simmons and Henderson[27] summarized results of this study as follows:

1. Professional and practical staff nurses are carrying approximately the same functions with the major difference appearing to be in the concentration of performance on either the professional or nonprofessional level of function.
2. The major portion of the time of both professional and practical staff nurses is devoted to patient centered activities.
3. Both professional and practical nurses are being used ineffectively in hospitals with professional nurses spending less than half their time on the level of functions for which they have been prepared and the practical nurses spending less than half their time on the level of function for which they have been prepared.[27]

Based on the preliminary studies, it was assumed that improvement of the process of nursing service administration would rest on information concerning the functions of nursing personnel, especially with growing specialization and employment of more auxiliary workers, and that professional nurses' functions and duties would relate to the *clinical elements* in patient care.

According to Abdellah and Levine,[3] some

studies had shown that nurses were dissatisfied with, as well as confused by, the existing allocation of duties among the professional nurses, the practical nurses, and the nurses' aides. Other studies[13] indicated agreement that some activities should be performed only by professional nurses, others only by licensed practical nurses, and some could be performed by both groups.

Action of The Joint Commission for the Improvement of Patient Care

Based on the recommendations of the studies just discussed, in 1953 The Joint Commission[30] agreed to direct its efforts toward defining the major functions of professional nursing. The commission's statement was accepted by the boards of trustees of the American Medical Assocation, American Nurses' Association, and the National League for Nursing and reads as follows:

Comprehensive nursing should be designed to provide physical and emotional care for the patient; care of his immediate physical environment; carrying out the treatment prescribed by the physician; teaching the patient and his family the essentials of nursing that they must render, giving general health instructions and supervision to auxiliary workers.[30]

The commission's report is an interesting one to review in relation to the nursing practice act of each state. (See Chapter 5, standards of nursing practice, 1974.)

American Nurses' Association special 5-year program on the nurse's function

Between 1950 and 1957, thirty-four studies were conducted in 17 states under the sponsorship of the American Nurses' Foundation and the American Nurses' Association. These studies included an investigation of nursing functions, job satisfaction, roles and attitudes and were summarized by Hughes and associates.[15,19]

It should be noted that the American Nurses' Foundation, a center for nursing research supported mainly by the American Nurses' Association, was established in 1955 by the board of directors of the ANA.

Several of the recommendations of the Brown Report (1948) were achieved with the completion and reporting of these studies. They furnish much information about what nurses actually were doing in the 1950s, how they regarded themselves and their work, how their colleagues regarded them, and how their patients and the public regarded nurses and nursing. The major goal of each study was directed toward more effective utilization of personnel, both professional and auxiliary, in light of the capacity, educational background, and experience of the staff.

The functional studies sponsored by the American Nurses' Association varied greatly in scope, approach, methods used, and depth of analysis. A large number focused on the activites carried out by the various categories of nurses in specified hospital settings.

Study of nursing practice in California hospitals

A study on nursing practice in California hospitals contributed much information on the methodology it utilized; the researchers endeavored to use standards of scientific objectivity and validity.[16,31] The study was accomplished by nonnurse surveyors[27] who were unable to judge nursing efficiency. This was interpreted as providing greater objectivity in the descriptive data and a receptive approach on the part of the personnel during direct observations. This study was composed of four different survey schedules: (1) a hospital survey of the organization, (2) a form and checklist for direct observations of staff nurses, (3) a diary form to be kept by nursing supervisors, and (4) a schedule to record interviews with auxiliary personnel.

Specific activities (439 separate nursing functions or operations) were classified under one of eight major divisions: (1) nursing care, (2) medications and treatment procedures, (3) housekeeping and messenger services, (4) time off, (5) stand by for assignment, (6) clerical and administrative duties, (7) care of equipment and supplies, and (8) special services.

Analysis of the many activities observed revealed that no clear-cut division between the functions of graduate nurses and those of other nursing personnel existed. There was much overlapping of duties. The surveyors[16] found little standardization of practice among the 40 hospitals studied and a wide variation in procedures both within nursing and in hospital practice. The information gathered from this study remains timely enough to be useful.

Study on patterns of patient care

With a grant from the Sarah Mellon Scaife Foundation in 1950 the School of Nursing at the University of Pittsburgh Medical Center attempted to find an answer to the question of how much nursing service is required by a group of nonsegregated medical and surgical patients in a large general hospital.[11] This study indicated that adequate nursing care could be provided for each patient when, and only when, the following conditions are met: (1) new patterns of hospital and floor management are established and (2) a sufficient number of nursing hours of care for each patient is available.

The following definition of "adequate" hospital nursing service was developed as a guide during the study:

Adequate hospital nursing service should provide for each patient, according to his individual needs, the kind and amount of care required to assist in 1. carrying forward the diagnostic, therapeutic, and rehabilitative plan prescribed by the physician; 2. preventing disease and deformity; 3. providing health instruction for the family as well as the patient and 4, giving the supportive care necessary to meet the psychological needs as well as the physical needs as they emerge.[11]

The major goal of the study was to provide optimum hospital nursing service for patients based on the kind and amount of nursing care required for each patient. The main objective of the study was to develop a plan whereby the patient would be assured continuity and adequacy of care and each worker's needs as a member of a nursing service team would be fulfilled.

Study on the function of the operating room nurse

In 1955 Stewart and Needham[29] did a comparison study based on the assumption that the function of the operating room nurse is sufficiently "different" from that of the other general duty nurses to merit separate consideration. In the ten hospitals in Arkansas that were chosen to represent variations in size, type, and kind of administrative control and educational programs, 20 operating room nurses were selected for interviews and observations. The duties performed by the operating room personnel were gathered from materials in these hospitals and divided into 207 categories. There were great time variations for the same activities in the different hospitals and considerable overlap in the nature of nursing technique and procedures in almost all of the hospitals.

They found that operating room nurses did not differ significantly from other general duty nurses in amount of education, professional orientation, interest, or morale. In relation to hospital status and physician-nurse relationships as compared to that of other nurses, the operating room service was recognized as separate and distinct in most hospitals. In many it was the only service with such recognition, and operating room nurses thus held a more favorable position than other nurses in the hospital. The work of the operating room provided closer contact with the surgeon, more attractive personnel policies such as more weekends off, and slightly better pay.

In the 1960s with the implementation of materials-management programs, improved facilities and equipment, and the use of trained technical assistants, the role of the professional registered nurse changed. With continued specialization, research, technical innovations in surgery, and approved technical programs for men and women who wish to be surgical technicians, the role and functions of the professional registered nurse have changed from so-called technical operations to teaching, supervising, directing, and coordinating functions of patient care.

Hospital and nursing administration, scientific management research, and the research staffs of manufacturers of equipment, sutures, and other supplies have contributed to better management of operating rooms. The founding of the Association of Operating

Room Nurses helped nurses to develop standards and training programs in operating room techniques.

Studies on activities of ancillary nursing personnel

The title "practical nurse" has been used to identify a large number of hospital workers.

The Stewart and Needham activity studies of auxiliary nursing personnel in 1955[28] indicated that the more education and experience the worker had, the less time she spent in the direct care of patients.

General hospitals employed an increasing number of practical nurses whose preparation ranged from that given in commercial correspondence courses to programs of 9 and 12 months and even 2 years in length. In 1947 a report was issued by the Office of Education, Federal Security Agency, under the title Practical Nursing. It was described as an analysis of the practical nurse occupation with suggestions for the organization of training programs based on the analysis.

The functional studies indicated that the auxiliary nursing personnel spent more time in maintaining supplies and equipment, housekeeping, and personal patient care activities than did the professional nurses, who spent more time performing indirect nursing care, including charting, hospital paper work, and conferences.

Application of scientific management to patient care

The study conducted at Harper Hospital, Detroit, under the direction of Marion J. Wright in 1954,[36] provided data on the efficiency of a central messenger service and managerial methods to release nurses from nonnursing functions and duties. It emphasized the invaluable contribution that the scientific management engineer made in the effective utilization of personnel in an efficient work-environment.

One of the first experiments on the use of a floor-manager plan in the patient units was carried out by Sinai Hospital in Baltimore with the guidance of the Division of Nursing Resources, United States Public Health Service, and a research grant from the National Institute of Health. The aim of this project was to determine a method of relieving nurses of material-management duties.

Improvement in administration of nursing services

In 1950 the W. K. Kellogg Foundation invited fourteen universities to participate in a 2- to 5-year program to improve the preparation of administrators of nursing services. Dr. Herman Finer,[10] the first project director, maintained that competence in nursing care results in efficient nursing administration. There was agreement that improved administration of nursing could be attained through greater knowledge and better control of the existing divisions of labor in nursing practice.

The government and nursing studies

In 1953 the United States Department of Health, Education, and Welfare, with the Public Health Service as one of its members, was organized under the jurisdiction of the executive branch of the federal government, with a chief administrative officer (Surgeon General) appointed by the President of the United States for a 4-year term. In 1949 Lucile Petry Leone, Chief Nurse Officer of the USPHS, was appointed by the Surgeon General to the grade of Assistant Surgeon General. Since then the USPHS has been a principal health agency of the federal government, contributing great leadership in the maintenance of high standards of practice, training, and research.

On September 1, 1960, surgeon general Leroy E. Burney announced the establishment of a division of nursing within the USPHS.[34] Margaret G. Arnstein was appointed head of the new division of nursing. The establishment of the division of nursing offered a better opportunity to create closer relationships among various groups, agencies, and others concerned with overall nursing services and resources in our country.

In 1960 the study group of the new division of nursing focused on the development of programs designed to meet the demands of nursing service, conduct and support nursing research, increase and improve the national supply of nursing personnel, and communicate with the general public and "special publics" to keep them informed about nursing.[34]

As a result of the recommendations presented by the Surgeon General's Consultant Group on Nursing entitled Toward Quality in Nursing, the Nurse Training Act became law in 1964. This act was designed to offset a persistent and critical shortage of nurses by providing funds for constructing new nursing schools, extending the traineeship programs for nurses, and establishing grants for recruitment projects, student loans, and refresher courses.

The 1975 Nurse Training Act provided some significant financial assistance in graduate and continuing education. However, Congress requested that it be kept informed regarding the supply and distribution of nurses. The 1977 provision indicates the need for nurses and others to continue their struggle to secure sufficient funds for nursing educational programs.

Relationship between nurse staffing and patient welfare

In 1951 the Division of Nursing Resources, in collaboration with behavioral scientists from the Institute for Research in Human Relations, developed a study design entitled A Design for a Study of Nursing Care and Patient Welfare.

Previous studies conducted in 1956 and 1957[1,25,26] had shown that patients and personnel may not verbalize their feelings about care. Often they express their feelings indirectly. In these studies the shortage of nursing personnel was found to be symptomatic of deep-seated problems.

Abdellah and Levine[3] also endeavored to find an explanation for the shortage of nurses. The researchers wanted to see whether differences in numerical staffing of nursing personnel in hospitals affect feelings about inadequacy of staffing. The findings indicated that no matter how much nursing care a hospital has available, some groups within

the hospital will comment that it is not meeting all the needs of its patients.

The State University of Iowa conducted multiple experiments in staffing patterns with patient welfare as a criterion measure. These experiments were conducted under the direction of Aydelotte.[5] The research team's objective was to test the validity of the hypothesis that increases in the amount or the quality of nursing care will produce improvements in patient welfare. The hypothesis was tested in two ways: (1) increasing the size of a floor nursing staff and (2) introducing an in-service education program designed to increase the amount and quality of nursing care given by the staff. The patient welfare measures were also categorized in major divisions such as clinical measures, scaled measures, and patient activity sampling measures.

The findings indicated that neither increasing the staff nor introducing an in-service program resulted in any noticeable improvement in patient care. However, the measures revealed differences among individual patients and among groups of patients classified by age and general condition.

The staffing study conducted by New and associates[23] at Kansas University Hospital in 1959 indicated that high levels of nurse staffing could have negative output in patient care and that too many nurses may be worse than too few.

Defining criterion measures in nursing

In a 1961 study Abdellah[2] suggested ways in which criterion measures in nursing could be developed. This study also provided useful guides in identifying major components of nursing care and defined operationally the terms from which the derivation of nurse staffing patterns might be traced.

Effects of the Progressive Patient Care system on patient welfare

In 1957 the Manchester Memorial Hospital in Manchester, Connecticut, began a project known as Progressive Patient Care to determine methodology for classifying patients based on an evaluation of many factors to make a determination of the best type of unit to which the patient should be assigned.[32] This study was sponsored by the United States Public Health Service's Division of Hospitals and Medical Facilities. A report of this study prepared by Abdellah and Strachan appeared in May, 1959, in the *American Journal of Nursing.*

In 1962, a research team composed of representatives of the health team, behavioral scientists, cost accountants, and others was established to conduct a hospital study to determine what factors, if any, affecting medical practices, nursing practices, dietary practices, costs, and patterns of patient recovery might be attributed to Progressive Patient Care (PPC).[32] PPC is defined as the organization of facilities, services, and staff around the medical and nursing needs of patients. The six elements of Progressive Patient Care were defined as (1) intensive care, (2) intermediate care, (3) self-care, (4) long-term care, (5) home care, and (6) outpatient care. These six elements correspond to the categories in a patient classification method.

These studies provided useful guidelines in classification of patients, bed allocation, creation of buffer beds, and specialty patient care units.

Study to determine quality of nursing care

Between 1950 and 1954 Reiter and Kakosh[26] of Teachers College conducted a field study to establish valid and reliable criteria to appraise the quality of nursing care. This study was financed by a USPHS grant and the Institute of Research and Studies in Nursing Education, Teachers College, Columbia University.

In this study the quality of direct nursing care is evaluated through the use of critical questions stated in terms of nurse operations and patient responses.

Nite and Willis[25] attempted to identify criteria that could be used to test the effectiveness of a special type of nursing care such as that given hospitalized cardiac patients.

As a result of these studies the membership of the American Nurses' Association agreed that there was a great need to define

more clearly the practice of professional nursing and the practice of practical nursing through state nurse practice acts. The 1957 Statement of the Functions of the Licensed Practical Nurse was approved by the Executive Board of the National Federation of Licensed Practical Nurses in October, 1963, and by the Board of Directors of the American Nurses' Assocation in January, 1964.

Survey and assessment of nursing research

In 1953 the National Committee on the Improvement of Nursing Services, under the auspices of Yale University, supported a survey and assessment of nursing research. The major purpose of the Yale survey was to find, classify, and evaluate the research in nursing during the past decade. Simmons and Henderson[27] headed this project.

To help those studying nursing, various bibliographies and indexes were developed. Under the direction of Virginia Henderson at Yale University the comprehensive Nursing Index and the journal *Nursing Research* were initiated.

Another important development in nursing was the establishment of the Institute of Research and Studies on Nursing Education at Teachers College, Columbia University, in 1953 under the direction of Dr. Helen Bunge. This was the first formalized mechanism within a university to carry out nursing research.

The Clearing House of the ANA and the journal *Nursing Research* began to publish a list of research projects in nursing.

Associate degree research program at Teachers College, Columbia University

To meet the demands for an increasing number of nurses and ensure society a high quality of nursing service, a project was initiated at Teachers College in 1952 to explore the junior community college as a potential source of nursing education. The researchers wanted to determine whether or not it would be possible to develop an education-centered program that would prepare nurses in less than the usual 3 years. Under the direction of Dr. Mildred Montag,[21] then Associate Professor of Nursing

Education at Teachers College, an experiment was conducted in close cooperation with seven junior colleges and one hospital school in six widely separated states. The project was completed by the Institute of Research and Service in 1957 to show that a carefully planned course within the organized system of education can produce technically well-prepared nurses in 2 years and that such a school can promote the movement of nursing education into institutions of higher learning and give impetus to a trend toward providing governmental funds for such nursing programs.

Since the establishment of associate degree nursing programs in 1952 there has been a steady increase in their size and number. This represents the implementation of one of the recommendations of the Brown Report of 1948.

SUMMARY

The results of the surveys and studies indicate that the categorical pattern in division of duties in nursing care has limitations.

Findings support the concept that a certain amount of functional overlapping may be an asset in attaining flexibility and in the application of individualized, personalized care of patients.

The many interpretations of the nurses' functions are the synthesis of many influences. Findings of the many studies completed during 1950 to 1960 indicate that the registered graduate nurses were not being fully utilized in relation to their knowledge, skills, and potential resources to meet the health needs of patients. It was concluded that nursing assistants could be trained to perform many of the care operations but would require professional nursing supervision.

In 1962, because of the increasing legal and professional problems facing nurses in practice, the American Nurses' Association proposed that committees on professional practice should be formed within each state nursing association. With acceptance of the proposal by the ANA House of Delegates, committees on functions, standards, and qualifications for practice were formed. The ANA Intersectional Committee on Nursing Practice was also formed to assist the state committees in their endeavors. (See Chapter 5, Standards of nursing practice and nursing services.)

During 1948 to 1960, nursing leaders, educators, and health organizations took an active approach in helping to devise ways to ensure society of adequate nursing care. With accelerated demands for health services, frustrations in the development of health systems, the need for trained health workers, and the desire to apply new knowledge to the cure and prevention of diseases, professional nursing made a tremendous contribution to the improvement of patient care.

In general, many more nurses than in past decades were intent on gaining knowledge, skills, and professional status. They looked forward to the years ahead in nursing as challenging and productive in the improvement of patient care. In today's complex health field, professional nurses face many different problems to assure quality of nursing care to consumer-patients.

REFERENCES

1. Abdellah, F. G.: Methods of identifying covert aspects of nursing problems, Nursing Research, 6:4-23, June, 1957.
2. Abdellah, F. G.: Criterion measures in nursing, Nursing Research, 10:21-26, Winter, 1961.
3. Abdellah, F. G.: and Levine, E.: Effect of nursing staffing on satisfactions with nursing care, Hospital Monograph Series no. 4, Chicago, 1958, American Hospital Association.
4. American Medical Association: Hospital services in the United States, Journal of the American Medical Association 149:13-16, 1952.
5. Aydelotte, M. K.: The use of patient welfare as a criterion measure, Nursing Research 11:10-14, Winter, 1962.
6. Brown, E. L.: Nursing for the future, New York, 1948, The Russell Sage Foundation.
7. Committee on the Functions of Nursing: A program for the nursing profession, New York, 1948, The Macmillan Publishing Co. (Note: commonly known as the Ginzberg Report.)
8. Cooper, B., and Worthington, N.: National health expenditures, 1929-72, Social Security Bulletin, Washington, D.C. 1973, United States Government Printing Office.
9. Ewing, O. R.: The nation's health—a ten-year

program, Washington, D.C., 1948, United States Government Printing Office.

10. Finer, H.: Administration and the nursing services, New York, 1952, The Macmillan Publishing Co.

11. George, L. F., and Kuehn, R. P.: Patterns of patient care, New York, 1955, The Macmillan Publishing Co., pp. 10-11.

12. Hamil, E. M.: Vice-president in charge of nursing. In Roles on today's health team, pub. no. 20-1392, New York, 1969, National League for Nursing.

13. Hanson, H. C., and Stechlein, J. E.: Nursing functions in general hospitals in the state of Minnesota, Minneapolis, 1955, University of Minnesota Press.

14. Hospital services in the United States, Chicago, The 1951-1967 Census of Hospitals, American Hospital Association.

15. Hughes, E. C., Hughes, H. M., and Deutscher, L.: Twenty thousand nurses tell their story, Philadelphia, 1958, J. B. Lippincott Co.

16. Kroeger, L. J., et al.: Nursing practice in California hospitals, San Francisco, 1953, California State Nurses' Association.

17. Lambertsen, E. C.: Nursing team organization and functioning, New York, 1953, Division of Nursing Education, Teachers College Press.

18. Levine, E.: Nurse manpower—yesterday, today, and tomorrow, American Journal of Nursing 69:291-296, 1969.

19. Lewis, C. E.: The team is in the doctor's bag. In Roles on today's health team: relationships, doctor, administrator, director of nursing (pub. no. 20-1372), New York, 1969, National League for Nursing.

20. Milo, N.: The care of health in communities access for outcasts, New York, 1975, The Macmillan Publishing Co., pp. 110-17.

21. Montag, M.: Education of nursing technicians, New York, 1951, G. P. Putnam's Sons.

22. Moxley, J. R., III: The predicament in health manpower, American Journal of Nursing 68:1486-1490, 1968.

23. New, P. K., Nite, G., and Callahan, J. M.: Nursing service and patient care: a staffing experiment, (pub. no. 119), Kansas City, Mo., 1958, Community Studies, Inc.

24. New York University, Department of Nursing Education: A study of nursing functions in 12 hospitals in the state of New York, New York, 1952, New York University Press.

25. Nite, G., and Willis, F.: Nursing care of the hospitalized cardiac patient, New York, 1964, The Macmillan Publishing Co.

26. Reiter, F., and Kakosh, M. E.: Quality of nursing care: a report of a field-study to establish criteria, 1950-1954, New York, 1963, Graduate School of Nursing, New York Medical College.

27. Simmons, L. W., and Henderson, V.: Nursing research, New York, 1964, Appleton-Century-Crofts.

28. Stewart, D., and Needham, C.: The auxiliary nursing personnel, Fayetteville, Ark., 1955, University of Arkansas Press.

29. Stewart, D., and Needham, C.: The functions of the operating room nurse in 10 Arkansas hospitals, Fayetteville, Ark., 1955, University of Arkansas Press.

30. The Joint Commission recommends: American Journal of Nursing 3:308-310, 1953.

31. University of California School of Nursing Faculty: A functional analysis of nursing service, San Francisco, 1950, E. A. Donahue Co.

32. U.S. Department of Health, Education, and Welfare, Division of Hospital and Medical Facilities: Elements of progressive patient care, USPHS pub. no. 930-C-1, Washington, D.C., 1962, United States Government Printing Office.

33. United States Department of Health, Education, and Welfare, Public Health Service: National Center for Health Statistics—vital statistics of the United States; Health Interview Survey, July, 1965 (pub. no. 1000, ser. 10, no. 37), Washington, D.C. vols. 2 and 2 for selected years, United States Government Printing Office.

34. U.S.P.H.S. creates division of nursing: American Journal of Nursing 10:1432, 1960.

35. West, M., and Hawkins, C.: Nursing schools at mid-century, New York, 1950, National League for Nursing.

36. Wright, M. J.: Improvement of patient care, New York, 1954, G. P. Putnam's Sons.

3 Nursing service in the hospital care system, 1970s

The current expansion of the sciences, technology, and philosophy has penetrated almost every aspect of man's life. Some health professionals now agree that comprehensive health care is closely associated with the social, cultural, and psychological, as well as the physical, needs of the individual. Some noted sociologists refer to the United States as a chaotic society faced with problems of transition from town to urban living in a technological age.

Apparently the social, economic, and political realities of our society are beginning to have a great influence on the delivery of health services in our hospitals. In planning, organizing, initiating, and assessing any health program, we must answer the questions *for whom? what type?* and *when, where,* and *how* will these services be rendered? One might safely predict that the hospital members—boards of trustees, physicians, hospital administrators, professional nurses, educators, sociologists, scientific managers, and consultants—will have a greater mutual understanding of their respective functions and apply the results of science and technology more effectively in future delivery of patient care. Professional nurses probably will function in a completely new system instead of the so-called traditional one.[7] As in the past, hospital health care will continue to change and adapt to the results of active societal forces. Historically, events indicate that the objectives of a hospital represent the responses of a society to existing socioeconomic challenges and guides for resolving new health problems.

When advances in industry became realities, man's socioeconomic status changed. Today many citizens believe that the hospital industry is obligated to use scientific technology for the benefit of all people regardless of race, creed, religion, or socioeconomic status. The processes of change have always been continuous in our society.

The language, tradition, concepts, expectations, and barriers that people live by, the customs, buildings, equipment, computers—all that man has created—form a culture. The hospital is, as it always has been, a social organization that represents the blending of people's responses resulting from their own life-styles, attitudes, values, and knowledge. The patterns and preferences that the boards of trustees, hospital administrators, physicians, nurses, and scientific managers have learned usually tend to make them resistant to change. Man's resistance to change, or his motivation to change, has always been based on his values. The concepts or objectives of a program thus become the vital part of any system. The concepts of health care held by the physician, the director of nursing and the nurse-practitioner represent an elaborate set of expectations and beliefs and a myriad of interactions that intertwine to form a reality.

Frequently when the nurse, physician, administrator, or patient confront each other, one of the primary problems they face is that they have been socialized differently. The socialization process of man has been compared to the programming of a computer. Like the computer, man can only give information based on what he understands. He may reject new ideas if he is not ready to accept them. A person's perceptions of his surroundings, experiences, or interactions are influenced directly by his expectations of them. We might agree that the only constant factor in life is change. As we assess the uniqueness of nursing care services and socialization processes or the humanization of patient care and compare it with all that went before, it becomes evident that some changes in concepts began centuries ago and that expectations become realities. Organizational behavior and communications cannot be treated as separate entities. They blend together in the system.

Consumers, government representatives, nursing service and hospital administrators, health practitioners, and nurse-educators are beginning to use new channels of communication and controls to provide for appropriate manpower resources and quality of care services. It is crucial that nurse-educators and nursing service providers at the local and state levels work together in determining the different categories of nursing personnel needed and the type of preparation each should acquire.

Hospitals are an essential component in medical care today. Until the late 1800s medical technology had little need for specialized facilities. The black bag of the physician was more than sufficient for his patients' needs. Hospitals today are complex institutions with elaborate policies and regulations and are operated by trained specialists in various occupations.

Until technology made specialization possible, most physicians and nurses were generalists, utilizing a range of techniques with varying degrees of complexity. Recent developments in biomedical research, advances in the basic sciences, and engineering refinements in electronic instruments and computers have made the hospital and its professional staff the guardians of complex hardware and techniques.[3,19,22]

FACTORS AFFECTING DISTRIBUTION OF HEALTH CARE

The distribution of health care resources in the United States is affected by four major problems: (1) the location of the resources, (2) patients' access to care, (3) specialization of physicians, and (4) patients' ability to pay for medical and hospital care.[2a,7,13,14]

Distribution of hospital resources

In the past decade in the United States, hospital beds per population units have been abundant in less affluent states. Tax funds that have financed hospitals, general clinics, and home health programs have been allocated on a population formula that favors poorer areas.[14,16]

Medical and health personnel are less available in rural areas than in more affluent urban areas. The overall physician-to-patient ratio in the United States is about 1:670. However, there are almost double the number of physicians and nurses in affluent states than in poorer states. Specialization by physicians aggravates the distribution problem since physicians tend to practice in more affluent urban areas rather than in rural and poorer areas. Specialists must practice where the population is concentrated to ensure a sufficient number of patients for their services. In 1970 the American Medical Association formally recognized 29 new specialties, increasing the total to 63, and thus increasing the number of specialists in urban communities.[7] Despite the high number of health professionals in cities, few of the urban poor have easy access to care.[14]

In 1970 over 50% of the 7,600 United States hospitals were owned by private, not-for-profit organizations. Hospitals are used primarily for the care of acute conditions and for chronically ill patients who are admitted because there are no other suitable facilities for them. Affluent patients with general health problems also are admitted to hospitals because they prefer hospital care to the existing ambulatory extended care services.

The impetus of Medicare in 1966 contributed to the closing of small hospitals that could not meet certification requirements of Medicare payments.[15,23] Medicare also contributed to an increase in larger hospitals. By 1969 there was a continuing decrease in the total number of hospitals, but an increase in both government and not-for-profit hospitals. Through governmental health care payments, hospitals of 150 to 500 beds have been able to survive.

The not-for-profit hospitals have received federal funds for construction and are eligible for other government funds. Hospitals through affiliation with university medical centers are eligible for additional grants to develop specialized services. To provide for better control of federal grants, the government recently passed new legislation. The Social Security Amendments of 1972 (PL92-603) require government review of all capital construction plans exceeding $100,000 in advance. On January 4, 1976 the National Health Planning and Resources Development Act of 1975 (PL93-641) established Health Service Areas (HSA) (see Chapter 4).

One reason for high hospital costs is the low utilization or misuse of services. In some hospitals about 30% to 40% of the beds in maternity and pediatrics departments are unused. W. McNeary's report[13] indicated that of the 360 hospitals with open-heart surgery units studied in 1969, 71% performed less than one operation per week, and 37 performed no services at all. Surgical statistics seem to indicate that the number of common surgical procedures performed in different parts of the country is related to the number of hospital beds and local surgeons rather than to medical need. The *New York Times* on January 25, 1976, in an article on physicians, advanced the idea that all surgery in not necessary, even though the patient may desire it.[17]

Overbuilding, underusing services, or overusing facilities increases costs, which must be met by all patients, rich and poor. Consumers of hospital services pay through rising insurance premiums and taxes for government programs and often pay for services that are not covered by Medicare or other insurance.

Underuse and overuse of services affect the utilization of nursing service resources, the cost of training programs, and the quality of nursing care.

Ambulatory services for primary care

Federal funds recently have been available for construction of ambulatory facilities. Ambulatory services could provide quality primary care if appropriate medical and nursing personnel were made available.[3,8]

In most hospitals the outpatient facilities and services have been neglected by both patients and professional staffs. It has been considered a minor subsystem of the hospital rather than a community-based health service. Traditionally ambulatory services have been provided on a segmented basis rather than on an integrated one combining professional inhospital and nonhospital health groups.

Milo[14] points out that people with acute illnesses such as upper respiratory infections and chronic illnesses such as heart disease, arthritis, and asthma, when not treated and cared for at home, require basic medical care such as diagnosis, physical examination, medications, laboratory tests, and counseling. Jacobs and Gavett[8] in a study of ambulatory patients in a group practice showed that only 9% needed either physician or dental specialists. In a similar study of hospital emergency departments, slightly less than 50% of the patients required specialists' services.

Emergency services as a part of the overall ambulatory facilities are being demanded by the public. According to Freese[6] and the United States Public Health Service and the National Safety Council, accidental trauma killed 114,000 persons and permanently impaired 500,000 more in 1971 alone. The public asks if it is a neglected epidemic of modern society. Recently hospitals have established effective ambulatory services employing trained nurse practitioners and medical assistants under the supervision of physicians.

Training programs for primary care

There are indications that the wide gap between specialization and primary care is closing. For example, some medical schools have established departments of family medicine and departments of primary care, and medical students are showing an interest in this new medical specialty.[11,22]

In 1970 a multidisciplinary HEW committee studied extended roles for nurses and outlined the elements of nursing practice in the delivery system.[9,12,18] These elements include primary care, acute care, and long-term care. Recently, family nurse practitioner training programs (PRIMEX) were offered in the United States to nurses to prepare for ambulatory care settings. The nurse practitioner in primary care must be able to provide general nursing care, have medical skills in diagnosis and patient management, give physical examinations, administer shots, do laboratory tests, diagnose and treat minor ailments, and counsel patients with chronic diseases or psychosomatic problems. By 1974 there were an estimated 14,000 nurse practitioners in primary care practice.[12] These nurses work in hospital clinics—general medical, pediatric, and obstetrical/gynecological. Others are employed in neighborhood community clinics or in physicians' offices. The nurse practitioner functions independently in accordance with the Nurse Practice Act, and establishes interrelationships with physicians.

Other programs include the Medex program offered to military corpsmen and the medical and surgical assistant programs. These assistants work with specialists and physicians in the hospital and ambulatory services. Some large city health departments offer programs to their public health nurses to function in neighborhood health centers as primary care practitioners.[1,5]

Most of the training programs in primary care have adopted the medical model and subdivide or segment basic health care for patients according to age, sex, or treatment types. This segmented approach is not likely to improve the redistribution of resources to isolated rural areas or urban ghettos. The approach now being used requires staffing many more practitioners in one area to care for children, adults, pregnant women, and chronically ill children and adults.[14]

Evaluation of practicing primary care practitioners indicates that they are providing service no less well, and sometimes better, than physicians and have not produced any significant problems of medical malpractice. However, it will take time for the public, physicians, and other health professionals to recognize the contributions that highly competent nurse practitioners can make in the delivery of primary care.[20,21]

The 1977 report of the National Joint Practice Commission established by the American Nurses' Association and the American Medical Association indicates that nurse-clinicians and physicians working together can meet consumers' health needs effectively and reduce the number of patient-hospital days and expenditures.[12a]

In 1977 the American Nurses' Association supported amendments of Title XVII of the Social Security Act that would give direct payment to nurse-practitioners and nurse midwives under Medicaid and Medicare.[2a]

INFLUENCES OF MEDICINE ON HOSPITAL STRUCTURE AND SERVICES

Medicine, assisted by technological engineering innovations and biomedical research, has developed various therapies that benefit many patients. The modern hospital and industrial man have placed their faith in the engineering technological approach, and the hospital has become a part of the scientific community.

The specialization process has increased the need for more medical specialty facilities, more trained nursing specialists, and more medical assistants. The engineering approach demands the use of newer hardware and more superspecialization by health practitioners. Widespread use of computers continues to increase the cost of treatment and care and promotes further specialization. In our society it is evident that medical practice and research cannot help but follow the development of new technology.

The pace of high technology and specialization in medical education and practice, as well as research through funding from the National Institutes of Health, have created a situation in which more and more resources are allocated for the cure of diseases that have a high death rate in our society. Carlson[3] points out a great amount of money has been spent on cures and little toward prevention.

The traditional organizational structure of hospitals remains a highly fragmented, costly, and labor-intensive industry despite rapid technological advances. The fragmentation of the delivery of health services stems from political, cultural, and socioeconomic forces in our affluent society.

The national health spending per person has more than tripled during the last decade from $212 to $638 in 1976. The total national health expenditures grew from $42.1 billion to $139.3 billion during this same period. The availability and use of new medical services and the increase in health cost inflation account for the rise in spending.[2a]

Medical care still is provided by physicians in their offices or by institutions including hospitals and nursing homes that are influenced and controlled directly or indirectly by physicians. The physicians who have not entered into formal arrangements with the hospital have a great influence on the hospital. In hospitals where physicians and hospital have joined together to provide services, frequently there is no powerful centripetal force to develop an effective participatory overall approach to the delivery of services. Hospital patient care is provided by an impressive group of physicians in various specialties assisted by professional nurses, an array of paramedical personnel, and others in many supportive services.

Within the traditional bureaucratic structure of the hospital the medical model divides the body of man (the patient) into parts, compartmentalizing the delivery system. Nursing services are organized on the medical model to include sex, age, and type of treatment. Nursing service is divided into departments based on the number and size of the various medical services; these departments are divided into various sections, and these sections are divided into units. The traditional bureaucratic nursing service structure is thus unwieldy and fragmented. It includes clinical nurse specialists, supervisors, nurse generalists, and an array of nursing assistants. The increasing medical sophistication of hospitals as an integral part of society has many implications for nurses and the nursing profession.[6]

The public demands competent nursing practice. Some patients are aware of the Patients' Bill of Rights (see Chapter 4). In our traditional hospital environment some nurses give up the right to make decisions that affect the nursing needs of their patients. They follow the old traditional approach that encouraged them to be subservient to physicians and hospital administration and their peers whom they regard as authority figures. Other nurses committed to raising the level of nursing practice and the nursing profession often accept decision-making responsibilities, sometimes with known personal or professional risk. This type of nurse is very much aware of her own capabilities and limitations and endeavors to establish colleagueship relations with other health professionals. Specialization, the assembly line processing of patients' needs and services, and nurses; attitudes and performance are factors that indicate that new approaches to delivery of quality nursing are needed. Shockley[21] wonders if the increasing medical sophistication of society will force nurses out of a job unless they define and support their professional role. There are indications that nurses and their professional associations are making efforts to do so, both in the hospital setting and through legislation and participation with other health associations.

A challenge for nursing leaders would be to examine the relationships of the nursing services to the philosophy and objectives of the hospital, as well as to examine the effectiveness of the management process of nursing in relation to the overall goals and objectives of nursing in the institution. Regardless of the size and the technical capacity of the institution, new ways must be found to enhance the practice of nursing, decrease consumer payments, and improve communications between nursing and the public, between nursing and other health disciplines, and between nurses themselves.[10] Organization, utilization of personnel, and staffing are discussed later in the text.

INCREASING COSTS OF MEDICAL SPECIALIZATION

To maintain a patient in a hospital bed in 1971 cost $36,000, which did not include the $50,000 for construction costs per hospital bed.[4] In 1975, construction costs per bed were estimated at $65,000.

The treatment and care of patients in specialty units such as coronary, intensive care, open heart, kidney dialysis, and burn units require highly complex hardware and many health practitioners with special knowledge and skills. According to the *New York Times* in an article written 11 January 1973, about $135 million was spent on kidney dialysis in the United States in 1972. This figure estimates that 5,000 dialysis patients, the estimated number of users by 1985, each will consume $200,000 per year, for a total of $1 billion per year.[3] With the invention of home-care kidney dialysis apparatus, newer methods of treatment, and training programs for patients, the expenditures should be reduced. Therapy breakthroughs, although complicated and costly, save many lives.

The United States revised 1978 health budget proposals include a nationwide program to hold down the rate of inflation in hospital costs, to improve health care for children in low-income families under Medicaid, and to reduce Medicare payments for the elderly.[2a]

Studies[24] indicate that acutely ill coronary, dialysis, and surgical heart patients require intensive professional care amounting to approximately 10 to 14 hours of direct nursing care per patient in a 24-hour period. This does not include nonnursing input performed by many other hospital personnel including pharmacists, laboratory and inhalation therapy technicians, and engineers. The nurse-to-patient ratio is thus approximately 1.8:1. Studies indicate that the physician-to-patient ratio is roughly 1:10 or 1:6 for coronary care patients. This means that high costs of human resourses are required to support specialty servces.

Moreover, specialization has increased the need to expand training programs for professional and paramedical groups. Between 1963 and 1973, 15 new types of training programs were approved by the AMA Council on Medical Education.[5,7,16] Many of these new assistants work for specialists. Hospitals have set up special training programs for nurses working in specialty units. Medical centers and universities affiliated with hospitals offer training programs in cardiovascular and pediatric nursing and other nursing specialties. The rapid pace of medical treatment has heightened demands for quantity and quality nursing care, although in many institutions, nursing service has not freed itself from nonnursing tasks as it has accepted new medical care responsibilities.

Personnel health care in hospitals doubled between 1965 and 1972. In 1972 hospital personnel of all types comprised about 60% of the hospital budgetary expenditures. Health is the second largest United States industry with over 1 million personnel.[1] The hospital is the predominant workplace of the health occupations, both in terms of its number of personnel and its health expenditures. In 1971, there were a total of 125 occupations with 250 alternate job titles.

The demands for special and primary care services, coupled with the rising costs of human and material resources and greater expectations of the public and personnel, require organization renewal, planning, and flexibility in decision making. Increased centralization and decentralization of decision-making areas within the institution, simplification in methodology of staffing services, adoption of hospital materials-management system, and accountability of nurses for nursing practices are just a few ways to improve the quality of nursing care in the modern hospital.

SCIENTIFIC APPROACH AND CARE ATTITUDES

Historically physicians not only practiced medicine in the care of their patients, but also functioned as counselors and confidants. However, medical education has emphasized how the future physician can utilize knowledge to examine, diagnose, and treat illness for the purpose of curing sick people. With the advent of complex medical hardware and biomedical research the technological aspects of medicine has been stressed.

Nursing education has focused on the emotional and social as well as the physical needs of patients. Linn[11] reports on a study entitled A Survey of the "Care-Cure" Attitudes of Physicians, Nurses, and Their

Students to look for differences in attitudes between the medical and nursing groups. The data indicate that the importance of the emotional components of illness was recognized by a significant number of both health professionals and their students. Medical students placed more value on care than their professors did. The findings seem to reflect a trend of increasing sensitivity among future physicians and nurses to nonmedical factors associated with illness. One hopes that nurses who assume more cure functions will continue to be sensitive to the care functions of patients, though historically, as a service profession becomes more professionalized, that service bureaucracy becomes less sensitive to social needs and more independent of social controls.

The public often views the hospital and its professional staff as cure-oriented. Many patients often are confused, frustrated, and feel helpless in the hands of experts. Some express their feelings in passivity; some become aggressive. Some people believe that the physician's role is becoming one of sickness care. The primary role of medicine comprises diagnosis and treatment: the "cure" process, whereas the primary role of nursing focuses on the "care" process. However, nursing and medicine have common goals: the preservation and restoration of health, but due to the past concept of physician and nurse relations within medical authoritarianism, the nurse's role has been constricted.

Hospitals are beginning to portray a new picture and are caring for the person with a disease. It seems logical that health practitioners should attend to the anthropological aspects of care along with the cure. The method of management of nursing care has a direct influence on how the patient feels about his treatment. Studies indicate when competent R.N.s are responsible for the total nursing care of patients, rather than many different workers, the patients' fears, frustrations, and negative feelings diminish.

It is evident that the complex technical aspects of patient care frequently are more manageable than the psychosocial and interpersonal aspects. Can nursing acquire sufficient knowledge and energy to develop and maintain its role? Can medicine develop a new approach that will result in more effective working relations with nursing?

How should nursing services programs in the modern American hospital be tailored within the overall system for the delivery of health care to patients? How should the various health career groups be educated and trained for specific nursing care services? In an era of specialization, can patients be assured that they will receive *personalized* care as it is rendered by various specialists and many different trained personnel?

As the information explosion continues, how will the nursing researchers work with others in related fields to assist the professional nurse-practitioners who must be depended on to implement the findings of research? These and many other questions face health leaders and nurse-practitioners who are dedicated to providing the answers to meet the preventive, curative health needs of our society.

Some historians may see the twentieth century ending the first period of hospital history and beginning a new approach to health care. Future historians may well describe our era as a period when man learned, or failed to learn, to use the results of his own knowledge and skills effectively and economically.

REFERENCES

1. American Hospital Association: 1973 Guide to the health care field, Chicago, 1973, The Association.
2. Budget of the United States Government: Fiscal year 1975, Washington, D.C., 1974, United States Government Printing Office, p. 197.
2a. Budget of the United States Government: Fiscal year 1978-budget revisions February 1977, Washington, D.C., 1977, United States Government Printing Office.
3. Carlson, R.: The end of medicine, New York, 1975, John Wiley & Sons, Inc., Chapter 3.
4. Comptroller General of the United States: Study of health facilities construction costs, Washington, D.C., 1972, United States Government Printing Office, pp. 98, 759, 847.
5. Department of Health, Education and Welfare: Summary of training programs: physicians support personnel, Washington D.C., June 1972, United States Government Printing Office.

6. Freese, A: Trauma—the neglected epidemic, Saturday Review, May 13, 1972.
7. Health Services Research Center: Medical manpower specialty distribution projections: 1975-1980, May 1971, Institute of Interdisciplinary Studies.
8. Jacobs, A., and Gavett, G.: Case classification of ambulatory care, American Journal of Public Health 63:721-26, August, 1973.
9. Januska, C., Davis, C. D., Knowmueller, R. N., et al.: Development of a family nurse practitioner curriculum, Nursing Outlook 22:103-108, 1974.
10. Kay, E.: The crisis in middle management, New York, 1974, American Management Association.
11. Linn, L: A survey of the "Care-Cure" attitudes of physicians, nurses, and their students, Nursing Forum 14(2):145-159, 1975.
12. Lubin, J.: Supernurses provide care for thousands helping doctors cope, Wall Street Journal, July 3, 1974, p. 1.
12a. National Joint Practice Commission: Together: a casebook of joint practice in primary care, 1977. NJPC/EPIC, 7383 Lincoln Ave., Chicago, Ill. 60646.
13. McNeary, W. J.: Why does medical care cost so much? New England Jounal of Medicine 282:1459-1465, 1970.
14. Milo, N.: The care of health in communities: access for outcast, New York, 1975, The Macmillan Publishing Co., pp. 93-102.
15. Myers, R. J.: Medicare. In McCahan, D.: editor: Accident and sickness insurance, Homewood, Illinois, 1970, Richard D. Irwin, Inc.
16. National Center for Health Statistics: Health resources statistics 1971, Department of Health, Education and Welfare, Washington, D.C., 1972, United States Government Printing Office.
17. New York Times, January 26, 1976.
18. Research Review, Chicago, Spring, 1973, Division of Allied Medical Education, American Medical Association.
19. Ryan, J. L.: The nursing administrator's growing role in facilities planning, Journal of Nursing Administration 5(9):22-27, 1975.
20. Schulman, J., and Wood, C.: Experience of a nurse practitioner in a general medical clinic, Journal of the American Medical Association, 219:1453-1441, March, 1972.
21. Schockley, J. S.: Perspectives in femininity: implications for nursing, Journal of Obstetrics, Gynecologic and Neonatal Nursing, 3(6):36-40, 1974.
22. Skipper, J. K.: Nursing implications (a discussion of R. Battistella article, The right to adequate health care), Nursing Digest 4(1):17-18, 1976.
23. Social Security Administration: Medicare: participating health facilities, July, 1972, Health Insurance Statistics, no. 48, July, 1973.
24. Warstler, M. E., editor: Collection of ten articles, a Journal of Nursing Administration readers' services, Wakefield, Mass., 1974, Contemporary Publishing Co., Inc.

4 | Clients' needs, medical costs, and legislation

Since the 1960s health institutions in the United States have assumed a more dominant and a broader role in patient services, health education, and research programs in cooperation with local, state, and national health agencies and associations.

The traditional health care system in the United States currently is being challenged to develop and implement new approaches that will result in quality health care services at a reasonable price. Consumer-patients, third-party insurers, and government representatives are demanding competent health care providers, more effective distribution of manpower resources, and the availability of "cure" and "care" services.

Professionals in the various health disciplines desire control over their own practices as they work to enhance their professional skills and their status in society. Professional nurses will be pressured to initiate new programs based on new objectives for providing quality nursing care at a reasonable price no matter what innovations and controls are introduced in our health care system and educational programs.

FACTORS AND ATTITUDES INFLUENCING THE HOSPITAL NURSING CARE SYSTEM

With the rapid expansion of medical specialization in the hospital industry and the lack of methods to consolidate services within and outside the hospital community, nurses in the fields of administration, education, and clinical practice, along with other groups associated with health services, have engaged in much introspection and are facing a number of provocative problems. Recent legislation in health services might be considered a prologue to a new health system.

The application of new scientific knowledge and techniques has forced health providers to adjust to a new concept of care and new operational methods and to learn new skills. Dubos remind us that:

Technological and social innovations are so numerous, extensive and rapid that they do not provide the conditions or the time for the spontaneous adaptive processes that used to be so effective in the past. This has been especially striking in the United States since the 19th century for the simple reason that growth and change then became dominant criteria in the American way of life.[29]

In light of hospital history and all the momentous current socioeconomic and technological events affecting the nurses' role in the care of patients, it is wise to look at the background against which we judge our successes and failures. This becomes necessary if we are to make changes to help resolve both old and new problems facing service workers in the care of patients.

General David Sarnoff made this comment when addressing the Board of RCA on the benefits of technological advances: "Our atomic age is like a knife; in the hands of a surgeon it can save a life, in the hands of an assassin it can take one. But to blame the knife is ridiculous." The philosophy of our society comes to life in words such as, "Let each become all he is capable of being," or, "Every man has a right to good health care."

With greater participation of the federal and state governments in health services, hospitals and other community agencies are now forced to find ways to work together more closely within a structured plan. Many planners of health care believe that adequate, continuing health care for all cannot become a reality unless everyone accepts some responsibility for health safety and the prevention of illness.

Man in the twentieth century has become a city-dweller. Urbanization is considered the pulse of economic and social development. The metropolis has become the habitat of modern man. Urban decay, air pollution, drug addiction, loneliness, and other phenomena are associated with today's health problems. Some believe that the innovations of a community-based health care system, which lead to the prevention of disease and correction of physical, economic, emotional, and spiritual problems that surround it, are more scientific and more comprehensive, even if less personalized.

According to Somers and Somers,[81] the four major forces influencing the demands for health services are technological expansion, a general high standard of living, the influence of youth, and the influence of the elderly.

Some authorities[54] indicate that the American public is reaching a threshold of tolerance concerning the quality of services and rising hospital bills. The hospital personnel are demanding higher wages, clarification of job functions, and more voice in the operational management system. The many bills enacted in the 1970s have forced health professionals and others to consider new concepts that will be acceptable to consumers, the government, and other groups in our society.

THE HOSPITAL HEALTH TEAM

With the predicted increase in consumer patient demands, the problems of chronic diseases in childhood, the increase in the chronically ill among the aged, and the ability to prevent and arrest cardiac and cancer diseases, initiate mental health, alcoholic, and drug abuse programs, and provide ambulatory care services in hospitals and the community raise provocative ques-

tions concerning the quantity and the quality of resources and costs. In this age of specialization the physician can no longer practice good medical care alone.

The physician, nurse, physical therapist, dietitian, social worker, minister, and others who assist the patient are beginning to see the value of the health team approach.[50] The role of the health team is more than just helping to eliminate, or at least control, the physical causes of the patient's disease. It is also being aware of his social, economic, and spiritual needs and understanding how they influence his health status.

The patient's physician as health team leader

Medical staff relations of the typical community hospital are a legacy from nineteenth century England. The rapid institutionalization of medicine, the increasing dependence of physicians on each other and on paramedical personnel, the use of expensive specialized equipment and facilities, and socioeconomic factors have changed the characteristics of hospital administration and operations. Professionalism and specialization have become the two hallmarks of the modern hospital. (See Chapter 3.)

In the late 1960s the National Commission on Community Health Services[60] stated the changing role of the personal physician:

Every individual should have a personal physician who is the central point for integration and continuity of all medical and medically related services to his patient. Such a physician will emphasize the practice of preventative medicine through his own efforts and in partnership with the health and social resources of the community. . . . His concern will be for the patient as a whole, and his relationship with the patient must be a continuing one. In order to carry out his coordinating role it is essential that all pertinent health information be channeled through him . . . and will mobilize them (all available health resources) for the patient. . . . To make the most efficient use of limited physician manpower, health care functions not requiring medical training should be delegated by the physician to other members of the health care team to the maximum extent that is practical.

Scientific management researchers, medical consultants, and other specialists currently are working with administrators, professional staffs, and trustees of institutions to develop the type of organizational system that could provide for effective group interaction in the operation of patient care services within the institution, and coordinate these services with related community programs.

Some hospital leaders and health researchers realize that the nursing service is a focal point providing efficient and economical patient services and at the same time humanizing the patient care process. This is true for several reasons: (1) it is the largest single health manpower group in the hospital; (2) it always has attempted to improve the functional organization and management aspects of care and support services; and (3) it has a continuous input in direct care activities and communication with patients, their families, and other health professionals.

Among members of organized nursing services and education there is a growing awareness that nursing as a health profession must select the kind of changes that will strengthen *nursing for people* rather than the kind that will continue to fragment and destroy it. Because nurses have had the "advantage" of being directly *available, accessible,* and *acceptable* to all groups, physicians, hospital administrators, and the public always have tried to help control and define the role and functions of nurses. In the midst of national and local crises, nurses have attempted to meet the nursing needs of patients and their families, usually working within a disorganized, fragmented, and obsolete system of management.

Many centuries ago, Cicero said, "Not to know what has transpired in former times is to continue always as a child. If no use is made of the labors of the past, the world must always remain in the infancy of knowledge." Members of organized nursing should be very much aware of what has taken place in order to help initiate and develop a new nursing system for the delivery of patient care.

During the 1970s nurses have taken a more confident position in communicating to the public and governmental representatives the appropriate and necessary role of nursing to assure quality nursing care services. Professional nurses need to understand recent health legislation, and if the profession of nursing is to have a part in major decision-making policies concerning the health care system and educational and training programs, nurses must work together toward achieving mutual goals within their professional organizations.

Changing perceptions of nurses as members of the health team

In past generations the nurse's role in providing patient care was perceived primarily as that of "handmaiden." Recently, nurses have been viewed as the "extenders" of medicine. In the pyramidal institutional organization, nurses have been accepted on health teams as functionary members, but have not had a part in the decision-making processes of planning and policy formation. Traditional nurses have not considered decision making an element of professional nursing practice.

In the past decade, nurses' approaches to their position, responsibilities, and nursing itself have been changing.[44,65] One major factor affecting these changes is the shift in nursing education from the hospital setting where programs focus on services and procedures to the university and college where programs are based on the sciences and philosophy. The increasing number of nursing programs in universities indicates that the image of the profession is changing and that nursing is becoming an appealing career.[80]

In reviewing recent professional literature and newspapers and in listening to recent graduate nurses, one realizes that a new aggressiveness exists among nurses. They are becoming more active advocates for their patients and are taking steps to personalize health care, rather than continuing to be "handmaidens" in the health system. The emergence of this "new" nurse in our technological and complex society should stimulate educators in nursing programs to structure future curricula to facilitate the development of skills essential to the roles of the future nurse.[79]

The competent nurse with a masters degree and adequate experience is articulate and confident in pressing to implement new approaches in the management of nursing care. These nurses seek positions that will permit them to use their knowledge and abilities to expand into more responsible roles in which they can account for their nursing practices. They want to establish effective colleagueship relationships as members of the health team and patient care system.

A second factor that has affected nurses is the women's liberation movement in our society. It has encouraged members of the nursing profession to recognize their own worth as persons and professionals. During the past decade more nurses recognized that they could gain more political power and status by working together through their professional associations. Nurses are directing their energies in a more sophisticated manner within their work environment and in community activities to enhance the practice of nursing. Recent developments in the formulation of nursing standards and peer review processes and participation in legislative actions are discussed later in this text.

Nurses who did not believe in the collective bargaining process for professional nurses now are realizing that it can be used effectively to improve the quality of care, as well as their status and salary.

Some hospital officials and educators are questioning the necessity in general for nurses to have a higher level of education in order to do their job. Moreover, the employment of educated nurses only increases the cost of health services. Sheldon, in his article "Are Problems in Graduate Nursing Education Unique?" states that advanced levels of education for nurses should be mandatory only when such educational requirement is proven necessary to improve the professional practice and the delivery of good health care.[79] In some institutions nursing service proves that cost con-

tainments can be controlled by employing competent educated nurses as well as by changing the structure of the nursing service system.

Competent nurses are more willing to take risks as members of the health team and are demanding a part in the planning and decision-making processes of patient care.[44] Nurse-practitioners and nurse administrators are confronted directly with making important decisions or selecting alternatives.[15] However, more nurses should understand that changes may not occur as desired.

Nurses in the work environment or as members of their organizations need to know what issues are at stake and be able to make decisions concerning compromises or agreements. Conflicts are created within the nursing staff concerning health groups and clients when decisions are made without adequate knowledge or expert guidance.

Professional nurses must be prepared to face the demands of cost containment, assurance of quality nursing care, and the control mechanism for the practice of nursing. Many debates continue in the nursing profession and with other professionals and out of the work setting over who shall accredit nurse-practitioner programs and certify professional nurses.

It is evident that in the health team structure no one provider has the knowledge and skills to give total health care to each client. All health care providers are important to patient care. Nurses have a right and a responsibility to participate in health planning and decision making after accepting this fact.

In the work environment, the community, or within their professional associations, nurses should be cognizant of the truism that conflict is an essential and expected part of human behavior and life.[52] However, if nurses want to shift from being functionaries in the patient care system to being professionals they must possess the knowledge and skills to make decisions. The nursing profession must prove that educated and competent nurses can improve the quality of patient care while containing costs.

CURRENT HOSPITAL AND HEALTH CARE EXPENDITURES IN THE UNITED STATES

Professional nurses should know about costs and expenditures of health care services of their own institutions and agencies as well as those of the state and nation. Awareness of these facts matters when one takes part in closing the gap between the supply and demand of health care services.

General perspective

The hospital may be viewed as a multiproduct service composed of many different service units that should be identified and their source and use completely understood by the providers, including nurses. Recent legislation provides avenues so that consumers can be kept informed (see Social Security amendments of 1972, and National Health Planning and Resources Development Act, 1974, discussed later in this chapter).

According to a study published by the Social Security Administration's Office of Research and Statistics, entitled National Health Expenditures,[88] health care spending in the fiscal year 1975 reached $118.5 billion, representing a 13.9% increase over the $104 billion spent in the fiscal year 1974. It is predicted that by 1980 the total health care service will be the largest service industry in the United States and that $1 of every $10 will be spent on health services.[91]

Between 1965 and 1972 about 10% of the total personal health expenditures in the United States was due to population increases, 38% resulted from the increased use and expansion of health services, and nearly 52% resulted from price increases for products and personnel. In 1975, inflation replaced the scope of services as a major reason for hospital cost increases.

According to the Department of Health, Education and Welfare's 1975 report,[87] the total death rate in the United States has remained about 1,000 per 100,000 population over the past few decades. Statistics indicate that the poor use a disproportionately large part of their income for health care services. For example, families with incomes of less than $2,000 spent 12.6% of their income in 1970 for care services, whereas families with incomes of $7,500 or more spent 3.5% of their income for similar services.[30]

The 1975 report on health in the United States indicates that through public funding health care for the poor has improved slightly. More persons were seen by physicians in 1974 than in 1964.[30] However, a wide gap still exists between the rich and the poor concerning the cost of services in relation to incomes, in addition to the uneven distribution of health resources for United States consumers as a whole.[57]

Personal health care expenditures in the United States

Personal health expenditures have risen steadily for the past 20 years with the expansion of medical services and specialization. Expenditures rose from $22.7 billion in 1960 to $59.1 billion in 1970. In 1973, all expenditures resulting from illness and injury totaled over $200 billion, with $80 billion of direct costs for personal health care services. In 1976 the total national health expenditure was $139.3 billion.[31a]

Government funding and private health insurance

In 1950 the consumer's out-of-pocket expenditures for health care was about 68% of the total bill in comparison to 1975, when only 33% of the total health expenditures was paid "out-of-pocket." Public funding now pays about 33% of the total hospitalization for persons under 65 years and 66% of the total expenditures for those over 65 years.[66] Currently, third-party insurance payments cover 90% of the total expenditures for hospitalization.

Hospital expenditures in 1974 accounted for 71% of Medicare funds and 37% of Medicaid funds. Such payments indirectly have given financial relief to medical centers and teaching hospitals with personnel budgetary costs, including salary increases for resident-physicians and their supervisors on the medical faculty. Public funding for the poor, the aged, and for biomedical research has assisted in the expansion of specialty services, inhospital coverage paid on an open-ended-cost reimbursement basis, and the open-ended fee for service reimbursement method for physician services.

According to Milo,[57] two major problems with third-party financing have been (1) incomplete and nonuniform coverage and (2) coverage that tends to encourage patient hospitalization and high cost care with lack of incentives to control costs.

Hospital facilities and revenues

The 7,000 hospitals in the United States have a total of more than 3 million beds and employ over 4 million people.[88] Between 1965 and 1975 the number of acute care beds increased and now totals about 850,000 beds. However, the total number of unoccupied beds increased by 28%. The average occupancy rate of hospitals ranges from 60% to 80%. The input utilization as measured by inpatient days has been decreasing since 1967. The problems of occupancy rate and the costs of speciality units are discussed in Chapter 3.

Hospitals are growing in size but not in number. It is estimated that over 40% of all hospitals will be over 400 beds by 1980. Small hospitals will become absorbed into larger units or shut down.

Since 1950 there has been a rise in costs and charges coinciding with the rise in expenditures. According to the HEW report,[87] hospital costs per admission rose from $127 in 1950 to $830 dollars in 1972. Likewise, semiprivate room charges rose from $30 in 1950 to $174 in 1972. Statistics show that the 44.8% increase in cost per adjusted hospital day in 1975 resulted from increases in the price of goods and services. The quantity of goods purchased contributed to 15.7% of this increase, and the personnel and average wages accounted for 28% of the total increase.[66]

According to the report, Health, United States 1975, 39% of the total care expenditures was for hospital costs and 26% was for physician services. One should note that insurance provisions governing reimbursement for nursing services tend to be totally inadequate or inappropriate. Institutions or physicians must authorize reimbursement for nursing services.[95] The consumer and nursing profession have had little control over the financing and the distribution of nursing care services.[49]

In our complex and changing society it has been predicted that the health care system will broaden its goals and begin to focus on health maintenance as well as on illness.[36,70,90] This could decrease costly medical care in inpatient hospital facilities and increase the health maintenance services offered in ambulatory and clinic facilities. With the establishment of newly designed facilities and services, the "new" nurses will establish themselves in the community in specialized settings such as burn care centers, respiratory centers, acute renal dialysis centers, and in modern nursing care facilities for the chronically ill and aged.

When the health system changes, the role of nurses will change.[16,74] This will have legal implications for the practice of nursing and will bring pressure to provide adequate insurance provisions governing reimbursement for nursing services.

Impact of governmental planning and financing of patient care

Government—federal, state, and municipal—has for many years assisted financially in hospital construction costs and services.[31a,54,58]

Government has participated in medicine to some degree since this country was born. The social legislation of 1935 had a powerful influence on the American way of life and hospital care. The passage of the Social Security Act in 1935 was the beginning of modern social reform.

In 1948 the 10-year health program prepared for President Truman by the Federal Security Administration aroused much controversy over the question of compulsory versus voluntary insurance as a method of paying for medical care.

Along with the increasing cost of hospital construction, there have been changes in hospital capital financing. In recent years, an increasing amount of money has come from government, for the most part in the form of federal (Hill-Burton and Hill-Harris Acts) monies. The NHPRD Act, 1974, is resulting in changes. This bill is discussed later in this chapter.

Introduction of Medicare for the aged

With the passage of the Social Security Amendments (Public Law 89-97) on July 30, 1965, and their signing by President Johnson, the Medicare program became a reality, creating a greater governmental stake in providing health care for people in the United States.

Medicare for the population over 65 years of age, with definitive hospital and related care services, was established under Title XVIII, with the Secretary of the Department of Health, Education, and Welfare given broad latitude as to the way in which payment rates are determined.[81]

The Medicare program became effective July 1, 1966, except for the posthospital extended care services, which became effective January 1, 1967.[58] The Social Security amendments of 1967 included changes and adjustments in the Medicare program. The Medicare program contains two major health insurance programs: (1) hospital insurance (Part A—Title XVIII) and (2) medical insurance (Part B—Title XVIII). The hospital insurance program provides for payment of covered services for hospital and posthospital care as set forth in the current title. The medical insurance program provides for payment of doctor's bills and certain other medical items such as outpatient therapy and a reserve of 60 days of coverage for inpatient hospital care. (See discussion of recent legislation.)

Through the Medicare program the United States has assumed responsibility for financing the health needs of a significant segment of the population using the mechanism of social insurance. Studies indicate that patients over 65 years of age in general hospitals required more general nursing care man-hours than those under 65. During the early 1970s the bed shortage that most hospitals feared did not occur. Medicare did not increase the admission rate, but it did increase the length of stay of individuals covered under the program.[58] The revised 1978 health budget of the President of the United States proposes Medicare program improvements to benefit 26 million Medicare beneficiaries. It aims to provide primary and rural health care by extending cost reimbursement to nurse-practitioners and physician-assistants practicing in rural health clinics.[31a]

Medicaid assistance (Title XIX)

The financing and utilization of Title XIX of the Social Security Amendment (Public Law 89-97) is also of importance to hospitals. This law authorized grants to states for medical assistance programs, with the federal government's share of such costs ranging from 50% to 83% according to a state's per capita income.

As of July 1, 1967, all Title XIX programs were required to minimally include (1) inpatient hospital services (except in hospitals for the care of patients with tuberculosis or mental diseases), (2) outpatient hospital services, (3) other laboratory services and x-ray services, (4) adequate home nursing services for individuals 21 years of age or older, and (5) physicians' services, regardless of where service was rendered.

Because Medicaid is a state program, each state establishes its own standards, policies, procedures, and interrelationships with other states and local health programs. This has created problems for hospitals.

The 1978 health budget of the President of the United States proposes a $180 million program of improvements in comprehensive health care for children in low-income families under Medicaid and $6 million for immunizations for disadvantaged children in rural areas. A 75% federal match is designed to give those states currently receiving reimbursements of less than 75% from the federal government a greater incentive to establish screening programs for children with medical problems.[31a]

The Federal Civil Rights Act

Since July 2, 1964, hospitals have been required to show compliance with the following nondiscrimination requirements as stated in Title VI:[83]

No person in the United States shall, on the ground of race, color, or national origin, be excluded from participation in, be denied the benefits of, or be subjected to discrimination under any program or activity receiving Federal financial assistance.

Regulations of the Department of Health, Education, and Welfare became effective January 3, 1965. From then on any applicant(s) for funds under any program of the department had to assure in writing that he or they would comply fully with the nondiscrimination requirements of the Civil Rights Act. All hospitals or health care institutions that are now receiving federal funds, as well as those requesting grants to remodel or build facilities or to conduct research or training, are required to submit form HEW-441 (assurance of compliance with the Department of Health, Education, and Welfare of the Civil Rights Act of 1964). The Civil Rights Act of 1964 also extended the nondiscrimination requirements to medical interns and residents and any other persons receiving training in the hospital such as nurses and technicians.

In accordance with the department regulations under Title VI of the Civil Rights Act, each state agency is responsible for informing hospitals and other health institutions throughout the state of the law and the regulations and seeing that such practices are carried out.

The Surgeon General of the Public Health Service published a list of questions for hospitals to review to determine their general compliance with provisions of the act. It appeared in *Hospitals*, August 1, 1965. Questions were listed under various headings such as admission policies, patient room assignment, availability of services and facilities, medical attending staff privileges, and training programs.

PATIENTS' BILL OF RIGHTS

Since the late 1940s, rapid technological innovations, application of biomedical research, health insurance coverage, an increased economy, and a better educated public have contributed to the expansion of medicine and the availability of hospital services. However, the use of health services by the poor has differed from other income groups because of the services available to them.[20]

Consumer-patients' demands

In general, health care providers were not very attentive to the preferences and choices of poor consumer-patients.[57] Hospital administrators and physicians have tended to determine patient choices by their own preferences and choices. Consumer-patients want to make their own choices when entering a hospital. They want to understand the treatments they may undergo, the risks that those treatments may entail, and what alternatives are available. They want information about their own bodies and clear answers to their questions.[3,10] Consumer-patients want access to information about themselves and their treatment in addition to control over any disclosures of that information to outsiders.[48,71]

Hospital administrators and physicians evaluate the quality of care in clinical terms. Patients view the quality of care differently, recognizing the value of basic sciences but believing that quality care also possesses humanistic concepts, including respect for the dignity of every man. Although more patients entered hospitals and recovery rates were greater in the late 1950s through the early 1970s, patients' rights received increasing attention by consumer groups and other citizens.

Patients' rights formally introduced

The beginning of the health care resolution was recognized by health providers. In 1959 the National League for Nursing published a public relations document entitled, What People Can Expect of Modern Nursing Service.[21]

The Committee on Health Care for the Disadvantaged of the American Medical Association developed the Patients' Bill of Rights (PBR).[20] This committee was composed of hospital administrators, hospital and planning agency executives, physicians, attorneys, and consumers. Unfortunately, nurses were not represented on this committee. In 1973 the American Hospital Association issued the PBR document in an effort to allay patients' fears concerning the unknown.

Consumer-patients, civic groups, and many hospital administrators, physicians, and legislative representatives in various states had reservations concerning hospital control and authority over medical and nursing actions. Questions arose concerning the ability to implement all twelve points of the bill and over the legal implications of these rights in written form. Some state legislatures adopted their own patients' rights bills; others, pressured by the AHA state association, passed a resolution encouraging the implementation of the PBR rather than mandating all hospitals to distribute the PBR to their patients.

In 1973 the Insurance Commissioner of Pennsylvania published his own bill of patients' rights to be used by Pennsylvania's insurance department.[24] This 12-point document, entitled Citizens' Bill of Hospital Rights: What the Patient and Public Can and Should Expect from Our Hospitals, is more explicit than the PBR. It presents statements that support recent legislative actions protecting such consumer-patient rights as economy of care, consumer input, participation in the decision process, access to information, answers about treatment, control of one's body and life, and action on complaints and problems.

The HEW secretary's Commission on Medical Malpractice stated in his 1973 report that to ignore the rights of consumer-patients would invite dissatisfaction that could lead to malpractice suits. The commission recommended (1) that hospitals and other health care facilities adopt and distribute statements of patients' rights in a manner that would most effectively communicate these rights to all incoming patients, (2) that functions of teaching hospitals be explained to all patients entering such hospitals and that those functions be emphasized in other forms of consumer education, (3) that those functions, where they exist, and distinctions in the treatment of patients in teaching hospitals based on the patients' race or socioeconomic status be eliminated.[87] The HEW secretary also offered a mechanism for consumer participation.

Federal legislation has supported the position of the consumer-patient through the amendments of the 1967 Freedom of Information Act (FIA) in the Primary Act (PL 93-579), that were enacted in September, 1975. This law is controversial, and interpretations of it are unclear, especially for hospitals receiving federal funds for medical care or research.[52a] Medical researchers are concerned about the effect of record availability in relation to other studies.

The HEW regulations require the patient to sign a very specific consent for research carried out under HEW auspices. The National Research Act of 1974 has established a commission to (among other functions) "identify the requirements for informed consent procedures for children, prisoners, and the mentally disabled, and determine the need for a mechanism to assure that human subjects are covered by HEW regulations are protected." Note the ANA Professional Code statement that "the nurse participates in activities that contribute to the ongoing development of the profession's body of knowledge" (see Chapter 3, code for nurses). The ANA document provides human rights guidelines for nurses.

It is necessary that patients near death be free of pain. There is a need for appropriate health care facilities for terminally ill patients and professional nursing care, resulting in more alert patients who would be able to make their own decisions about what to do and how to die. In such institutions patients would not be subjected to experiments with anticancer drugs or other extensive surgical and medical treatments. They only would be given treatment to keep them as comfortable as possible.[52a]

Informed consent

The trend is to view the physician and patient as a partnership in decision making rather than as a medical monopoly.[3,10,24] The informed consent contains several basic elements: (1) an explanation of the condition, (2) a fair explanation of the procedures to be used and the various possible consequences, (3) a description of alternative treatment or procedures, (4) a description of the benefits to be expected (not assured), and (5) an understanding that the patient will not be coerced to agree and may withdraw if he changes his mind.

A consent is a free and rational act that presupposes knowledge of the thing to which consent is given by a person who is legally capable of consent. Nurses, as a patient's advocate, should be aware of signs that the patient does not understand clearly what is involved. Nurses should notify the physician of patient's withdrawal of consent and see that the patient is not treated. It should be noted that in such cases both physician and nurse are liable. There is a growing trend among nurses to assume accountability for their own actions in caring for patients and to act as informed advocates on patients' behalf. Will nurses also assert their rights to be colleagues in health care?

Through recent legislative action new opportunities have opened up, enabling consumer citizens to participate in the planning and controlling powers of our health delivery system. The 1972 amendments of the Social Security Act grant access to public information and the performance of state agencies, insurance carriers, and other intermediaries who administer programs. The Occupational Safety and Health Act and the National Health Planning and Resources Development Act, 1974, which will be discussed later, offers legal tools to press for the necessary changes to maintain health services for all people. Collective bargaining legislation (NLRA) offers options to professional nurses inside the health organization for internal formal decision making.

Milo,[57] in discussing consumers as patients, emphasizes that continuous bargaining and decision making in and between organizations on the local, state, and national levels results in improved distribution of funds, facilities, personnel, and access to information. Such actions give citizens, patients, and professional nurses a greater voice in the decisions that affect them.

AREAWIDE AND REGIONAL PLANNING FOR PATIENT CARE

The Regional Medical Program (the Heart Disease, Cancer and Stroke, Amendments of 1965, Public Law 89-239) resulted from the DeBakey Report. Initially the plans were to build regional centers around a university-medical school nucleus, these were revised, with less emphasis placed on the medical school as a nucleus.

The comprehensive Health Planning and Public Health Service amendments of 1966 (Public Law 89-749) provided a mechanism through which regional health programs could become a reality and produce an effective health industry. Hospitals encountered many problems concerning overall planning and government reimbursements.[84]

The major objectives of Public Law 89-749 were (1) to provide for comprehensive planning for health services, health manpower, and health facilities on the state and local level, (2) to strengthen and improve existing public health plans and project grant programs, (3) to provide for the interchange of federal, state, and local health workers, and (4) to provide greater flexibility in participative planning to support health services in the community.

In 1973, after approximately 5 years of development, comprehensive health planning (CHP) agencies existed on a statewide level with about 200 related areawide level agencies. Most of the areawide agencies were unable to develop a master plan, which was their mandate.[73]

A number of states passed certificate-of-need statutes, a mechanism of cost control directed primarily at controlling health facilities' construction. These statutes gave the agencies review-and-approval authority over applications from hospitals and nursing care facilities for expansions costing from $50,000 to $350,000. With this authority CHP agencies generally were able to prevent unnecessary expansion and the construction of new facilities.

Under the 1972 Social Security amendments, states could name a designated plan agency to carry out capital expenditures, control overall health care providers except for individual practitioners, and receive social security financing when such expenditures exceeded $100,000. This actually was a national certificate-of-need law. Comprehensive health planning agencies thus, moved from an initial voluntary planning concept toward a mandatory cost-control focus, first by the state and then by the federal government. (see discussion, on the NHPRD Act, 1974, later in this chapter).

SOCIAL SECURITY AMENDMENTS, 1972

The Social Security amendments of 1972 (PL 92-603), often referred to as Hr 1, established changes in service care payments for Medicare, Medicaid, maternal and child health, and the disabled, as well as methods to control costs, utilize resources, construct facilities, and assure quality care.[90,96] Of the 97 separate sections affecting Medicare and Medicaid, the two problems of cost containment and assurance requirements for health care practitioners (section 1160 of the act) have important implications for nursing.

Congress inserted a provision (section 222 of Public Law 92-603) authorizing experimentation and demonstration projects "to determine under what circumstances payment for services would be the most appropriate and equitable amounts of reimbursement . . . for services which are performed independently by an assistant to a physician, including a nurse practitioner." Third party reimbursement for nurses has become a high priority professional issue in the 1970s. The ANA has worked vigorously for direct-fee-for-service reimbursement for nurse-practitioners by both public and private third party payors. There are indications that some nursing services will be reimbursable in the near future.

Major organizational changes

The former Title XVIII Medicare is now called Health Insurance for the Aged and Disabled under the supervision of the Health Insurance Benefits Advisory Council. The former Medical Assistance Advisory Council was terminated and its functions under Title IX were added to the new council's functions.

The provision that each state develop a comprehensive medical program by July 1, 1976, was repealed.[96] The Act mandates that hospitals and skilled nursing facilities participating in Medicaid and child health groups, with few exceptions, use the utilization review (peer review) of the Medicare program. Family planning services become a part of the basic Medicaid program.

Under section 1122 of the 1972 amendments, health facility planners will examine proposals for expansion and modernization projects and make recommendations to institutional providers in relation to community needs for new facilities. The National Health Planning and Resources Development Act, 1974, has established additional changes of comprehensive care planning.[14] This new act is discussed later in this chapter.

PROFESSIONAL STANDARDS REVIEW ORGANIZATION

According to the Department of Health, Education, and Welfare report entitled Foward Plan for Health, fiscal year 1977-81,* the quality assurance plan will provide a framework for integrating the many different health functions of the federal government into a coherent program and thus improve the quality of health services throughout the United States. It could become a national operational quality assurance system of a national health insurance program.[36,85]

This organization is mandated under B, Title XI of the 1972 Social Security amendments. It provides for the establishment of PSROs within the states for the review of the professional activities of physicians and other practitioners and of institutional and other

---

*United States Public Health Service, Department of Health Education and Welfare: Forward plan for health FY 1977-81; Washington, D.C., 1975, United States Government Printing Office, p. 22.

providers of health services to consumers in designated geographical areas.

The act mandates that state and local PSROs be established by July 1, 1978. State-wide professional standard review councils will report findings and problems to its national council.

The National Council on Professional Standards Review is under the direction of the assistant secretary of the Department of Health Education and Welfare. HEW, assisted by the Bureau of Quality Assurance, is responsible for writing regulations and policies in accordance with Congressional intent. A new office of Professional Standards Review has been established in the assistants' office. The National Council of PSRO is composed of 11 physicians. This type of representation is similar to the Foundation of Medical Care (FMC).

The statewide councils and their supportive local units consist of both physicians and nonphysicians. The term nonphysicians includes registered nurses, dietitians, pharmacists, and physical therapists. The nonphysician health providers are charged to participate in the development of appropriate criteria and standards, using the national council's guidelines for review of their services rendered to clients.[62]

Several provisional statements on reporting requirements for the PSRO program have ben issued since 1975, but those requirements still are subject to change. As of 1977, each PSRO is responsible for defining its own data set that makes up the uniform hospital discharge data set (UHDDS). The PSRO hospital discharge data set (PHDDS) incorporates the UHDDS and other specific data required for federally reimbursed care. The Bureau of Quality Assurance (BQA) has started to apply pressure on PSROs to perform other mandated activities such an ancillary and ambulatory services.

Implications for nursing

The Department of Health, Education, and Welfare agrees that there is no one definition of quality health care.[90] It has developed the working definition, "Quality health care offers the patient the greatest achievable health benefit, with minimum unnecessary risk and use of resources in a manner satisfactory to the patient."

The American Nurses' Association has participated in developing guidelines to review nursing care as contracted by the Bureau of Quality Assurance (BQA).[62] As of January, 1976, the ANA's two documents were endorsed by the National Council of PSRO. The one document is entitled Recommendations for Involvement of Nurses in PSRO Review and is used by the BQA. The other document, Guidelines for Review of Nursing Care, has been prepared for those in state and local quality assurance programs.

The nursing criteria were developed by nurse-practitioners and tested by nursing experts throughout the nation. The design of a quality assurance program for a nursing department is discussed later in this text. At recent forums for nurse educators and nursing service pertinent papers were presented on quality assurance.[12,25,26]

It is true that the present PSRO policy does not define clearly the expanded role of the professional nurse.[56] Many nurses wonder if PSRO will permit them to function at the level for which they are prepared. Others wonder if physicians will regard the nurse-practitioner as competing for organization support, a reasonable wage, and a voice in the decision-making process. Institutional providers and other professional colleagues ask if nurses will accept their responsibility for accountability in the quality assurance program.

As professional nurses, we should recognize that in this mandate society has given us the permission to perform services for our clients and recognizes them as legitimate.[49] Aydelotte[12] reminds us that along with our right to practice nursing, we are expected to account for the quality and the effects of our services. Through PSROs, nurses have an opportunity to evaluate and document the input and outcome of nursing care against defined criteria and standards.

Professional nurses should seek membership on state councils and supportive units where they will have opportunities to evaluate the PSRO process and make recommendations for improvements. Nurses as members of their professional association should work as a group through local, state, and national channels to create closer colleagueships to improve the system, and to increase communications with the public regarding nursing roles in the health care delivery system.

HEALTH MAINTENANCE ORGANIZATION

The HMO Act, 1973 (PL 93-222), demonstrates support of a health system that provides a wide range of health maintenance and treatment services to a voluntarily enrolled population in return for a previously determined fixed sum of money per year. The HMO amendments of 1975 (Hr 9019) liberalized requirements for participation under a HMO, reduced the basic health service package offered to every HMO enrollee, and changed physician employment policies.[37,92]

HMOs may be organized as a nonprofit, profit, sponsored, or independent system. Even though HMOs may differ slightly in their management and objectives, they are basically similar: (1) an HMO is an organized health care delivery system composed of health practitioners and others who work in the facilities and who are capable of providing or arranging for all services that enrollees may require; (2) an HMO serves the enrollees who agree to get most of their medical care from HMO; and (3) the HMO determines the price of the total health package in advance and agrees by contract with enrollees to provide such services. The HMO determines a fixed monthly charge for each enrollee, regardless of the amount of services used. Thus, income is no longer tied to services.

In an HMO, nurses and physicians should become partners in the economic strategy of the system. This requires a closer look by professional health providers at the costs of care to help determine what services should be offered and what would be the outcomes: what methods and techniques could be initiated that would not jeopardize the quality of care and at the same time maintain and control costs.

Implications for nursing

Nurse-practitioners and nurse-administrators in HMOs should have an opportunity to participate in quality care assurance and cost containment processes. The act does not mention nurse leadership positions within HMO.

The HMO concept of care emphasizes prevention of disease, health maintenance, and treatment.[37] Primary care is an integral part of the program. In the Harvard Community Health Organization the nurse provides desired and needed health care for a group of consumers and their families.[17,93] In most HMOs the organizational structure resembles the traditional pyramid hierarchy with the medical practitioner in control of medical and other professional practices. In the present health care crisis and with an uneven distribution of physicians, competent nurse-practitioners are becoming effective health team members.

The HMO program does not define nursing services as one of its basic services. The medical group is defined to include physicians, doctors of osteopathy, and other licensed health professionals. Nurses should be defined as members of the group practice. They can share in the formal partnership as they share in the care and treatment of HMO subscribers.

NATIONAL HEALTH PLANNING AND RESOURCES DEVELOPMENT ACT, 1974

This complex health service planning act (Public Law 93-641) aims to augment and restructure area and state planning for health care services, manpower, and facilities based on recommendations for a national health planning policy. This act combines into one statewide health authority all federal mechanisms used for local health planning and resource development: the regional medical program, comprehensive health planning, Hill-Burton state hospital planning councils, and area health education centers.[90,91]

The objectives of the act include (1) increasing the access to health services, (2) maintaining continuity of care, (3) restraining increases in health care costs, (4) preventing unnecessary duplication of services, and (5) assuring effective utilization of manpower resources.

Organization plan

Health systems agencies (HSAs) serve in various geographical areas in each state. Each HSA has been given responsibility for collecting and analyzing data concerning the health care status of the residents in their designated health service area, the status of the area's health care delivery system, its use by the people in the area, the effect of health services rendered, the number, type, and location of the area's health resources, and the patterns of utilization of those health resources.[51,70]

Each HSA is responsible for developing health systems plans (HSP) and an annual implementation plan (AIP). It is anticipated that these documental guides will stimulate hospitals and other providers to develop their own plans and programs to serve their designated community areas.

The majority of health systems agencies that will supplant existing areawide comprehensive health planning agencies are expected to be private, not-for-profit organizations with governing bodies of between 10 and 30 health service area residents. A majority of residents must be consumers of health care. They must broadly represent the areas' social, economic, linguistic, and racial populations. The remaining members of the HSA will represent health care providers, insurers, government authorities, health professional schools or allied health professions, and the local government. The governors have been charged with setting up HSAs in their states with the approval of the Department of Health, Education, and Welfare.

The HSAs are responsible for implementing their plans, coordinating their efforts with other planning organizations, making recommendations to the state advisory agency, and assisting the state in determining the appropriateness of existing institutional facilities in their respective areas.

Each state is required to establish a state health planning and development agency (SHPDA) and a state health coordinating council (SHCC) that serves as advisor to the state agency. The SHPDA is delegated to conduct state health planning and functions related to both state and HSA. The SHCC prepares state health plans for budget reviewing.

The state council is composed of at least 16 members appointed by the governor, and 60% of the council's members must be HSA members.

The national council is responsible for developing guidelines for the state councils and for interpreting the act and keeping the councils informed of technological innovations that would affect the delivery health care system. This council is under the direction of the secretary of the Department of Health, Education, and Welfare.

Recent HSA regulations include the development of a memorandum of understanding (MOU) between HSAs and PSROs within 6 months after an HSA has been established. The data requirements of PSROs and HSAs and the plan for these programs aim to support each other. This will undoubtedly affect the hospital information systems. The data now being requested are forcing integration and interrelationships of data bases involving clinical and management operations.

Implications for nursing

Competent professional nurses should endeavor to become members of HSA and the councils. By joining HSA nurses have an opportunity to work with consumers of health services as well as with other health providers. Nurses can contribute a great deal in the development of good functional data regarding nursing manpower, available nursing services, and the determination of facilities to meet community needs. A good data base of the area could provide documentation of current usage patterns in forecasting and setting priorities for health care in various areas in each state. Nurses who work in hospitals and agencies and those in nursing education can contribute in determining priorities in the care of clients with acute and chronic health problems as well as in maintenance of health, training and educational programs for health care personnel, and utilization of resources.

Many issues will surface in the implementation of this act. It is true that nurses must unite to identify their goals and plans of strategy, assume responsibility, and be willing to take risks. Power does not exist in a vacuum.[14] Participation and evaluation of both actions and outcomes are necessary to help make decisions.

NONPROFIT HOSPITALS AND THE NATIONAL LABOR RELATIONS ACT, 1974

Thirty-nine years elapsed before the National Labor Relations Act was amended to make nonprofit hospitals and their employees subject to its provisions. The revision of the Wagner Act in 1947, later known as the Taft-Hartley Act, includes a provision charging that professional employees could not be organized in the same collective bargaining unit with nonprofessionals, unless a majority of the professional employees voted for such inclusion. The act also exempts nonprofit hospitals from coverage.

American Nurses' Association's position and goals

Since 1896 the membership of the professional nursing organization has endeavored to improve the working environment and welfare of nurses so that consumers would have quality nursing care. With the passage of the Landrum-Griffin Act in 1959, both the ANA and the SNA officially declared themselves and registered as labor organizations.[97]

Since 1946 the SNAs have expanded their programs to protect new nursing roles and the practice of nursing. The ANA maintains that the SNAs should represent nurses because they, as professional organizations, are most knowledgeable about the nursing profession and nurses' abilities, skills, and economic needs.[19]

The state associations use the ANA commission's guidelines in developing suitable economic and general welfare (EGW) programs or in adopting state policies. The goals of the EGW programs stress that such programs are utilized to effect, maintain, and upgrade educational standards and professional practices. Nurses should be aware of the full meaning and implications for nursing in both the Code for Professional Nurses (see p. 2) and the ANA goals of the EGW program.[19]

GOALS

- *To provide quality nursing care*
  1. At the place of employment, to implement the standards enunciated by the professional association that affect nursing care.
  2. To secure conditions of employment and a climate for practice that foster a lifetime career attachment to nursing.
  3. To secure conditions of employment that will attract able persons to careers in nursing.

- *To promote professional self-determination*
  1. To involve nurses actively in determining the conditions of employment under which they practice, through collective action.
  2. To represent nurses at their place of employment utilizing collective bargaining.

- *To protect and advance the economic and professional status of nurses*
  1. To attain wide understanding and recognition of the scientific and social contribution of nurses to the health and welfare of the community.
  2. To achieve an employment status for nurses commensurate with their preparation and qualifications and with the intellectual and technical nature of their services.
  3. To promote social, economic and health legislation beneficial to the economic and general welfare of nurses.*

Fundamental principles of the 1974 National Labor Relations Act

The major concept of the 1974 National Labor Relations Act is based on our society's respect for the dignity of both man and his work. The NLRA encourages the utilization of collective bargaining as a means of establishing wages and conditions of work for nonmanagerial and nonsupervisory em-

*Commission on Economic and General Welfare of the American Nurses' Association: Philosophy, goals, policies, and positions, pub. no. EC-119, 10/7510M, Kansas City, Mo., 1975, The Association.

ployees. It now provides a way through which most health care professionals and nurse-educators have the right to freely form or join a union and bargain collectively to meet their goals.[89]

Employees seeking to organize or refrain will be protected from undue interference or coercion from their employer or an organized union. The act charges that both management and union will bargain in good faith.

Determination of employee grouping and unit representation

The NLRA authorizes employees to organize and choose freely their own representation through secret ballot elections. Although the majority vote of employees determines acceptance for unionization, problems may arise in grouping employees in different positions into units. For example, if the grouping of a unit was determined along functional lines, the hospital would be obliged to deal with many bargaining units. The act states that professionals may not be grouped with nonprofessionals unless a majority of the professionals vote for their inclusion.

In some institutions and agencies the administration tries to include registered nurses and paramedical employees in one unit as done at the Mercy Hospital in Sacramento, California.[45] In this case the decision handed down by NLRB stated (1) that nurses are professionals and are entitled to a separate bargaining unit and that (2) the definition of a nursing supervisor is one who supervises in the interest of providing patient care as opposed to the employer's management interests. This decision and others have enabled the ANA and state associations to represent the interests of its membership more effectively.

In accordance with the 1974 Massachusetts Public Employee Collective Bargaining Law, the regional administrator of the state health agency divided its employees into ten collective bargaining units replacing over one hundred unions. The Massachusetts Nurses' Association became the representative for over 3,100 state health care pro-

fessionals, including physicians, nurses, dentists, and other professionals. The nurses wanted to be represented by the MNA, and the others voted to accept the MNA because they preferred representation by a professional organization in which they would have more influence rather than in a large employee union. The 1977 MNA state contract includes clauses improving clinical supervision, professional evaluation, and in-service education programs.

In some hospitals a group of employees other than registered nurses may ask the SNA to be its bargaining representative, and the employer of that group supports their request. In general, the SNA endeavors to give the asserted group assistance that is compatible with the law. However, the SNA recognizes always that the primary responsibility of the professional nursing organization is to registered nurses who pay dues to support the professional programs.

Collective bargaining for nurse-educators and instructors

Faculty participation in university decision-making policies occurs through the established senate that operates within a defined limit of power and functions. In the 1960s most senates dealt with such issues as curriculums, admissions, and educational policies.[42,76] A few senates discussed economic issues, faculty appointments, and promotions. However, personnel and economic issues generally were considered secondary. Employment conditions for educators and teachers were favorable, permitting them to move up the academic ladder if they so chose.

In 1971 The American Association of University Professors' (AAUP) National Council voted to accept collective bargaining as another means to maintain the association's goals in higher education. The National Education Association (NEA) and the American Federation of Teachers (AFT), an AFL-CIO affiliate, have organized faculties in colleges and universities.[76]

It is evident that professional nurses in education and nursing practice are becoming more active about what happens to the nursing profession, to themselves, and to students who will be the future practitioners, educators, and administrators.[72,80] Professional nurses are realizing that the power of nursing in providing quality nursing care to various client groups depends on how effectively educators and practitioners work together.

Role of the National Labor Relations Board

Prior to the enactment of the 1974 amendments of the NLRA, industry requested that Congress provide standards of unit determination in the act.[59] Congress refused to do so but instead established a legislative historical guide for the board. The board was advised that consideration should be given to prevent proliferation of bargaining units in health institutions and agencies.

The board, utilizing its past experience and gathered facts, decides whether the asserted unit of a particular institution or agency is an appropriate unit. The board endeavors to find mutual interest and similarities among the employees of the asserted group in their responsibilities, skills, their integration and coordination of responsibilities, and the interchange of employees, as well as among their work patterns, working conditions, and wages. It considers the history and pattern of preexisting bargaining relationships in the institution or agency.

Although professionals have the right to separate themselves from nonprofessional units, the board can decide which professional employees will be in each unit. Since 1974 the board has considered many unit determination cases, and in the years ahead they will have many more test cases to add to their files. Nurses are beginning to see the value of using collective bargaining and collective action to improve both economic and practice conditions. However, the board will look for true professionalism of nursing care in determining if most nurses should be members of a collective bargaining unit.[18]

Implications of professional nursing in accordance with the NLRA

The professional employee, as contained in the NLRA, section 2(12) is defined as (a)
any employee engaged in work (1) predominantly intellectual and varied in character as opposed to routine mental, manual, mechanical, or physical work, (2) involving the consistent exercise of discretion and judgment in its performance, (3) of such a character that the output produced or the results accomplished cannot be standardized in relation to a given period of time, (4) requiring knowledge of an advanced type in a field of science or learning customarily acquired by a prolonged course of specialized intellectual instruction and study in an institution of higher learning or a hospital, as distinguished from a general academic education or from an apprenticeship or from training in the performance of routine mental, manual, or physical processes, or (b) any employee who (1) has completed the courses of specialized intellectual instruction and study described in clause (4) of paragraph (a), and (2) is forming related work under the supervision of a professional person to qualify himself to become a professional employee as defined in paragraph (a).[18,89]

The definition of a professional as defined by the NLRA should encourage nurses to upgrade effectively the practice of nursing in accordance with the nurse practice act of their state. It could become a powerful force in relation to individual professional accountability to clients and in restructuring the management of nursing services in institutions.[27]

Recent implementation of peer reviews and professional standards review organizations (PSRO) will strengthen professionalism in nursing as well as enhance the status and economic interests of nurses.[12,61]

Peer review of the professional nurse's competence should be a part of the professional model of collective bargaining. The use of merit increases is one way to reward nurses for excellent performance. Nursing has followed the hospital tradition established by labor unions. To base all salaries on job title, earned degrees, and length of service is truly an escapist technique.[18] Under the peer review system the nursing practice council in consultation with the nurse-employer committee (if one existed) could determine on a percentage basis who rated a high performance, who rated an average performance, and who rated the lowest. Those rated lowest would receive a warning. Cleland emphasizes that a contract for professional nurses must not interfere in any way with the use of clinical judgment by the registered professional nurse.[18]

Implications of supervisory nurses in accordance with the NLRA

Professional nurses' philosophies and goals in the management of patient care, regardless of position, are different than those in other industries. When a factory worker is promoted to foreman or supervisor, he ceases to identify with the workers he supervises in the same way. In his new position he becomes a part of the management team that works toward a different set of goals and values. All nurses work toward common goals and objectives that will improve their own expertise and that of others so that patients will receive a better quality of nursing care. Nurses as members of their professional organization, regardless of their employment position work together to meet the goals of the organization's programs.

Can supervisors, head nurses, and staff nurses practice professionally in hospitals that function as bureaucratic authority structures? In most hospitals, position titles emphasize managerial functions rather than the independent functions of nursing, thus minimizing the importance of professional practice.[45,97] In many hospitals the roles of supervisors and clinical specialists, or clinical coordinators with preparation and expertise in a clinical nursing specialty, are defined by administration without the consent or counsel of the nursing staff. Nurses have allowed themselves to depend on others for permission to perform their independent professional functions.

In recent years, based on bedside research, professional management of care has been established to permit nurses to practice a mode of nursing that promotes both a professional level of individual responsibility and comprehensive care concepts in the care of patients. When administration removes

bureaucratic controls and frees nurses from administrative and managerial duties, nurses in supervisory positions are able to perform professionally, as defined by the legal definition of nursing practice. More "new" prepared nurses are using collective bargaining to help meet their professional goals and determine their interdependent relationships with other health professionals.[80]

The nurse-administrator and collective bargaining

A director of nursing service should work for the recognition of nursing as an autonomous and significant profession in the delivery of health services to society. Some directors are frustrated by the duality of their role: their membership on the hospital administration team and their professional responsibility to provide quality nursing care to all patients.

Many directors have been concerned about their relationship with the SNA if that body is the collective bargaining representative in the institution.[31] In some situations, hospital administrators have required the director of nursing to forfeit membership in the ANA as a condition of employment. Other directors believe that as administrators, their loyalty belongs to administration rather than to the nursing profession.[75]

At the 1976 ANA convention the House of Delegates agreed with the Commission of Nursing Services and its Council of Nursing Service Facilitators that they should be permitted full active membership. They rejected the concept of job categorization as manager or nonmanager as the basis for electing delegates, board members, and nominating committees. The ANA, its constituents, and many directors agree that management nurses should be excluded from the state's council on economic and general welfare.[28]

The NLRB has recognized that collective bargaining is only one function of the professional nursing organization and that administrators of the profession have a right to belong and participate in those other programs. The ANA and SNA expect the director of nursing to sit at the bargaining table as a member of the hospital management team.[13,28]

A review of recent collective bargaining cases indicates that professional nurses consider the collective bargaining process primarily as a means of reacting to constraints in the nursing profession rather than an aggressive action against the director of nursing. Many nurses want a director who accepts a leadership role in the nursing profession.

It is well known that directors of nursing services have been discharged because of their efforts to maintain acceptable standards and establish effective communications between nurse administrators, supervisors, and staff nurses for the establishment of effective nursing practices, peer evaluation, service standards, continuing education, and research programs. Directors of nursing and their immediate assistants are vulnerable to conflicts with the medical staff if they wish to determine staffing measures and define nurses' functions without nurses consultation or consent. In these cases many administrators will support the medical staff because it is the physician[34] who admits patients to the institution and helps keep the hospital operationally solvent.[18]

In the absence of a collective bargaining unit the nursing staff has little power to confront the issue, except to resign en masse. In recent instances nurses have sought the assistance of the SNA in establishing a collective bargaining unit. Some directors who were discharged had the courage to challenge their employers for violating their civil rights. Most directors have no employment contracts and can be discharged without notice. The ANA's goals in relation to economic and general welfare should include all members, and the ANA should take legislative steps to get the NLRA amended to reflect the differences between a professional and an industrial organization.

Strikes

Nurses do not want strikes. However, the right to strike is defined as the moral and political right of employees to withdraw or withhold labor in order to gain concessions from their employers.[9,97] During the 18 years when nurses agreed to the no-strike policy, nurses generally bargained with their employers from a position of weakness. Both public and private employers refused to negotiate to resolve nursing issues. They took advantage of nurses' dedication and loyalty to their profession. In recent years many nurses have felt they can identify no longer with administration or expect reasonable action to be taken in resolving their problems.[16,55]

As a result, nurses have sought the establishment and utilization of formal collective bargaining procedures. Representatives of an employing agent meet with representatives of nurses employed by a particular institution to determine economic conditions under which the professional nurses carry out their agreed upon responsibilities. Considering the number of nurses employed in the United States, few strikes have occurred.

Nurses do not strike in the same fashion as employees in other industries.[9,13] They recognize their responsibility to the patient and provide emergency nursing care to those patients who are critically ill and permit nurses who are willing to cross the picket lines to do so. Strikes under these conditions disturb physicians, who are the traditional power structure of the hospitals. They are inconvenient although not dangerous to consumers. Nurses desiring to institute changes view the right to strike as a necessary condition for providing quality nursing care. As advocates of the patient they want a clearer mandate governing care. One hopes that strikes are only a temporary solution to nurses' problems. It is apparent to nurses, employers, and the public that a strike is more harmful to patients than to employers.

How can nurses resolve their problems with employers and fulfill their ethical and moral obligations to patients? Nurses should strengthen their professional responsibilities in nursing practice. With support from their professional organization and with guidance from nurse-administrative leaders, nurses should create a professional model that includes standards of nursing practice. Peer review of hospital administration should establish a patient care committee composed of administration, medicine, and nursing representatives in addition to a joint medical-nursing practices committee.

In short, the bureaucratic complexities of the institutional health system must be changed to permit health care professionals participation and involvement in evaluating policies that affect and control both the practices and the management of the patient care system.

The number of "new" prepared nurses willing to take risks in order to resolve issues and create changes in the traditional nursing service organization is increasing.[44] Bloom,[13] in "Strike With Honor," gives some very pertinent guides that directors, physicians, administrators, and staff nurses should consider. The use of a collective bargaining contract holds the nurses and the hospital administration accountable to the consumers. Nurses should remember that complacency and inactivity are the only unacceptable strategies in a profession.

Arbitration

From a practical viewpoint, arbitration resolves problems. Arbitration involves a legal contract between two parties, and noncompliance means breaking the law.[9,45]

Voluntary arbitration is decided by employees and employers when they make the contract, and it stipulates that an arbitrator will be called when a dispute cannot be resolved through negotiations. Both parties agree on the selection of an arbitrator when one is needed. Voluntary arbitration presupposes the existence of collective bargaining, for without it the mechanism for voluntary arbitration cannot be set up to the satisfaction of both parties.

Compulsory arbitration rather than collective bargaining may be utilized to settle contracts and disputes. It requires the arbitrators to be a government employee who is knowledgeable concerning the particular industry involved. Compulsory arbitration also may occur when collective bargaining is utilized as the primary way to resolve issues and in drawing a contract. Compulsory arbitration forces both parties to turn their unresolved problems over to a government arbitration for resolution.

Arbitration of nurse-employer issues eliminates the need for strikes. If hospital and health agency administrations want to avoid strikes and their consequences, they may accept voluntary or compulsory arbitration as the best method for settling disputes.

Fact-finding

In fact-finding both parties agree to call in an impartial person or persons to hear both sides. The fact-finder will prepare a series of recommendations based on the facts presented. The parties are not required to accept these recommendations even if they are under pressure to do so. In 1966 Cailfornia nurses voted to use the fact-finding procedure rather than to go on strike, and the fact-finders recommendations were effected.

Mediation-arbitration

In mediation-arbitration a neutral and experienced arbitrator sits in during the contract negotiations or disputes. If difficulties arise, he endeavors to mediate between the parties and secure a voluntary agreement. If he cannot achieve an agreement by mediation, at whatever point he thinks appropriate, he assumes the role of an arbitrator and issues a decision that both parties must accept as the settlement of the issue.

CNA and hospitals in the San Francisco Bay area used this procedure and prevented a strike.[9] The nurses covered by collective bargaining were satisfied with the results of the mediation, but hospital representatives returned to collective bargaining procedures in 1974 negotiations. The result was a three-week strike by nurses, primarily over issues of patient care.[13] The settlement requires all hospitals to develop a system to determine nurse staffing with staff nurse participation in assessing patients' daily nursing care needs. The system must be reviewed by SNA. Hospitals agreed that nurses without appropriate training or experience would not be assigned to special care units except in emergencies.

Mediation and conciliation

Mediation and conciliation are used in traditional bargaining. The mediator is called in and tries to achieve voluntary agreement. The experienced and responsible negotiator with a knowledge of health institutions and nursing has a opportunity to resolve the disputes and prevent a strike.

Perhaps the consumers of health services who now are participating in planning health services through legislation will gain a greater understanding of the issues between nurses and their employees, promote corrective action to resolve these issues, and make it unnecessary for nurses to strike.[52]

CREDENTIALING IN THE NURSING PROFESSION

Licensure, certification, and accreditation processes comprise credentialing. All are closely interrelated. This system is being scrutinized critically by consumers, professionals, and others in our society. During the past 10 years increased federal funding has supported education and training programs for the development of health manpower resources. The consumer-patients want quality care at a fair price.

Good health care is considered the right rather than privilege of every U.S. citizen, and public accountability in our health care system is becoming a reality. All health professionals are responsible for establishing a meaningful partnership between professions for credentialing that will be in the public interest.[4,35,78] The credentialing system of the immediate future has implications for all registered nurses and involves the nursing practice act of each state.

Definitions

The Department of Health, Education and Welfare defines the various aspects of credentialing[59,78] as follows:

licensure a process by which a governmental agency grants permission to individuals who have met predetermined qualifications to engage in a given profession or occupation, use a particular title, or grant permission to institutions to perform specified functions.

certification or registration the process by which a nongovernment agency or association grants recognition to an individual who has met certain predetermined qualifications by that agency or association. (Certification means that those licensed have attained the minimal degree of competency necessary to ensure safety and welfare and that public health will be reasonably protected. It is used by health professionals and other organized occupational groups to test for a level of knowledge, or practice, or for entry into practice.)

accreditation the process by which an agency or organization evaluates and recognizes an institution or program of study as meeting certain predetermined qualifications or standards specified by that agency or association. This process applies only to institutions and their programs of study or their services.

These evaluative credentialing systems were established independently of one another to meet functional and social needs.

Credentialing system challenged

The entire credentialing system, especially health licensure in the United States, has been closely scrutinized by professionals, consumers, and government reforms. The number of those defining nursing practice and those interested in nursing practice acts are both escalating rapidly. The increasing demands of more consumers seeking health care services have caused many new occupational groups to become members of the health manpower system.[74] Some reformers are challenging the utilization of manpower resources in addition to educational and training personnel costs.

Some consumers believe that the health credentialing system is more responsive to the desires of health professionals than to the interests of consumers. These consumers want to participate in the decision-making policies that affect them: the quality and the price of health services.

Positions of health organizations and the government

Government reformers and others maintain that the system should be updated. Viewing the system's problems, the American Medical Association and the American

Hospital Association in 1970 adopted resolutions calling for a nationwide moratorium on the licensure of any additional health personnel categories.[46,86] The American Public Health Association, the American Nurses' Association, the National League for Nursing, and others supported this resolution.

The Department of Health, Education, and Welfare in its 1971 report[86] supported this resolution and emphasized that the concept of institutional licensure could exist as supplement or as an alternative to current individual licensure mechanisms.

In 1973 the Report of the Secretary's Commission on Medical Malpractice recommended that studies be undertaken to determine the effect of the institutional licensure mechanism (excluding registered nurses) on the quality of care.[87] In 1973 the assistant secretary of HEW requested a continued moratorium on new licensure at least until 1975 and indicated that credentialing processes would have high priority.[11,25]

Changes in definition of nursing practice acts

Since 1972, nurses in most states have been determining changes or introducing revisions in their nursing practice acts.[27,47] In many states the nursing practice act has been updated to assure both quality of care and legal protection for professional nurses as they assume added responsibilities and independent decision making for more complex patient care.

The legal posture of nurses in many of their new roles is ambiguous since practice is based on complex biomedical and technological principles. For more than 10 years nurses have carried out complex techniques involving independent decision making. These often are called the gray areas between medical and nursing practices. Policy statements by hospital committees and joint statements on a state level gave nurses a superficial feeling of confidence in their new roles. However, the development of the nurse-practitioner roles, especially in primary care, has gained much attention concerning the legality of nursing practices.

In some states the nursing practice acts[1]

amendments involve rules and regulations concerning medical diagnoses and treatments. Other amendments focus on the composition of the state examining board and the regulations of the nursing practice acts. The definition of nursing practice contained in the law is the essential ingredient.

The New York State Nursing Practice Act, amended in 1972, emphasizes the distinction between professional nursing and medicine and promotes the concept of nursing as a separate profession. Section 16902 of the act states:[65]

The practice of the profession of nursing as a registered professional nurse is defined as diagnosing and treating human responses to actual or potential health problems through such services as case finding, health teaching, health counseling, and provision of care supportive to or restorative of life and well-being, and executing medical regimens prescribed by a licensed or otherwise legally authorized physician or dentist.

The New York State Nurse Practice Act of 1972 clearly outlines and legally establishes the independent and accountable practice of professional nursing. The definitions of the amended 1972 New York State Nursing Practice Act are defined clearly. The act states that:

. . . *diagnosing* means that identification of and discrimination between physical and psychosocial signs and symptoms essential to effective execution and management of the nursing regimen. Such diagnostic privilege is distinct from a medical diagnosis. *Treating* means selection and performance of those therapeutic measures essential to the effective execution and management of the nursing regimen, and execution of the prescribed medical regimen.

Arizona, Nevada, and New Hampshire have made regulation amendments in recent years that permit acts of medical diagnosis and treatment if authorized by rules and regulations agreed on by both the medical and nursing boards and implemented by the nursing board of the state. In Idaho,[41] consistent with the rules and regulations, qualified professional nurses can be employed to provide primary medical care. In 1973 the State of Washington[94] amended its nursing practice act to eliminate the prohibition against medical diagnosis or the prescription of therapeutic or corrective measures by nurses and to permit professional nurses to perform additional acts requiring education and training.

With the introduction of the physician's assistant, many nurses became concerned about possible infringements on nursing practice. Rothberg[74] states that "the physician's assistant is the *symptom* of both medicine's and nursing's inability to define their individual roles, to respect each others' competencies, or to deliver an acceptable level of care."

There is much conflict and confusion over the distinctions between the role of the physician's assistant and the expanded roles of professional nurses, but in no sense is the physician's assistant considered an independent health practitioner. He carries out some tasks of medical care usually performed by a physician but under the supervision and direction of a physician. Throughout the centuries the professional nurse's scope has broadened in keeping with medical, scientific, and technological advances. In some states, legislative developments indicate that the nurse-practitioner's role is to pursue a professional nursing role.

In 1974 the National Practice Commission recommended (1) that those practice acts broad enough to provide flexibility should not be changed and that joint-practice statements be used to define role realignment and (2) that those medical and nursing practice acts having narrow definitions should be restated to provide breadth and flexibility with joint-practice committees, and these appropriate statements be issued without legislative endorsement.

Mandatory and voluntary licensure

State licensing laws are mandatory for physicians, pharmacists, and nurses in most states. Mandatory licensure means that all individuals who practice medicine for compensation must be licensed. In some states voluntary licensure is required; that is, only individuals holding a license are authorized to use a designated title such as R.N. or L.P.N. Unlicensed individuals may work in a field, but they cannot use the protected title.[68]

As of early 1975 only the District of Columbia and Georgia had voluntary (permissive) laws with no definition of nursing in the practice act.[46] Other states such as Indiana have statutes making it unlawful to practice as a registered nurse without a license. Clauses in nurse practice acts, as in the Indiana law, tend to legalize the tasks of ancillary workers. In such cases the employer may interpret the clauses loosely, resulting in unqualified personnel's performing nursing practices in the care of patients. Such actions do not assure quality care for consumer-patients.

Some employers do not support mandatory licenses for the R.N. and L.P.N. since they find the voluntary law less restrictive in the employment of unlicensed nurses. Other fear that under the mandatory law unlicensed practicing nurses could find it difficult to earn a living in nursing. The mandatory licensure law does permit unlicensed nurses a limited time to secure a license without fulfilling all the qualifications, providing that they can show appropriate evidence of their competence in nursing.

Criteria and qualifications for nurse licensure

Each state's nursing practice act mandates the criteria required of individuals who take licensing examinations. Nursing is one of the few professions utilizing national standards examinations for the licensure of registered and practical nurses in jurisdictives. This allows nurses mobility from one state to another. All states license nurses coming into the state through the endorsement or reciprocity process, provided that the nurse fulfills the second state's requirements.

The legal practice of foreign nurses has been a major concern to the nursing profession.[77] In some states the hospital association and others have encouraged the employment of unlicensed foreign nurses, recommending that such nurses be permitted to perform nursing practices without a license as long as they practice under the control, supervision, and instruction of a licensed individual of that state and secure the approval of the state medical association.

Various critics believe that the nursing practice acts, criteria for admission are too inflexible. Some reformers suggest that criteria be based on the workers' skill and job performance. (See institutional licensure.) In some states barriers to career mobility are being reduced. For example, in 1969 the State of California enacted legislation to the effect that (1) medical corpsmen's training shall be recognized when seeking entrance to become a registered nurse and (2) credit for vocational training shall be given to facilitate upward mobility of the practical nurse to become a registered nurse. Studies indicate that the educational preparation for an R.N. is quite different from that of an L.P.N.; and both differ from a military corpsman's training.

The new "open curriculum" program permits students to move quite rapidly through the nursing process and still receive the necessary orientation to patient care. In this program there are units in which an R.N. or L.P.N. curriculum could be learned through experience or by individual study, and a passing grade on a proficiency examination could exempt students from these requirements.[67]

To assure quality care and utilize effectively prepared professional nurses in the delivery of health services, some state associations believe it necessary to make a distinction between the professional nurse and the so-called technical nurse by means of the nursing practice act. The New York State Nurses Association proposed legislation to change the qualifications for professional nurse licensure.[63] It recommends a baccalaureate degree in nursing as the base for licensure effective in 1985. The proposal identifies two distinct careers in nursing: professional and technical. It is recommended that legislation provide a regulation that would waive these requirements for individuals already holding an R.N. or L.P.N. license.

Various professional health groups have voiced opposition to revision of this practice act; others have supported the SNA proposals.

In most states licensure is a political, uncoordinated, and confused process.

Composition and responsibilities of state licensing boards

The nursing licensing boards are responsible for enforcing standards of practice for the profession of nursing. They grant licenses, periodically collect fees for registration, issue regulations and standards of practice, examine applicants' credentials, and investigate schools.

Originally nurse leaders followed the model of other health organizations and worked together through their own associations to establish standards that would improve the quality of care, gain the public's respect, and enhance the status of nursing. With more individuals entering different health occupations, professional associations could not adequately carry out a licensing system. Thus, the Constitution delegated power to the states to enact licensing laws and practice acts of health occupations and professions. There were few established health professions with a licensure system when nursing licensure laws first were enacted. In recent years some states have changed the traditional appointment by the governor of nurses only. Other states have advisory committees of mixed membership, including nurses, physicians, and hospital administrators.

Various educators and other professionals recently advocated that state examining boards be made up of experts representing the academic field, clinical specialties, and research fields of nursing.[35,78] With many more individuals seeking licensure and the concomitant expansion of the state government bureaucracy, some reformers propose centralizing the licensing functions of all health professions in one licensing agency composed of various representatives of the health professions. Others advocate the formation of a federal commission to assist organized health settings in establishing an operational plan that will evaluate quality of care in accordance with specified criteria. To assure that quality care and objective policy decisions are made in the public interest, consumers are demanding to participate in all areas of policy making.

Based on a 2-year study, the 1975 NLN Position Statement on Nursing License[68] recommends that (1) nurse licensure should remain the prerogative of state governments; (2) policy decisions regarding the practice of nursing require nursing expertise and should continue to be made by a separate nursing licensure board composed of a majority of R.N.s; (3) consumers should be appointed to serve on nurse licensing boards; (4) a national, standardized licensing examinations should be administered by all state licensing boards; (5) applicants for the registered nurse or practical nurse licensure examination should be graduates of their respective state-approved programs of nursing; and (6) a continuing education requirement for the licensure of nurses should be carefully planned and gradually implemented.

Mandatory continuing education and voluntary continuing competence

Under the present licensure regulations in most states a licensed health practitioner only has to pay a periodic renewal fee to maintain licensure. In our technological society this renewal regulation contributes to professional obsolescense. Consumer and some professional groups are encouraging the adoption of mandatory continuing education for professional nurse relicensure.[8,53] Other groups are challenging this position.[23,33,82] The Joint Commission on Accreditation of Hospitals (JCAH) standard V states that "There shall be continuing programs and educational opportunities for the development of nursing personnel.[43]

The statutory requirement of the State of California Nurse Practice Law has been amended, stating that "after January 1978, all R.N.s and L.V.N.s licensed by the state must prove to the proper licensing authority at the time of license renewal that he/she is current." This regulation neither requires the licensee to undertake continuing education nor provides a mechanism to measure or ensure competency.[33,38]

The American Hospital Assocation and the American Nurses' Association have developed mechanisms to assure quality of care in response to societal pressures for accountability for the care delivered to consumer-patients.[2,12] A 1972 AHA manual, *Quality Assurance Program for Medical Care in Hospitals,* states that "By law, society delegates to the hospital the authority and accountability for the organization and delivery of hospital services . . . to assure the public of optimal quality of all care delivered by all professionals within the institution."[4]

The American Nurses' Association has developed standards of practice for the divisions of practice (see Chapter 5). The Association developed the appropriate nursing criteria for peer review under the federally mandated PSROs and initiated a certification program for excellence in practice and other actions to assure quality of nursing care.

A bill to initiate mandatory continuing education for all health professionals was defeated in legislature in the 1973. Most state nurses' associations and continuing education recognition programs (CERP) are using ANA guidelines as a basis for the approval of programs.[2] The majority of states favor or have initiated voluntary programs. In Oregon, South Dakota, and Colorado the practice act permits the state board of nursing to set up a mandatory program if necessary. In California and New Mexico mandatory programs are in the planning stages.

Some professionals are against mandatory continuing education. Cooper,[23] Stevens,[82] and others believe that legal requirements downgrade professional autonomy and each practitioner's right to determine what learning experience is best suited to his or her professional needs. It is evident today that many professional nurses accept personal responsibility for maintaining competence and value opportunities to participate in continuing education programs.

When the health care system and credentialing mechanisms are undergoing rapid changes the mechanism adapted for continuing education will not guarantee the future competence of each practitioner. In the final analysis, professionals should account for their own performances. A nurse-practitioners level of competency should be determined and monitored periodically by a peer review mechanism.

Trends in nursing certification and registration

In accordance with HEW's definition of certification as previously stated, the American Nurses' Assocation developed and initiated a certification program. Certification of nurses specializing in several fields of practice is a recent innovation.[11,32,78]

Each of the five divisions of practice in the ANA has its own certification board. The ANA certification program is designed to recognize excellence in clinical nursing practice rather than to endorse entry into practice.

In 1976 the ANA proposed a revision of its certification procedure to set up two levels of credentialing: (1) certification for competence in specialized areas of practice with distinctive eligibility requirements and (2) certification for excellence in practice and diplomate status in an American College of Practice for certified nurses who meet additional criteria.

The ANA certification proposal has met with hostility by some nurses because of qualifications, requirements, and the cost for certification examinations.

Criteria have been developed by each ANA division on practice based on the guidelines established by the ANA Congress for Nursing Practice. An educational testing service is employed to administer the examinations, although the content of the examinations is developed in the ANA structure.

Because ANA does not certify for entrance into the profession an agreement could not be reached between ANA and many clinical specialty groups in nursing as to criteria and procedure for certification, some groups joined with medical specialty organizations and received certification. Some SNAs established their own certification program with their own criteria. The 1977 HEW report recommends that a national voluntary system for "allied health" certification be established using national standards. Nursing is not included in the "allied health" certification system.

Accreditation

Professional health organizations and others who have been studying the problems inherent in the system recognize that accreditation cannot be viewed apart from other components of credentialing. Reformers recognize that licensure, certification, and accreditation are interrelated and that changes in one will influence the others. The restructuring of the credentialing mechanism must establish interlocking relationships. The system must reduce credentialing costs and duplication as well as enhance career mobility and close the gaps in the quality assurance mechanisms.

The Study of Accreditation of Selected Health Educational Programs (SASHEP) was initiated by the American Medical Association's Council on Medical Education and the council's Advisory Committee for Allied Health Professions and Services.[4] This study was conducted in cooperation with the Association of Schools of Allied Health Professions and the National Commission on Accrediting.[78]

This study states that in our society nongovernmental accreditation of specialized health educational programs should be oriented primarily to society's needs rather than toward the protection of a particular profession. It should be a major means of providing surveillance and help, particularly in the health field. The commission also advocated that physicians should be involved in the process of accrediting study programs in all of the selected allied health fields. Approval of standards and accreditation of such programs must be subject to the final authority of a body that represents no single profession.

Selden,[78] in discussing credentialing, suggests that a strong agency be developed through the proposed merger of the National Commission on Accrediting and the Federation of Regional Accrediting Commissions of Higher Education. He believes that accrediting agencies today may be obliged to modify their structure and functions to permit greater participation from all interested groups.

The American Nurses' Association

The initial ANA participants who planned the study of credentialing included representatives of AACN, NLN, ANA, and other health professions, the United States Office of Education, and other accrediting bodies.

The ANA in April, 1976, announced the major aims of this study and its methodology.[32] It will critically examine, compare, and evaluate the current credentialing system in nursing and develop alternative models for a credentialing system for practitioners in nursing, nursing education, and service agencies. The NLN, the accrediting agency for nursing education programs as of February, 1976, declined the ANA's invitation to cosponsor this study.

The ANA credentialing study to be initiated in late 1977 may present new data and directions. One question is, Who should accredit nursing programs?

Institutional licensure

Under institutional licensure a single license would be issued to the employing agency, replacing the licensure of the individual health provider.[46] The institution or agency would be permitted to determine which individuals met certain qualifications and possessed certain competencies for work in that institution or agency.[6,68,69] HEW recommended that studies be conducted to determine the potentials of institutional licensure as an alternative to individual licensure.[87]

Hershey,[39,40] an early advocate of institutional licensure, proposed a licensure model that would (1) establish state institutional licensing bodies with consulation from qualified individuals in the health field; (2) delegate the formulation of job descriptions to the state licensing bodies for positions in hospitals and health agencies as well as qualifications in terms of education and experience required to hold each position; (3) delegate power to institutions within the bounds established by the state licensing bodies to regulate and control their health

workers in the various positions, employers to place workers in positions in terms of levels and grades.

The American Hospital Association's licensure model originating from the AHA's Ameriplan was presented in 1970; later this proposal was withdrawn. In 1971 the AHA issued a policy statement advocating review and study of alternatives to the individual licensure system.[5] It recommended that health care corporations be delegated specific responsibilities for quality and effective delivery of care rendered by all health practitioners, including physicians.

The AMA Council on Health Manpower presented a more limiting definition of health institutions. The council's statement made a distinction between independent and dependent practitioners, classifying nurses as dependent employees. The dependent employees would be unlicensed and accountable to the employing agency. Physicians, dentists, and the independent osteopaths, to whom the public has direct access, would retain their present licensed status and would be held accountable for personnel working under their supervision. In June, 1973, the AMA's House of Delegates opposed the extension of institutional license in lieu of individual professional licensure to physicians and nurses.

The resolutions of the ANA's House of Delegates in 1972 reaffirmed commitment to individual licensing and individual accountability essential for providing safe, high quality nursing care.[6] The NLN statement in 1972 stated its opposition to the concept of extending institutional licensure to include the regulation of nursing personnel. The NLN's 1975 position statement supports individual licensure by state and presents recommendations for changes to update the licensure mechanism.[68]

According to the 1977 HEW report, institutional licensure is temporarily dead as a substitute for or adjunct to individual licensure.[87a]

Summary

It seems evident that the credentialing of health education and services will become more integrated nationally, more accountable publically, and linked more closely to government agencies. Nursing is facing new challenges. To participate actively in decision making concerning the delivery of quality care to consumer-patients, nurse-practitioners, nurse educators, and nurse administrators must take an active role through their organizations for the standards of nursing practice, peer review, and the legislative programs that will assure the public of quality care at a reasonable price.

REFERENCES

1. Agree, B. C.: The threat of institutional licensure, American Journal of Nursing 10:1758-1763, Oct., 1973.
2. AJN reports: Recognition for continuing education, American Journal of Nursing 5:878-880, May 1974.
3. Alfedi, R. J.: Informal consent, Journal of the American Medical Association 216:1225-1329, May 24, 1971.
4. American Hospital Association: Quality assurance program for medical care in the hospital, Chicago, 1972, The Association, sections 1 and 2.
5. American Hospital Association: Statement on licensure of health care personnel, Hospitals 45:125-27, March, 1971.
6. American Nurses' Association: Resolution on institutional licensure, American Journal of Nursing 72:1106, June, 1972.
7. American Nurses' Association: Human rights guidelines for nurses in clinical and other research, Kansas City, Mo., 1974, The Association.
8. American Nurses' Association: Continuing education in nursing: an overview pub. no. COE-10. Continuing education in nursing: guidelines for staff, pub. no. COE-11, Kansas, 1975, The Association.
9. Amundson, N. E.: Alternatives to the strike in collective bargaining, Journal of Nursing Administration 5:11-21, Jan., 1975.
10. Annas, G. J.: The rights of hospital patients (American Civil Liberties Union Handbook), New York, 1975, Avon Books.
11. Arnold, P.: ANA certification program expands, The American Nurse 8:18-19, Feb. 15, 1976.
12. Aydelotte, M. K.: quality assurance programs in health care agencies. In Quality assessment and patient care, New York, 1975, Division of Community Planning, National League for Nursing, pp. 1-11.
13. Bloom, I.: Strike with honor, Journal of Nursing Administration 4:19-20, May, 1975.
14. Bowman, R. A., and Culpepper, R. C.: National health insurance; some issues, American Journal of Nursing 75:2017-2021, Nov., 1975.
15. Bowman, R. A., and Culpepper, R. C.: Power, Rx for change, American Journal of Nursing 74:1053-1056, June, 1974.
16. Brown, G. Feldsine, F., and Piemonte, R.: Implementing the definition of nursing practice, Journal of New York State Nurses' Association 6:6-9, March, 1975.
17. Callow, B. M.: An RN's view of the health maintenance organization, Journal of Nursing Administration 3:39-41, Sept.-Oct., 1973.
18. Cleland, V.: The professional model, American Journal of Nursing 75:288-292, 1975.
19. Commission on Economic and General Welfare of the American Nurses' Association: Philosophy, goals, policies and positions, pub. no. EC-119, 10/751OM, Kansas City, Mo., 1975, The Association.
20. Committee on Health Care for the Disadvantaged: A patient's bill of rights, Chicago, 1972, The American Hospital Association.
21. Committee to Draft a Patient's Bill of Rights: What people can expect of modern nursing service, New York, 1959, The National League for Nursing.
22. Committee to Survey Cooperative Multi-Hospital Management Engineering Programs: Report Cooperative multi-hospital management engineering program, Chicago, 1968, Hospital Management Systems Society.
23. Cooper, S. S. Continuing education should be voluntary, Journal of the Association of Operating Room Nurses 18:471-477, Sept., 1973. (Condensed in Nursing Digest Focus on Professional Issues, Wakefield, Mass. 1975, Contemporary Publishing, pp. 28-32.)
24. Denenberg, H. S.: citizens' bill of hospital rights—what the patient and public can and should expect from our hospitals, Harrisburg, Penna., 1973, Insurance Department, State of Pennsylvania.
25. Department of Baccalaureate and Higher Degrees: Quality assurance—a joint venture, pub no. 15-1595, New York, 1975, National League for Nursing.
26. Division of Community Planning: Quality assessment and patient care, pub no. 52-1572, New York, 1975, National League for Nursing.
27. Driscoll, V.: Liberating nurse practice, Nursing Outlook 20:24, Jan., 1972.
28. Driscoll, V.: The myth of two hats, Journal of New York State Nurses' Association 4:36-39, Nov., 1973.
29. Dubos, R. S.: Life: An endless give and take with earth and all her creatures, particularly including man. Washington, D.C., 1970, Smithsonian, Smithsonian National Association.
30. Editoral: Percentage of income spent on health care still highest for the poor, Hospitals 2:18, Feb., 1976.
31. Edwards, M. L.: The role of the director of nursing in implementing the new definition of nursing, Journal of New York State Nurses' Association 4:8-11, 1973.
31a. Executive Office of the President—Office of Man-

agement and Budget: Fiscal year 1978, budget revisions, February 1977, Washington, D.C., 1977, United States Government Printing Office.

32. Fondilla, S.: ANA to initiate credentialing study, The American Nurse **8**:1, 1976.

33. Forni, P. R.: continuing education vs. continuing competence, Journal of Nursing Administration **34**(9):34, 1975.

34. Friedson, E., and Lorber, H.: Medical men and their work, Chicago, 1972, Aldine Publishing Company.

35. Green, J. L.: Accreditation in nursing education: New trends and responsibilities, Nursing Forum **13**(1):5-15, 1975.

36. Greenberg, D. C.: National health insurance forever imminent, New England Journal of Medicine **293**:461-46; Aug. 28, 1975.

37. Gumbiner, R.: The health maintenance organization—HMO—putting it all together, St. Louis, 1975, The C. V. Mosby Co.

38. Hatfield, P.: Mandatory continuing education. Journal of Nursing Administration **3**:35-40, Nov.-Dec., 1973.

39. Hershey, N.: Alternatives to mandatory licensure of health professionals, Hospital Progress **50**:73, March, 1969.

40. Hershey, N.: Expanded roles for professional nurses, Journal of Nursing Administration **3**:30-33, Nov.-Dec., 1973.

41. Idaho State Board of Medicine and State Board of Nursing: Minimum standards, rules and regulations for the expanding role of the registered professional nurse, Boise, June, 1972, The board.

42. Jacax, A.: Collective bargaining in academe, Nursing Outlook **21**:700-703, Nov., 1973.

43. Joint Commission on Accreditation of Hosptial Nursing Service Standards 5, Accreditation Manual for Hospitals, Hospital Accreditation Program, Illinois, Chicago, 1971, The Commission, p. 52.

44. Judge, D.: The new nurse: a sense of duty and destiny, Modern Health Care **2**(4):21-27, 1974. Reprinted in Nursing Digest **3**:20-24, Nov.-Dec., 1975.

45. Kane, J. J.: Nonprofit hospitals and the national labor relations act, Journal of Nursing Administration **5**:15-17, July-Aug., 1975.

46. Kelly, L. Y.: Institutional licensure, Nursing Outlook **21**:566-572, Sept., 1973.

47. Kelly, L. Y.: Nursing practice acts, American Journal of Nursing **74**:310-319, July, 1974.

48. Kelly, L. Y.: The patients' rights to know, Nursing Outlook **24**:26-32, Jan., 1976.

49. Krizay, J., et al.: The patient as a consumer, Lexington, Mass, 1974, Lexington Books, pp. 27-30, 177.

50. Larson, R. C.: Administration, Hospitals **43**:69-73, 1969.

51. Lash, M. P.: Current legislation enhances health care planning prospects, Hospitals **59**:59-61, Dec., 1975.

52. Leininger, M. M.: Conflict and conflict resolutions: theories and processes relevant to the health professions, American Nurse **12**:17-22, 1974.

52a. Levine, M. E., et al.: Ethical dilemmas in nursing, American Journal of Nursing **77**:845-876, May, 1977.

53. McGriff, E. P.: Mandatory continuing education for nurses, Journal of the Association of Operating Room Nurses **18**:479-485, Sept., 1973. (Condensed in Nursing Digest Focus on Professional Issues, Wakefield, Mass; 1975, Contemporary Publishing, Inc., pp. 33-37.)

54. McNerney, W. J.: Changing the health care system, American Journal of Nursing, **69**:2428-2435, 1969.

55. Miller, M. H.: Nurses' right to strike, Journal of Nursing Administration **5**:35-39, Feb., 1975.

56. Miller, M. H.: PSRO—boon or bust for nursing? Hospitals **49**:81-84, Oct. 1975.

57. Milo, N.: The care of health in communities: access for outcasts; New York, 1975, The Macmillan Publishing Co., pp. 118 and 231.

58. Myers, R. J.: Medicare. In McCahan, D., editor: Accident and sickness insurance, Homewood, Ill., 1970, Richard D. Irwin, Inc.

59. National Commission on Accrediting: A report on the study of accreditation of selected educational programs (SASHEP), Chicago, 1972, The American Medical Association.

60. National Commission on Community Health Services: Health is a community affair, Cambridge, Mass., 1967, Harvard University Press, pp. 21-22.

61. Newmark, G. L.: PSRO future ensured with dual funding policy, Hospitals **50**:28, Feb., 1976.

62. News: ANA, PSRO document stated for publication by federal agency, American Journal of Nursing **76**:91, Jan., 1976; **76**:126, Feb., 1976; **76**:347, March, 1976.

63. News: Controversy flares over baccalaureate as licensure base, American Journal of Nursing **76**:14, Jan., 1976.

64. News: Nursing's role under new health planning act emerges at HEW departmental briefing, American Journal of Nursing **75**:336-337, May, 1975.

65. New York State Nurses Association: Nurse practice act 1972, New York State Nursing Association publication, Albany, 1972, The Association.

66. National League for Nursing Committee on Perspectives: Perspectives for nursing, pub. no. 11-1580, New York, 1975, The League.

67. National League for Nursing: Open curriculum conference, pub. no. 19-1586, New York, 1975, The League.

68. National League for Nursing: Position statement on nursing licensure, New York, 1975, The League.

69. Peterson, P., and Guy, J. G.: Should institutional licensure replace individual licensure? American Journal of Nursing **74**:444-447, March, 1974.

70. Phillips, D. F.: Ambulatory care has come of age, Hospitals **50**:537, Feb., 1976.

71. Quinn, N., and Somers, A. R.: The patients' bill of rights—a significant aspect of the consumer rev-

olution, Nursing Outlook **23**:240-244, April, 1974.

72. Reilly, D. E.: Why a conceptual framework? Nursing Outlook **23**:567-569, Sept., 1975.

73. Roseman, C.: Problems and prospects for comprehensive health planning, American Journal of Public Health **42**:16, Jan., 1972.

74. Rothberg, J.: Nurse and physicians' assistant: issues and relationships, Nursing Outlook **21**:154-158, March, 1973.

75. Rotkovitch, R. R.: The director of nursing and the hat of administration, Journal of New York State Nurses' Association **4**:40-43, Nov., 1973.

76. Saxton, D. R.: Collective bargaining in academe, Nursing Outlook **21**:704-707, Nov., 1973.

77. Schmidt, M. S.: New York State's experience in licensing foreign educated nurses, Journal of New York State Nurses' Association **5**:7-13, Nov., 1974.

78. Selden, W. K., Frey, D., and Ginley, T.: Health occupations credentialing: three views—a report on SASHEP. In Nursing digest focus on professional issues, Wakefield, Mass., 1975, Contemporary Publishing, pp. 16-24.

79. Sheldon, W. K.: Are problems in graduate nursing education unique? Nursing Outlook **23**:622-624, Oct., 1975.

80. Smith, R. A.: Why college graduates choose nursing, Nursing Outlook **24**:88-91, Feb., 1976.

81. Somers, H. H., and Somers, A. R.: Medicare and the hospitals, Washington, D.C., 1967, The Brookings Institution.

82. Stevens, B. J.: Mandatory continuing education for professional nurse relicensure. What are the issues? Journal of Nursing Administration **3**:25-28, Sept.-Oct., 1973.

83. Terry, L. L.: Hospitals and Title VI of the Civil Rights Act, Hospitals **39**:34-37, Aug., 1965.

84. United States Department of Health, Education, and Welfare: A guide to federal financial aid for the development of medical care, Washington, D.C., 1966, United States Government Printing Office.

85. United States Department of Health, Education, and Welfare: PSRO program manual, Rockville, Md., 1974, Office of Professional Standards Review.

86. United States Department of Health, Education, and Welfare: Report on licensure and related health personnel credentialing, pub. no. HSM 72-11, iii., Washington, D.C., 1971, United States Government Printing Office.

87. United States Department of Health, Education, and Welfare: Secretary's Commission on Medical Malpractice: medical malpractice report, pub. no. OS 73-88, Washington, D.C., 1973, United States Government Printing Office, pp. 71-74.

87a. United States Department of Health, Education, and Welfare: Credentialing health manpower, Washington, D.C., 1977, United States Government Printing Office.

88. United States Health Services Research and Health Statistics: Health, United States, 1975, United States Department of Health, Education, and Welfare, United States 1976, Washington, D.C., United States Government Printing Office.

89. United States National Labor Relations Board: Text of Labor Management Relations Act, 1974, as amended by labor management. Reporting and Disclosure Act, Washington, D.C., 1959, United States Government Printing Office.

90. United States Public Health Service: Executive summary of the United States forward plan of health for fiscal years 1976-1980, United States Department of Health, Education, and Welfare, 1975, Washington, D.C., United States Government Printing Office.

91. United States Public Health Service: Forward plan for health, Feb., 1977-81, Department of Health, Education, and Welfare, June, 1975. Social Security amendments 1972, pp. 19-27. Health Planning Act 1974, pp. 183-187, Washington, D.C., United States Government Printing Office.

92. Wagner, D. L.: American Nurses' Association—statement on health maintenance organization Senate subcommittee on health, Kansas, 1971, American Nurses Association.

93. Wagner, D.: Nursing in an HMO, American Journal of Nursing **74**:236-239, Feb., 1974.

94. Washington State: Laws regulating the practice of registered nurses, 1973, State of Washington, chapter 202, section 7.

95. Welch, C. A.: Health care distribution and third-party payments for nurses' services, American Journal of Nursing **75**:1844-1847, Oct., 1975.

96. Wilson, F. A., and Neuhauser, D.: Health services in United States, Cambridge, Mass., 1974, Ballinger Publishing Company, pp. 121, 138-147.

97. Zimmerman, A.: Taft-Hartley Amendment—implications for nursing—the industrial model, American Journal of Nursing **74**:284-288, Feb., 1974.

5 | Standards for health care institutions

The major role of a health institution is to provide quality care to consumer-patients, ensure a safe environment for patients, visitors, and employees, and initiate programs and standards through an organized structure.

A hospital or medical center holds a unique position in the community because of its moral and legal responsibilities concerning the health care of the public.[3,9,32,46] The hospital is quite different from other industrial services in that it is generally a self-contained industry. Primarily a health care service, it also provides hotel, laboratory, pharmacy, library, chapel, gift shop, educational, and training services. Moreover, it has medical, nursing, and other specialty staffs, assisted by many different categories of personnel (see Chapter 3).

On the current local, state, and national level, health professional business and industrial associations, government and community agencies, and commissions assist health institutions in improving the quality and quantity of available resources needed to provide adequate care.

THE AMERICAN HOSPITAL ASSOCIATION'S STANDARDS FOR SAFE PATIENT CARE

The American Hospital Association and the American College of Hospital Administrators have accepted their roles in the improvement of patient care. In 1963, with the increasing number of different types of hospitals, the Board of Trustees of the American Hospital Association established requirements [46] for the acceptance of hospitals for registration. To be eligible for an accreditation survey under the Hospital Accreditation Program of the joint commission, a hospital must be registered or listed as a hospital by the American Hospital Association. It must have a current unconditional license to operate as required by the state and have a governing body, organized medical staff and nursing service, and other supporting services. Nurses should be familiar with the current standards set forth by the Joint Commission on Acreditation of Hospitals.[39]

In 1965 the American Hospital Association formulated and issued a statement that identifies *six major characteristics of optimum health services* in areawide community planning.[9] This statement focuses on the essential elements of any modern health system. They are as follows:

Optimum health care in the contemporary world must of necessity have certain characteristics. It must be based on the scientific method, be applied in a personalized manner with full recognition of and attention to personal dimensions in patient needs, and be carried out within a framework of social responsibility. Each of these components must be continuously redefined in the light of new knowledge, as soon as it becomes available. Optimum health care should be accessible to each person in his own community or through regional arrangements. Although the content of modern medicine constantly changes, as does the manner in which certain of its techniques are applied, it is recognized that a balance among the scientific, personal, and social components is always essential at every level of organization of health services.[9]

Essential elements of optimum health services are:

1. A team approach to the care of the individual, in which the health professions providing services are integrated and coor-

dinated under the leadership of the physician.

2. A spectrum of services that includes diagnosis, specific treatment, rehabilitation, education, and prevention.

3. A coordinated community and/or regional system that incorporates the full spectrum of health services and provides for coordination of care from the time of the patient's primary contact with the system through the community hospital to the university hospital and/or medical center and other health agencies. Each should provide the portion of the total spectrum of health services that is feasible in terms of the type of community it serves and the overall pattern of health facilities of the region in which it exists.

4. Continuity among the hospital aspects of patient care, the community, the physician, and the health agencies rendering particular services.

5. Organization of the hospital care of both ambulatory and bed patients into a continuum with common or integrated services.

6. Continuing programs of evaluation and research in the quality of the services provided and in their adequacy in meeting needs of the patient and the community.

These elements are essential to the optimum care of all patients, regardless of their socioeconomic situation.

The hospital, with its medical staff, is now the major health resource in most communities. To meet the expanded responsibilities of this position it is essential that it widen its concerns to include the totality of health services and, with others, to provide leadership in their attainment. The hospital should be prepared to assume a primary position in the implementation of community health plans. Each hospital, then, through its governing body, medical staff, and administrators has a clear mandate continuously to examine its organization and facilities in the light of this central role in coordinating the principles of optimum health services.*

FUNCTIONS OF A HOSPITAL NURSING SERVICE DEPARTMENT

In 1962 the American Hospital Association Board of Trustees approved the State-

---

*Reprinted, with permission, from American Hospital Association: Statement on role of American Hospital Association in interrelated areawide health care planning, Chicago, 1965, The Association.

ment on Functions of a Hospital Nursing Service Department as defined by the NLN Department of Hospital Nursing. The American Hospital Association first issued this statement in August, 1963. The statement defines the role and functions of the nursing service department, focusing on three distinct aspects off patient care: (1) patient-family services, (2) personnel services, and (3) institutional management services. As the role and functions of nursing change, this document has less value as a guide. With the implementation of business and clinical specialization and the expansion of the professional nurse's role in medical care, the functions of nursing service departments have changed.

The 1962 Statement of Functions of a Hospital Department of Nursing Service is as follows:

The department of nursing service carries out its functions according to the philosophy, objectives and policies of the hospital established by the governing board. Accordingly, the director of nursing service is responsible to the administrator of the hospital. Within this organizational pattern, the functions of the department of nursing service are:

1. To provide and evaluate nursing service for patients and their families in support of medical care as directed by the medical staff and pursuant to the objectives and policies of the hospital.

2. To define and implement the philosophy, objectives, policies and standards for nursing care of patients and related nursing services.

3. To provide and implement a departmental plan of administrative authority which clearly delineates responsibilities and duties of each category of nursing personnel.

4. To coordinate the functions of the department of nursing service with the functions of all other departments and services of the hospital.

5. To estimate the requirements for the department of nursing service and to recommend and implement policies and procedures to maintain an adequate and competent nursing staff.

6. To provide the means and methods by which the nursing personnel can work with other groups in interpreting the objectives

of the hospital and nursing service to the patient and community.

7. To participate in the formulation of personnel policies, to implement established policies and evaluate their effectiveness.
8. To develop and maintain an effective system of clinical and administrative nursing records and reports.
9. To estimate needs for facilities, supplies and equipment and implement a system for evaluation and control.
10. To participate in and adhere to the financial plan of operation for the hospital.
11. To initiate, utilize, and/or participate in studies or research projects designed for the improvement of patient care and the improvement of other administrative and hospital services.
12. To provide and implement a program of continuing education for all nursing personnel.
13. To participate in and/or facilitate all educational programs which include student experiences in the department of nursing service.*

Statement on nursing role and functions of the registered nurse supported by AHA

The AHA issued a Statement on Functions in Health Care Institutions that Require the Competence of a Registered Nurse in November, 1968.[7] The statement reaffirmed the fact that registered graduate nurses have a distinct, unique role in providing quality patient care. This document focused on the clinical judgmental and assessment functions necessary to plan, provide, and evaluate nursing care; on the functions of supervision, teaching, and directing all those who give nursing care; and communication and coordinating functions in planning, initiating, and assessing patient needs through the health team approach.

The statement on the role and functions of a registered nurse in a health care institution is as follows:

One of the goals of every hospital is to meet the health care needs of the public it serves at the lowest possible cost consistent with high stan-

dards of quality. Since the quality of care depends largely upon the number, competence, and ability of those who staff the hospital, the judicious utilization, deployment, and retention of personnel are major factors in achieving this goal.

In order to help the administrator in his efforts to improve the utilization of hospital personnel in all departments, the American Hospital Association has identified the following functions as those it believes require the competence of a registered nurse[5]:

1. *Planning of nursing care pursuant to the medical care plan of the physician.* Assessment of patient needs for nursing and establishment of objectives for nursing actions on a continuing basis.
2. *Implementing plans of nursing care in accordance with objectives of the nursing care plan.* Organization, direction, and supervision of nursing personnel in giving nursing care. In the assignment of nursing personnel, registered nurses give care to patients whose condition requires their professional competence and skills.
3. *Evaluating the quality of nursing care in terms of the extent to which objectives of the nursing plan are met.* Appraisal of the quality of nursing care, the performance of nursing personnel, and the proper use of equipment and supplies in rendering nursing care.
4. *Coordinating patient care activities.* By virtue of the strategic position the registered nurse occupies as the most constant figure relating and communicating both with the patient and with members of the professional staff in providing patient services— the coordination of activities to achieve to the greatest extent possible a unified approach to the care of the patient.
5. *Teaching to nursing personnel the nursing care of patients in relation to the objectives of the nursing care plan.* Determination of specific nursing knowledge and skills that need to be learned by nursing personnel.

The above functions are those which, at this point in time, are within the general perimeter of nursing practice and which registered nurses generally have the competence to perform. It is anticipated that, as scientific and technical advances are made in the care and treatment of patients, as physicians delegate greater responsibility to nurses for initiating and performing treatment procedures, and as nurses become increasingly competent in specialized fields of

---

*Reprinted, with permission, from American Hospital Association: Statement on functions of a hospital nursing service department, Chicago, 1963, The Association.

practice, the functions of the registered nurse will expand in terms of patient care. Consequently, hospitals in the future will have increased responsibility for providing or monitoring new types of educational experiences for registered nurses, for safeguarding their patients, and for meeting their legal obligations by assuring the competence of the registered nurses who perform these new functions.*

The concluding paragraph of the AHA statement concerning the role and function of the registered graduate nurse does differentiate between the professional and the technical nurse.

With the expanded roles of professional nurses in the practice of nursing, I believe that a registered nurse with only an associate degree or diploma in nursing is not prepared to make clinical nursing judgments. In today's care of patients the assistant nurse becomes a valuable member of the nursing care staff as an assistant to the professional nurse. The team or primary nursing concept cannot become a reality without prepared professional nurses responsible for a group of patients' clinical care.

Today the professional nurse has an expanded role in comparison to the traditional role of assistant to the physician and the performer of routine tasks.[67] This new role encompasses increased responsibility and accountability for nursing care along with tasks previously considered the physician's responsibility. It is the use of special nursing skills in the management of clinical nursing that distinguishes the professional nurse from the assistant nurse.[10,40] Likewise, in the clinic or ambulatory setting the special knowledge and skills of the nurse-practitioner distinguish this nurse from the physician's assistant.

To assume a leadership role in team nursing, primary nursing, or as a nurse-practitioner, the professional nurse needs to be educated in a setting that provides interdisciplinary educational opportunities, and advanced scientific knowledge in nursing care,

resulting in the use of this knowledge in the delivery of health services. It is gratifying to see special nursing programs being offered to college graduates. The college graduate seems to be aware that modern nursing offers opportunities for independent decision making and creative action, as well as for team work. With more college graduates entering the nursing profession, the public image of nursing will be enhanced.

In support of the ANA's 1965 position paper,[11] the New York State Nurses' Association in the late 1975 presented to the assembly a legislative proposal to implement the resolution on entry into professional practice through revision of Article 1939, Title VIII of the education law.[57,63] The proposed changes in the New York State Nurse Practice Act are (1) requirements for license as a registered professional nurse by 1985 would be a baccalaureate degree in nursing and (2) requirements for license as a licensed practical nurse would be an associate degree in practical nursing. There would be two legal categories of nurses. Professional nurses would have the right to function autonomously and make independent nursing decisions based on a theoretical body of knowledge acquired during formal education, and the practical nurses would be responsible for making judgments within the scope of their knowledge while assisting the professional nurse in the primary or team nursing model. This bill would strengthen and standardize educational qualifications for the two currently licensed careers in nursing. Other state associations are studying similar legislation (see Chapter 4).

PURPOSE AND MEANING OF STANDARDS

Every professional nurse should keep in mind that the essential reason for a department of nursing service is to provide quality nursing care to patients.[14,53] The experienced and qualified nursing service director and staff work toward the achievement of quality nursing care. Health care professionals, consumers, and others currently are striving to answer the question of what constitutes adequate nursing care and

---

*Reprinted, with permission, from American Hospital Association: The statement on functions in health care institutions that require the competence of a registered nurse, pub. no. S-55, Chicago, 1969, The Association.

how it is to be provided at a reasonable price to consumer-patients (see Chapter 4 on recent legislation).

Many professional nurses do not believe that the standards prepared by licensing agencies and accrediting bodies are sufficient for a quality assurance program in nursing.[52] In recent years professional nursing asssociations have developed precise criteria and statements of what they consider to be the minimum essentials of quality nursing care (see PSROs, Chapter 4, and peer review and nursing audit, Chapter 16).

Setting standards is the first step in structuring an assessment system.[10,30] A standard may be viewed as a model establishment by an authority. It is a level or degree of quality considered adequate for a specific purpose. Standards define what should be done and identify conditions under which one reasonably can expect quality care to be given.

However, standards and statements do not assure that quality care is given.[18,49] For example, the written organizational plan and chart may appear effective, but such a plan does not of itself assure effective communication between staff members, or a consistent flow pattern of manpower during each 24-hour period for a particular group of patients with various nursing needs.[16]

The Joint Commission on Accreditation for Hospitals, the American Nurses' Association, and the National League for Nursing have chosen a structure to identify necessary conditions for quality care. The statements are directed toward evaluating the structures through which nursing care is managed and delivered.

JCAH STANDARDS FOR NURSING SERVICE

Nursing consultants participated in developing the JCAH section on nursing service. The nursing consultants used the material produced by the ANA and the NLN as a frame of reference.

The 1976 JCAH standards for nursing service are as follows:

Standard 1: The nursing service shall be under the direction of a legally and professionally qualified registered nurse. There shall also be a sufficient number of duly licensed registered nurses on duty at all times to plan, assign, supervise and evaluate nursing care, as well as to give patients the nursing care that requires the judgment and specialized skills of a registered nurse.[39]

The director of nursing is delegated to develop and execute a staffing program. To do this the director must understand the elements of a staffing program and the mechanisms necessary for its planning, implementation, and evaluation.[13,17,43] The effectiveness of a stable staffing program depends on the manpower provided and on whether the nursing practice will be directed toward providing a minimal or a high quality of care. *Standard 1* of JCHA expects nurses to focus on a staffing program that uses the knowledge and skills of the nursing staff in appropriate numbers and that promotes clinical nursing leadership.[29,71] Principles and methodologies of staffing programs are discussed in Chapters 13 and 14.

Standard 2: The nursing service shall have a current written organizational plan that delineates its functional structure and its mechanisms for cooperative planning and decision-making.[39]

Before an organizational plan can be designed it is necessary to define the essential elements in providing quality nursing care to meet the needs of patients.[14,35,50] Patients' needs for nursing care therefore must be identified. Many variables of specialized treatment, age, and ethnic, educational, and economic backgrounds of the patients and their problems, as well as the patient population expected, must be determined.[44] There are important factors in designing the functional structure of a nursing service department[37] (see Chapters 9, 10, and 12).

Development of a manpower division in the management of nursing care is the primary consideration, with the development of necessary top management a secondary task, and the structure therefore must be designed from the bottom up. To utilize effectively the nurses' professional judgment and clinical expertise the organizational plan must be flexible enough to permit decision making in the direct care of patients.

Standard 3: Written nursing care and administrative policies and procedures shall be developed to provide the nursing staff with acceptable methods of meeting its responsibilities and achieving projected goals.[39]

To develop effective and meaningful policies nurses should seek answers to the following questions. Why is the policy required? Does it help achieve department objectives? Does it prevent incidents from occurring?[45,51]

To determine the appropriateness of policies one should determine the degree that they facilitate quality care.[12] It is evident in some areas of direct patient care that activities, procedures, and policies are required and serve as guidelines for the personnel (see Chapters 7 and 8).

Standard 4: There shall be evidence established that the nursing service provides safe, efficient and therapeutically effective nursing care through the planning of each patient's care and the effective implementation of the plans.[39]

Since the 1940s, there has been much controversy among nurse educators and nursing service staffs on what a nursing care plan is and on what it should contain.[40,44,65] All involved agree that nursing care must be planned, but the literature indicates various purposes and methods for this organizational tool. Kramer[40] reminds us that written nursing care plans are a means to the end of quality patient care rather than an end in themselves.

Nursing care planning should be accomplished by those involved in the care of each patient. The patient and his family should actively participate in the planning. Nursing care plans could become a valuable tool in evaluating programs of care and practice[55,62,65] (see Chapters 11 and 12).

Standard 5: There should be continuing training programs and educational opportunities for the development of personnel.[39]

With the increased application of new technological innovations and the use of new therapies, there is a need for in-service education and training for nurses.[25,28] New graduates generally are not prepared to perform on a nursing staff without receiving special preparation in the care of a particular group of patients. Nurse assistants and attendants require preservice training before they can perform nursing care tasks.

The training and in-service educational programs must not be viewed as a separate entity but rather as an integral part of the total quality control system (see Chapters 4 and 12).

ANA STANDARDS FOR NURSING SERVICE

The American Nurses' Association, the National League for Nursing, and other health agencies have developed statements in an effort to help nursing improve patient care. The ANA Committee on Nursing Service formulated standards for organized nursing service to help implement them through appropriate channels in accordance with the 1964 ANAs Certificate of Incorporation. In 1965 the ANA published its first statement: Standards for Organized Nursing Services. The 16 standards and assessment factors were supplements to the ANA statements of standards for the individual nurse-practitioner issued previously by the occupational sections within the ANA organization.

The Nursing Service Standards were revised in 1973 by the ANA's Commission of Nursing Services.[14] The standards and their guidelines directed health health administrators and nurses in developing a nursing care system in any modern health institution.

The 12 standards are as follows:

Standard I: Nursing administration has a philosophy and objectives which reflect the purposes of the health care organization and give direction to the nursing care program. [See Chapter 7.]

Standard II: Nursing administration has the responsibility and authority for the quality of nursing practice within the health care organization. [See Chapters 6, 9, and 12.]

Standard III: A nursing service has a designated leader who is a qualified Registered Nurse and a member of the operational policy-making bodies of the health care organization. [See Chapters 10 and 17.]

Standard IV: The nursing care program is integrated into the total program of the health care organization. [See Chapters 11 and 13.]

Standard V: Nursing administration determines the budget necessary to carry out the nursing care program and administers the approved budget. [See Chapters 15 and 16.]

Standard VI: A nursing service organization plan delineates the functional structure of the department and shows established relationships among nursing personnel and with other services. [See Chapters 10 and 17.]

Standard VII: The nursing administration has written personnel policies which assist in recruiting and maintaining a qualified staff. [See Chapter 8.]

Standard VIII: Nursing administration shall detail guidelines for utilization of nursing personnel. [See Chapters 13 and 14.]

Standard IX: The nursing administration provides programs for orientation and continued learning of nursing personnel. [See Chapters 15 and 17.]

Standard X: A nursing service has the responsibility to participate in the education of students in the health care field.

Standard XI: A nursing service supports research in the health care field. [See code for nurses, p. 2.]

Standard XII: A nursing service evaluates its clinical and administrative practices.* [See Chapters 16 and 17.]

These standards are designed for use in any health care system that is relevant to contemporary health care ends. The Commission of Nursing Services is charged with the continual evaluation of standards and revisions to meet nursing service objectives and functions in keeping with society's health needs.

ANA'S STATEMENT ON NURSE-ADMINISTRATOR OF NURSING SERVICE[15]

In keeping with the ANA. 1964 Certificate of Incorporation previously mentioned, the ANA Commission of Nursing Services was delegated to assume a leadership role to refine and implement nursing service standards with the assistance of its members and other related health groups. In June, 1969,

*From American Nurses' Association: Standards for organized nursing services in hospitals, public health agencies, nursing care homes, industries, and clinics, Kansas, 1973, The Association. Reprinted with the permission of the American Nurses' Association.

the Commission issued the statement: The Position, Role and Qualifications of the Administrator of Nursing Service.[15] The major functions of the nurse-administrator is organized nursing services of a health care system were defined as follows:

The administrator of nursing services carries ultimate administrative authority and responsibility in one or more health facilities for the nursing services provided individuals and families. As a member of the administrative staff, the administrator of nursing services participates in formulating agency policy, in devising procedures essential to the achievement of objectives, and in developing and evaluating programs and services. She has full authority and responsibility for the development of nursing service policies. The responsibilities of the position are to plan, organize, direct, coordinate, and evaluate activities of the nursing service staff. The nature of the position implies accountability for creating a social system which fosters the participation of nursing staff in planning, implementing, and evaluating practice to insure safe, efficient, and therapeutically effective nursing care. The functions of the administrator of nursing services are derived from A.N.A.'s Standards for Organized Nursing Services.

The competence of the administrator of nursing services involves an ability to facilitate and coordinate a diverse staff of nursing specialists who are making decisions about nursing needs of individuals, families, and other social groups and an ability to make decisions about the organization and delivery of nursing services. Two requisites for this leadership role are an understanding of the social, political, and economic influences affecting programs of health care and competence in dealing with any problems in the relationships of professional practitioners and within the complex social system in which nursing is practiced.

Abilities essential to the administrative leader of a program of comprehensive nursing care are the following:

1. The ability to think and act in terms of the total system of health care and to recognize the need for adapting that system to the needs of people.
2. The ability to think and act in terms of the distinctive and contributory role of the nursing profession.
3. The ability to use pertinent knowledge and methods of working with and through people who are concerned with, or affected by, health care.

4. The ability to use the knowledge, methods and techniques pertinent to directing, guiding, and assisting nursing staff members in fulfilling their responsibilities for nursing services.

Basic to these skills is the ability to coordinate, integrate, and reconcile the needs of nursing practitioners, and their goals for nursing service, with organizational requirements, and objectives.

Minimum educational qualifications for administrators of nursing services should include completion of a baccalaureate program which has prepared them for professional nursing practice, and completion of a master's degree program with a focus on clinical nursing practice and on administration of organized nursing services. Professional experience should have contributed and enhanced the development of the competencies described above.*

Since 1970 the ANA's Commission on Nursing Services and the NLN Council of Hospital and Related Institutional Nursing Services have held regional conferences to give members an opportunity to refine statements and to find better ways to use nursing personnel. Questions have been raised concerning the role and functions of the nurse-administrator and the minimum qualification requirements for the position. As the hospital industry expands and changes its system, the role and functions of the nurse-administrator and nurse-practitioner will change, along with those of other hospital personnel.

To work effectively with people in nursing services and with other professionals, the director and department heads in nursing services must avail themselves of the heritage of the humanities and behavioral sciences to assist in the humanizing processes of patient care services. They should possess the energy to turn problems into opportunities and a tremendous capacity to manage, that Howard Johnson, President of Massachusetts Institute of Technology, defines as the "art of studying the facts and then reaching firm decisions."

---

*From American Nurses' Association: The position, role and qualifications of the administrator of nursing service, New York, 1969, The Association. Reprinted with the permission of the American Nurses' Association.

REALITIES OF THE NURSING SERVICE DIRECTOR'S ROLE

Amid the increased complexity of medical technological functions, automation, computers, systems approach and the demands of professional nurses to use their knowledge and skills in clinical nursing care, the director of nursing services is challenged in many ways as the head of the largest department in the institution.

The major responsibility of the director of nursing services is to provide a high quality of nursing care to all patient-consumers at as reasonable a price as possible. Nursing's responsibilities lie in all areas of nursing practice concerning the health and care of patients/clients. Thus, directors of nursing and their roles in creating a conducive environment for providing quality nursing care are so broad in scope that any job description becomes a simple guide requiring interpretations.[45,60,64,71]

The role of the nurse-director is perceived in various ways by different directors, administrators, physicians, and consumer groups.[59] It is vital that the role perceptions of the nurse-director be viewed openly and carefully, and either accepted or changed. In selecting a director of nursing, administrators no longer use the Peter Principle and allow people to rise to their level of incompetence.[58] There is growing evidence that there are more academically prepared nurses. However, too many directors of nursing services with a background only in nursing services function under the traditional structure, policies, and procedure of the institution without the confidence, knowledge, and skills to effect change. Likewise, the faculty members have separated themselves from the nursing practice environment in many situations and do not seem knowledgeable either about nursing care or the role of the director.

To enhance the quality of nursing care and prepare future graduate nurses to care for their patients, the director should try to unite nursing education and nursing practice in the clinical setting. Society allocates resources to prepare nurses to meet their health and nursing care needs. Some directors accept a nursing leadership role in creating a partnership between nursing education and nursing practice.

Several health institutions recently divided top administrative control of organized nursing service. In such cases the department of nursing has a clinical nurse-director and a nonnurse manager. This division of responsibility (power) aims to keep the nurse, expert in the clinical role, providing quality nursing care and to leave management responsibilities such as staffing, equipment, and finances to the nonnurse.

In my opinion this division of responsibilities quickly results in loss of control over the quality of nursing practice.[10] Finances and decision-making powers go hand in hand. Since clinical nursing depends on the allocation and distribution of monies and the regulation policies, the clinical nurse-director eventually becomes dependent on the decisions of the nonnurse manager who controls the level of nursing care to be delivered.

Administratively, the goals, objectives, and resources of organized nursing must be brought into appropriate balance. This is an important function of the director and the professional staff. Staff creativity and ability can reduce deficiencies to a degree. The director assists top administration to effect economic and efficiency goals without compromising the quality of care. In educating the administrator, the board of trustees, and the medical executive committee about the objectives and the meaning of quality nursing care, the director must draw on facts and data based on continued analysis and research, as well as appraise data on the effectiveness of nursing care given to patients. It is the director of nursing who should innovate efficiency programs, such as the unit management system, that result in high quality of care and other services without cost increases.

Directors should understand their roles in negotiating labor contracts with the nursing staff, or in settling grievances, especially when the bargaining agent is the local nurses' association. At the bargaining table the director is a member of the hospital's administrative team but must not abdicate the standards and principles of nursing during negotiations. During these negotiations the director should recognize that conflicts are inherent in the role of director of nursing services and should not be taken personally. It is advisable for directors to seek the guidance of professional negotiators, especially if they are unfamiliar with the contractual process (see discussion on collective bargaining in Chapter 4).

The director of nursing must understand the values inherent in cost benefit analysis and systems approach and use such innovations in collecting necessary data. Nurse-directors should be confident in their leadership roles as members of the top administration team and endeavor to establish effective colleagueships with nurse educators, physicians, and consumer groups in the community. In the competitive world of a health institution, directors need to acquire political skill and utilize all possible resources to compete productively for the nursing department. The 1977 government cost containment proposals bring new challenges to directors of nursing services. With their fund of information on problems and issues that influence the quality of institutional care, they must articulate to others what professional nursing is and define a nursing system in cost effectiveness terms.

Accountability may be defined as being responsible for the services one provides or makes available. It is the nurse-director's support, motivation, and leadership that promote nurses to function autonomously and be accountable in all areas of practice in the care of their patients. Despite the everyday pressures to compromise the quality of care, the prepared and confident director has a challenging opportunity to improve the patient care system.

ANA STATEMENT ON NURSING STAFF REQUIREMENTS FOR IN-PATIENT HEALTH CARE SERVICES

The ANA Statement on Nursing Staff Requirements for In-Patient Health Care Services prepared by the committee on nursing service[13] and issued in May, 1967, did not propose the use of one specific formula, ratio, or numerical staffing system; it recommended that each nursing service director and staff member take into consideration facts and statistical hospital data such as the number of patient days of recent years, those projected for the coming fiscal year, nursing service man-hours rendered per category of worker during the fiscal year, number of patients in various nursing classifications, and manhours required to render safe, adequate care. The statement also recommended that statistical data on personnel turnover, sick time, and vacation time allowances be considered and that periodic assessment tools be used for continual review of the input and output of resources.

The major points of this staffing statement, taking into consideration Standards for Organized Nursing Services, specifically standard No. 6 and its four assessment factors, include the following:

The nursing department promotes safe and therapeutically effective nursing care through implementation of established standards of nursing practice.
  A. Registered nurses review and revise nursing care programs as necessary.
  B. A registered nurse plans, supervises, and evaluates the nursing care of each patient.
  C. A registered nurse assigns the nursing care of each patient according to the needs of the patient and the preparation and competence of available staff.
  D. A registered nurse gives nursing care to patients who require her judgment and specialized skills.*

With these standards as a basis, the administrative staff should make decisions for each situation such as (1) for how many patients in a particular area can one registered nurse plan, supervise, and evaluate nursing care simultaneously? (2) how many auxiliary personnel can one registered nurse direct, supervise, and evaluate? and (3) how many patients will require the direct care of

a registered nurse and how many nursing man-hours will be involved in this care?

The ANA statement enumerates those policies, practices, and factors that should be determined prior to setting nurse staffing requirements as follows:

1. The purposes and objectives of the health care facilities and the nursing service department, including the standard of patient care established and supported by the health care facilities.
2. The assigned responsibilities and functions of each department and its employees in relation to services to patients, especially as these affect the amount of nursing time spent on activities not directly related to nursing care.
3. The number of physicians referring, visiting, and directing the medical care of patients within the health care facility.
4. The level of activity throughout the hospital and within each nursing unit, such as patient turnover, number and complexity of operations, diagnostic procedures, treatments and medications.
5. How often and for how long does the patient have to leave the nursing unit for special procedures and treatments?
6. The intensity of illness, the nursing needs, the degree of dependence, and the age distribution of patients cared for within the health care facility and the placement of these patients within the various nursing units.
7. The physical layout of the total institution, the relationship of individual departments to each other, the size, geographical layout, number of beds, type of accommodations, the proximity to other hospital departments of each nursing unit, and the number and type of specialized nursing units.
8. The quality and availability of supplies, equipment, supportive personnel and services to the patient care units over the 24 hours of the day and 7 days of the week.
9. The number, level of preparation, and assigned functions of all nursing personnel and the time required to bring new nursing employees to the level of their job expectations.
10. The method of patient care assignment employed by the nursing department.
11. The quality of nursing administration and supervision available.

---

*From American Nurses' Association: Statement on nursing staff requirements for in-patient health care services, New York, 1967, The Association. Reprinted with the permission of the American Nurses' Association.

12. The method of assignment and the number and level of competence of private duty nurses normally available and employed by patients or the health care facility.
13. The amount of time spent by nursing service personnel in teaching and research activities.
14. The amount of nursing time spent in planning for continuity of patient care.*

The various designs of a nursing service staffing system, staffing composition, budgeting for the nursing service department as an element of planning, preparation of the nursing service payroll budget, and analysis methodology of input and output systems are discussed later in the text.

ANA STANDARDS OF NURSING PRACTICE

The American Nurses' Association's first priority for the 1974-76 biennial convention states, "Improving the practice of nursing through assisting by implementation of standards of practice enunciated by ANA."

This priority was adapted by the ANA Board of Directors and endorsed by the 1974 House of Delegates. The Standards of Nursing Practice,[10] developed by the ANA's Congress for Practice, is one step in enabling the profession to assure clients/patients that quality nursing care can be identified, measured, and delivered, and that professional nurses are responsible for the outcome of their own professional acts.

The ANA's Congress for Nursing Practice states:

Nursing practice in all settings must possess the characteristics identified by these standards if clients/patients are to receive a high quality of nursing care. Each Standard is followed by a rationale and assessment factors. Assessment factors are to be used in determining achievement of the Standard.

Standard I: The collection of data about the health status of the client/patient is systematic and continuous. The data are accessible, communicated, and recorded.

Standard II: Nursing diagnoses are derived from health status data.

Standard III: The plan of nursing care includes goals derived from the nursing diagnoses.

Standard IV: The plan of nursing care includes priorities and the prescribed nursing approaches or measures to achieve the goals derived from the nursing diagnoses.

Standard V: Nursing actions provide for client/patient participation in health promotion, maintenance and restoration.

Standard VI: Nursing actions assist the client/patient to maximize his health capabilities.

Standard VII: The client's/patient's progress or lack of progress toward goal achievement is determined by the client/patient and the nurse.

Standard VIII: The client/patient's progress or lack of progress toward goal achievement directs reassesment, reordering or priorities, new goal setting and revision of the plan of nursing care.*

ANA Standards of Medical-Surgical Nursing Practice

The statement defines medical-surgical nursing practice as the nursing care of adults who have a known or predicted physiological alteration as follows:

In order to implement the nursing process effectively, nurses who are engaged in the practice of medical-surgical nursing should (1) base nursing practice on principles and theories of biophysical and behavioral sciences; (2) continuously update knowledge and skills, applying new knowledges generated by research, changes in health care delivery systems, and changes in social profiles; (3) determine the range of practice by considering the patient's needs, the nurse's competence, the setting for care and the resources available; and (4) insure patient and family participation in health promotion, maintenance and restoration.

Standard I: The collection of data about the health status of the patient is systematic and continuous. These data are communicated to appropriate persons and recorded and stored in a retrievable and accessible system. Data are obtained by interview, physical examination, review of records and reports, and consultation. Priority

---

*From American Nurses' Association: Statement on nursing staff requirements for inpatient health care services, New York, 1967, The Association. Reprinted with the permission of the American Nurses' Association.

---

*From American Nurses' Association: ANA standards of nursing practice, Kansas, 1974, The Association. Reprinted with the permission of the American Nurses' Association.

of data collection is determined by the immediate physical condition of the patient.

Standard II: Nursing diagnosis is derived from health status data. Nursing diagnosis is a concise statement identifying the patient's problem(s). It is not a summary of all abnormalities.

Standard III: Goals for nursing care are formulated. A goal is the end state toward which nursing action is directed.

Standard IV: The plan for nursing care prescribes nursing actions to achieve the goals. The plan for nursing care describes a systematic method to meet the goals.

Standard V: The plan for nursing care is implemented. The plan must be applied to achieve the goals.

Standard VI: The plan for nursing care is evaluated. Patient response is compared with observable outcomes which are specified in the goals.

Standard VII: Reassessment, reordering of priorities, new goal setting and revision of the plan for nursing care are a continuous process. The steps of the nursing process are used concurrently and recurrently.*

As mentioned in Chapter 4, the medical-surgical division of nursing practice has issued additional standards concerning its subspecialties. These standards serve as basic guidelines for nurses to develop criteria for the evaluation of nursing care.

ANA Standards of Maternal-Child Health Nursing Practice

The maternal and child health nursing practice is a direct service. The ANA statement developed by the Executive Committee and the Standards Committee of ANA's Division on Maternal-Child Health Nursing Practice and setting forth the Standards of Nursing Practice "is a direct service to individuals, their families and the community during childbearing and childrearing phases of the life cycle." Maternal and child health nursing practice includes independent, dependent, and interdependent functions. The way that the nurse uses knowledge and skills depends on awareness and self-understanding as a therapeutic agent as well as on the

*From American Nurses' Association: Standards of medical-surgical nursing practices, Kansas, 1974, The Association. Reprinted with the permission of the American Nurses' Association.

ability to mold knowledge and skills into effective practice.

These standards are based on 14 premises, 11 aims, and include 13 standards, each with rationale and assessment factors. It behooves nurses in maternity-child health settings to study these standards carefully and evaluate nurses' actions by means of the assessment factors.

ANA Standards of Psychiatric–Mental Health Nursing Practice

The ANA Executive Committee and its Standards Committee of the Division on Psychiatric–Mental Health Nursing Practice state that:

Psychiatric nursing is a specialized area of nursing practice employing theories of human behavior as its scientific aspect and purposeful use of self as its art. . . . the dependent area of psychiatric nursing practice is implementation of physicians' orders . . . independent areas are assessment of nursing needs and development and implementation of nursing care plans. . . . Psychiatric nursing is practiced largely in collaboration and coordination with those in a variety of other disciplines, who are working concomitantly with the patient.[10]

The aims of the standards, characteristic aspects of the practice of psychiatric nursing, and the rationale and assessment of the 14 standards are stated clearly.

ANA Standards of Community Health Practice

The ANA Executive Committee and Standards Committee of the Division on Community Health Nursing Practice state that:

Nursing practice is a direct service, goal directed and adaptable to the needs of the individual, family and community during health and illness. Community health nursing is a synthesis of nursing practice and public health practice applied to promoting and preserving the health of populations. . . . In community health nursing practice the consumer is the client or patient. . . . Consumers include individuals, groups and the community as a whole. . . . Professional practitioners of nursing bear primary responsibility and accountability for the nursing care consumers receive.[10]

This document presents eight standards with accompanying rationale and assessment factors for each standard.

ANA Standards of Gerontological Nursing Practice

The term *gerontological* rather than *geriatric* reflects the change in the division's title and describes more accurately the scope of nursing practice in the care of the older adult.

Gerontological nursing is concerned with assessment of the health needs of older adults, planning and implementing health care to meet these needs, and evaluating the effectiveness of such care.[10]

Each of the nine standards is accompanied by a statement of rationale and assessment factors that are to be used in determining achievement of the standard.

FORMATION OF ANA COUNCIL OF NURSING SERVICE FACILITATORS

The first meeting of the Council was established in May, 1974, and held in June, 1974, during the ANA biennial convention. The Council's purpose is to advance sound nursing practices, implement the ANA Standards of Nursing Services, promote the exchange of ideas, and recognize excellence in nursing service administration.

The functions of the council are defined as (1) advancing the quality of nursing care for consumers; (2) promoting communication among nurses who are responsible for nursing service administration; (3) devising methods to implement the ANA Standards for Nursing Services; (4) devising methods to work cooperatively with nurses to implement the ANA Standards of Nursing Practice; (5) delineating problems and issues in nursing service administration and seeking involvement of appropriate groups for deliberation and resolution; (6) recommending solutions to problems and positions on issues to the Commission of Nursing Services; (7) providing recognition of excellence in nursing service administration; and (8) developing and maintaining working relationships with other units of the association and with related professional and community groups as appropriate to the responsibilities of the Council.

The membership includes nursing service administrators and their associates and assistants for service and education employed in health care agencies. The Council has an executive committee composed of five council members. The chairman of the council of nursing service facilitator serves as the official liaison to the Commission on Nursing Services.

NATIONAL LEAGUE FOR NURSING ACTIONS TO IMPROVE HOSPITAL NURSING SERVICES

In June, 1964, the Department of Hospital Nursing of the National League for Nursing issued In Pursuit of Quality—Hospital Nursing Services,[56] a statement of objectives for nursing service. In the statement hospital nursing service leaders formulated goals of nursing care that only can be achieved through effective administration, organization, and utilization of health workers. The statement reflects and expands the 1959 statement that was the basis for the pamphlet "Your Nursing Services Today and Tomorrow," published in 1961. In Pursuit of Quality included the statement on functions of a hospital department of nursing, which was approved by the NLN Department of Hospital Nursing and the American Hospital Association Board of Trustees in 1962.

Committee on Quality of Patient Care

During 1962 to 1964 the Nursing Steering Committee of the National League for Nursing sponsored a series of regional conferences referred to as Blueprint for Action for the purpose of interpreting and reinforcing the statement on the quality of nursing care. These conferences were the first of their kind ever to be undertaken by the League and were co-sponsored in each region by the regional councils of state leagues of nursing.

In 1966 the NLN Committee on Quality of Patient Care, Department of Hospital Nursing, issued the booklet "Quest for Quality: a Self-Evaluation Guide to Patient Care"[55] to help hospital nursing services evaluate the quality of patient care provided and initiate ways to improve care of all patients. The guide is divided into major sections corresponding to the stages a patient goes through as he progresses along the health continuum. The indices represent the elements of care—physical, mental, psychosocial, spiritual, educational, vocational, financial, safety, and legal.

The NLN Committee on Quality of Patient Care developed a survey questionnaire that was submitted to hospital nursing service departments to help determine what kinds of organizational patterns existed in hospitals in the United States. In 1968 the results gathered from the survey were published by Aydelotte,[18] chairman of the NLN Committee on Quality of Patient care. The collected data demonstrated that (1) medical care and hospital support services had increased, (2) nursing service departments were taking on additional duties as well as keeping the old ones, and (3) nursing service administration and supervisory staff were responsible for carrying out operational duties of other hospital departments, usually during holidays and weekends, but sometimes on a daily basis.

The collected data from this NLN survey indicated that few changes had been made between 1966 and 1968 to relieve nursing personnel of hospital service tasks. This survey also brought to light the inadequacy of the hospital health management team to solve problems because of inadequacies in the social structure and management of the hospital departments and ineffective utilization of prepared professional and technically trained graduate nurses.

Criteria for evaluating hospital nursing services

In 1965 the Department of Hospital Nursing, National League for Nursing, issued the statement Criteria for Evaluating a Hospital Department of Nursing Services.[55] The ten criteria and their interpretation provide a tool for self-evaluation and program improvement. Directors and supervisors of hospital nursing service should use this guide in working with nursing service personnel, hospital managers, and interested

groups who share functions in providing efficient, safe patient care.

The basic criteria or general guides may be summarized as follows:

The department of nursing service
1. Defines tenets of philosophy and objectives
2. Establishes a plan of organization consistent with the objectives of nursing care and goals and objectives of the hospital
3. Develops and initiates written administrative nursing service policies
4. Develops nursing service management in keeping with hospital personnel policies and procedures
5. Develops and implements programs for providing nursing care
6. Develops and presents to the hospital executive officers a fiscal budget for its operation
7. Initiates and operates a system for control and use of equipment, facilities, supplies, and manpower
8. Maintains an effective system of clinical and administrative records and reports
9. Participates in a program of in-service education for all members of the staff
10. Conducts a systematic appraisal program by which it evaluates its progress toward attainment of established objectives

During the 1970s the divisions of the NLN published several presentations on nursing service community health planning, quality assessment of patient care, approaches to staff development, and accreditation of nursing educational programs. In 1977 the NLN issued reports on staff development for departments of nursing and on the role of the director of nursing service. The NLN's Council of Associate Degree Programs agreed to initiate a study beginning in November, 1977, on the competencies of graduate nurses with an associate degree in nursing.[57]

The four NLN education councils for nursing endeavor to promote and improve nursing education in the United States. Since 1972 the NLN has participated in evaluating the existing credentialing process with educational and health service groups and health associations (see Chapter 4 on credentialing).

SAFETY STANDARDS AND GUIDES FOR HEALTH CARE INSTITUTIONS

Health institutions today are required to develop, initiate, and evaluate their safety programs, policies, and procedures in accordance with existing legislative acts and standards established by state and national regulatory bodies. A health care institution is legally as well as morally responsible for protecting patients, visitors, and all individuals working in the institution.[3,39,61]

Employers' growing responsibility to provide a safe work environment for employees

Prior to the Industrial Revolution, most industries were protected by common law rules indicating that employees and not their employers[21] were responsible for their own safety. Before 1910 in almost every state the laws determining employers' responsibility for industrial injuries had been handed down from the preindustrial period in England and the United States. The common law rules of liability attempted to determine who was at fault. If the employer properly performed all of these duties he could not be held liable for a work-related injury to an employee. It was not easy for an employee to prove breach of employer's duty[19] in court, and fellow workers who witnessed a worker's injury usually were reluctant to testify against the employer. With the expense of litigation and other responsibilities the injured worker faced many obstacles in pressing a claim. Court decisions provided the employer with considerable protection, reflecting the doctrine of individualism and a laissez-faire philosophy. The slightest lack of ordinary care on the part of the injured worker that contributed to his injury kept him from recovering any damages. If the employee contributed 1% of the factors that led to the accident and his employer 99%, he still could not recover. For many decades countless numbers of workers suffered without justice regarding occupational injuries.

The enactment of employer liability statutes developed out of the public's agitation to remove some limitations on the employee's right to recover.[19] With the introduction of technology and changes in organization, the inequities of the common law principles of employers' liability became evident. The employer liability acts did not attempt to create a new system of liability but followed the concept that the employee must bear the economic loss of an industrial injury, unless he could show that some other person was directly responsible through a negligent act or omission for the occurrence of the accident.

By 1917 the United States Supreme Court held that compulsory compensation laws were constitutional, thus setting the pattern of elective statutes. About 66% of state compensation laws are compulsory. Workmens' compensation, the first social insurance program to be accepted in the United States, was organized by the administrative practices and philosophy of the early twentieth century.

Workmen's compensation benefits now include four separate types of payment: (1) permanent total disability, (2) permanent partial disability, (3) temporary total disability, and (4) death.[61]

In the 1960s the courts and legislators in most states held that hospitals, although charitable institutions, were basically service corporations and as such were subject to the regulations and penalties imposed on industries and businesses.

Hospitals recently have been a party in suits involving injuries to workers and in malpractice suits involving patients. The potential threat of legal liabilities prompted hospitals to develop policies and procedures in accordance with legislative safety acts and standards established by regulatory bodies. Such actions aim to reduce the costs of medical expenditures, compensation, and malpractice, and the indirect costs of losses in services, training, materials, and equipment and to keep public esteem.

Safety Standards of the Joint Commission on Accreditation of Hospitals

Since the JCAH was incorporated in 1952, it has established safety standards to assure a safe physical environment for patients, visitors, and persons working in a health care institution.[39] Over the years the commission has broadened its standards in keeping with the operations of hospitals and long-term care facilities.

With the tremendous advances in medical treatment and the application of advanced technology, hospital services are accomplished with the aid of complex electronic equipment, many different kinds of mechanical devices, flammable and combustible chemicals, and radioactive materials.

Note that the JCAH standards set forth in its manual are minimum, not optimum. For many years the American Hospital Association,[3,9] the American Medical Association, and other professional groups have advocated criteria and the need for safety and health programs in hospitals. However, the literature provides little information on how effective such programs are in reducing the injuries and illnesses of employees. In connection with the 1970 safety legislation hearing, the Labor Standards Bureau conducted a study on work-injury. Data indicated that 8% of disabling injuries went unreported each year, and injuries that were not disabling were not reported.[61]

Accident prevention is an important issue in any health institution. Hospitals and insurance companies always are looking for new ways to reduce the number of patient and employee accidents. Insurance companies promote safety services through associations that maintain cooperative relationships with hospitals.

The nursing staff of a hospital has a vital role in providing a safe environment to assure quality care to patients. Safety is a constant concern of health professionals as they use different pieces of equipment and materials in patient care and as they supervise the care and services rendered by other workers. The nursing service department also employs the largest number of personnel. Professional nurses are a liaison between many departments and functions of the hospital and the patients themselves and thus have opportunities to motivate and guide the personnel to practice safety prevention and to help maintain an effective safety and health program.[26,33]

Many of the JCAH standards are associated closely with nursing practices, techniques, and procedures. Nurses should evaluate critically existing safety policies and procedures and make recommendations to improve environmental conditions.

The JCAH standards that pertain to the nursing care of patients, to visitors, and to personnel are as follows:

Standard I: The hospital shall be structurally constituted in a manner that protects the lives and ensures the physical safety of its patients, its personnel, and its visitors.[39]

Fire safety includes prevention, detection, confinement, evacuation and, extinguishment. The NFPA life-safety code (NFPA No. 100) usually is revised every 3 years.[54] This code is based on the theory of compartmentalization, and it provides regulations and procedures concerning operating features with information on clothing, bedding, maintenance, smoking, housekeeping, and the personnel training program.

It is important that new employees receive appropriate instructions concerning hazardous areas and fire safety in their orientation program. Periodic fire practice drills are an important prevention measure.

The chairman of the safety council and the director of the buildings and ground department should make periodic inspections. Nurses who are members of a facility planning committee should know about construction regulations and safety codes so that designs will meet the purposes of the unit and allow for good quality care, conserve manpower resources, and provide a safe working environment.

Standard II: The hospital shall be equipped, operated, and maintained so as to sustain its safe and sanitary characteristics and to minimize all health hazards in the hospital for the protection of both patients and employees.[39]

The interpretations given for this standard involve a safe, controlled, and adequate ventilation system. The safety council provides a written preventive maintenance program in accordance with current NFPA standards. Critical areas such as the surgical suite, the recovery room, the nurseries, the respiratory and burn units, and the isolation rooms require a controlled and regularly inspected filtered air supply that is supervised by the building department.

The preventive maintenance program establishes regulations concerning the facilities required to render quality care to patients in isolation areas and to assist in the control of the disease.[22] The maintenance program focuses on reducing potential injuries resulting from faulty or incorrect use of electrical equipment, instruments, and other appliances. For example, new electrical equipment should be tested by an authorized electrician and tagged with the date the equipment was tested and any special precautions to be followed, such as proper grounding and safety device requirements, to protect patients and personnel.[66]

To create an optimal safe environment for the delivery of patient care, G. Michaelsen[47] uses a rating form based on a systems approach as an administrative tool for environmental controls. The total facility is divided into geographical or functional areas. Each is assigned a weight factor (0 to 4) depending on the degree of hazard associated with the environment. For example, the ventilation of the isolation unit is given a higher factor (4) than the rehabilitation unit (0). Accident prevention is assigned a higher factor in the laboratory than the pharmacy. On inspection, the appraiser determines if the hazard is related to a deficiency in structure, equipment operation, or both. The head of the department is responsible for reducing or eliminating the hazard. Data gathered by the appraiser is used by the safety maintenance committee.

Every 3 months a written analysis of job injuries should be given to the hospital staff. The report should indicate the number and types of all injuries regardless of the degree of disability. Such information can generate action to eliminate the most frequent types of injuries.[34]

Some hospitals use a safety action sheet.[24] The supervisor at the place of the employee's accident or illness fills in the sheet and sends it to the health service department. Workmen's compensation insurance and the Oc-

cupation Safety and Health Act require that all facts be documented at the time and place of the incident. These sheets are used to determine factual data for the safety committee and to initiate the necessary policies, procedures, or in-service training to reduce the incidents. These sheets are kept on file for 5 years. Frequently occurring accidents can be prevented. The aim of the OSH Act[23] is to reduce employee accident rate by 45% in 3 to 5 years.

In many hospitals, back disability is the major reason for compensation payments. Hospitals that include the basic principles for lifting and handling patients or equipment in its in-service training programs have reduced such injuries.[38]

Standard III: Responsibility for the control of infection within the hospital, and for the evaluation of the infection potential of the related environment, shall be vested in a multidisciplinary committee of the medical staff.[22,26]

Every hospital is required to report and evaluate hospital infections in order to identify and control potential epidemic situations,[32,33] but simply recording and evaluating data on many laboratory cultures does not constitute an effective infection control program.

Many suggestions for an infection control program are published in current hospital medical and nursing literature.[33,41] In acute-care hospitals, many administrators appoint a physician in the field of microbiology who knows current infection practices as the infection control officer. In hospitals of 200 beds or more the officer is assisted by a qualified bacteriology technologist and a nurse-epidemiologist. An effective surveillance and prevention program must include investigation and follow-up.

A team approach and qualified personnel are essential for an effective infection control program. The patient is the focal point of infection control.

Standard IV: The hospital shall have written plans for the proper and timely care of casualties arising from both external and internal disasters, and shall periodically rehearse these plans.[23,69]

In our technological society the hospital

must be prepared to care for casualties resulting from motor or airplane crashes, floods, fire, explosions, or bombs.[2]

The disaster plan should be developed in conjunction with the police department and other emergency facilities in the community so that adequate logistical provisions are made for the expansion of the hospital's activities in coordination with the activities of these facilities.[3,39] The planning and development of a written plan involves hospital administration, public relations, and local civil authority representatives of other medical agencies. The disaster-site triad distribution of patients and the extent of each hospital's resources should be identified for use by local police, rescue squads, and ambulance teams. The medical and nursing service department heads have an important role in planning such a program.

The safety committee or council of the hospital is responsible for planning and initiating an internal disaster plan. Internal disaster and fire plans include evacuation procedures, the assignment of personnel to specific tasks, and instructions in the use of alarm systems, signals, and other provisions. These plans should be made available to hospital personnel and posted in appropriate places throughout the hospital. Evacuation drills should be held periodically, although patients need not be moved to safe areas during the drill. The chairman of the safety committee should submit an administrative written report and evaluation of all drills. The internal disaster program should be a part of the in-service orientation program for new personnel.

Multidisciplinary approach to implement safety standards

The hospital administrator delegates responsibilities and authority to qualified staff members for the effective functioning of a safety surveillance program, infection control, and a disaster program.[3,27]

The structure of the total safety program depends on the size and the operations of the hospital. Regardless of the committee structure, department heads, supervisors, and all professional health providers are delegated within their functions to endeavor to protect patients and personnel from unnecessary risks that may result in accidental injuries, from acquiring infection, or from fire-related injuries.

A safety committee or council should include qualified, informed representatives from patient services, medical and nursing staffs, electrical engineering, building and grounds, material-management, personnel, hospital in-service training, and medical and nursing school and student dormitories if they are associated directly with the hospital. Ths task force should make full use of consultants and specialists on a local and state level.

Nonprofit organizations such as the National Safety Council, the National Fire Protection Association, the American Hospital Association, the United States Public Health Service, and the Industrial Hygiene Services offer services and publications containing technical assistance and research programs designed to protect individuals and reduce accidents. The functions of the safety committee should relate to the JCAH standards and the regulations established by the Occupational Safety and Health Act.[61]

The primary purpose of the safety committee is to discover and remedy unsafe environmental conditions and practices, to observe and correct unsafe acts and performances, and to document results of the total program and communicate information to the hospital personnel.

The committee should formulate a statement of policy and procedures on safety and fire prevention, a methodology for reporting accidents of patients, visitors, or employees, for reporting illness of employees, for investigating incidents, for communicating information to hospital personnel, and for initiating and evaluating in-service training safety programs.

The federal Occupational Safety and Health Act

Before 1969, legislation containing universal safety standards had been proposed but ignored. In 1969, different bills were proposed by Congressman James O'Hara, Senator Harrison Williams, and by William Ayers and Senator Jacob Javits. These bills are similar in nature and are based on the concept of compulsory federal standards.[19] Much debate focused on the duty of employers to ensure job safety and on the rights of both employers and employees. As a result of the disagreements, a compromise bill entitled the Occupational Safety and Health Act, (Public Law 91-596) was passed in 1970.[23,61] This law covers almost all workers in the United States except persons with jobs covered by other federal safety legislation and persons employed by federal, state, and local government. The Department of Labor was authorized to issue rules based on existing federal standards and consensus standards.

The act states that "it is the general duty of each employer to furnish each of his employees employment and places of employment that are free from recognized hazards causing or likely to cause death or serious physical harm to his employees."[1,61]

Enforcement. The enforcement of the standards under the act is the responsibility of the Department of Labor. This department is required to conduct repeated inspections without advance notice. Both employer and employee representatives may accompany the inspector.[19,61]

Any employee or employee's representative may request a special inspection if he believes a particular condition threatens physical health. The Department of Labor will conduct a special inspection as requested if it finds reason for doing so. The employee's name is kept confidential.

If a violation is discovered during any inspection, a written citation describing the violation and the expected correction date is posted at or near the violation site. Monetary penalities are authorized for each serious or continuing violation.

To appeal a citation or penalty, an employer is required to notify the Department of Labor, who then notifies the Occupational Safety and Health Review Commission. The commission's only function as an independent government agency is the review of appeals from the Labor Department's ci-

tations and penalties. This commission has no regulatory powers. The decisions of the commission can be appealed to the United States Court of Appeals.[3,61]

Records and statistics. The act mandates comprehensive record-keeping requirements. The three major parts of the record system are (1) a log (OSHA form No. 100) of recordable occupational injuries and illnesses, or any private equivalent; (2) a supplementary record (OSHA for No. 101) of recordable occupational injuries and illnesses or an alternative, such as a workmen's compensation report containing all the information required in the supplementary record; and (3) an annual summary (OSHA form No. 102) of occupational injuries and illnesses, based on the information recorded in the log.[3]

Explicit rules for filing logs and reports are defined in the *AHA Safety Guide for Health Care Institutions*, Chapter 11.[3]

The Department of Labor initiated a new injury and illness statistics program to be used in evaluating the effectiveness of federal safety standards.

Research and training. The act charges the Department of Labor and the Department of Health, Education, and Welfare with conducting educational programs in occupational safety and health to ensure a sufficient number of qualified professional specialists and enforcement personnel. These departments are directed to conduct research in any aspect of occupational safety and health that leads to the provision of criteria for new and improved standards, in studies of psychological aspects of occupational safety and health, and in the epidemiology of latent diseases associated with occupational stress.

State role under the 1970 act. The 1970 act encourages states to assume responsibility for administration and the enforcement of the law by means of grants for planning, research, and operating. Several criteria must be met by states for approval to administer and enforce the law.

Conclusions on the federal role. Some administrators and others have voiced both positive and skeptical opinions of the act's potential. Some of the standards have been challenged as unrealistic or inappropriate. Regardless of the outcome, the act presents a significant change in government's role toward industrial safety.[1,23]

REFERENCES

1. Althouse, H.: How OSHA affects hospitals and nursing homes, American Journal of Nursing **75:**450-451, March, 1975.
2. American Hospital Association: Principles of disaster planning for hospitals, Chicago, 1967, The Association.
3. American Hospital Association and the National Safety Council: Safety guide for health care institutions, Chicago, 1972, The Association.
4. American Hospital Association: Nursing services, principles and standards for hospital accreditation, practical approaches to effective functioning of the department of nursing service, Chicago, 1972, The Association.
5. American Hospital Association: Statement on functions in health care institutions that require the competence of a registered nurse, pub. no. 55, Chicago, 1969, The Association.
6. American Hospital Association: Statement on functions of a hospital nursing service department, pub. no. 516, Chicago, 1971, The Association.
7. American Hospital Association: Statement on a hospital employer's minimum expectations of a registered nurse, pub. no. S-34, Chicago, 1972, The Association.
8. American Hospital Association: Statement on the position of the administrator of the department of nursing service in hospitals, Chicago, 1971, The Association.
9. American Hospital Association: The changing hospital and the American Hospital Association: statement on optimum health services, pub. no. 5-17, Chicago, 1965, The Association.
10. American Nurses' Association: ANA standards of nursing practice—standards of community health nursing practice; standards of gerontological nursing practice; standards of maternal-child health nursing practice; standards of psychiatric-mental health nursing practice; standards of medical-surgical nursing practices, 1974; standards of cardiovascular nursing practice; standards of emergency nursing practice; standards of nursing practice: operating room; standards of orthopedic nursing practice, 1975; standards of urological nursing practice; standards of neurological and neurosurgical nursing practice, 1976, Kansas City, Mo., The Association.
11. American Nurses' Association: A position paper, Kansas, 1965, The Association.
12. American Nurses' Association: Standards of nursing practice, Kansas, 1973, The Association.
13. American Nurses' Association: Statement on nursing staff requirements in patient health care services, New York, 1967, The Association.
14. American Nurses' Association: Standards for organized nursing services in hospitals, public health agencies, nursing care homes, industries, and clinics, Kansas City, Mo., 1973, The Association.
15. American Nurses' Association: The position, role, and qualifications of the administrator of nursing service, New York, 1969, The Association.
16. Aydelotte, M. K.: Staffing for high quality care. Hospitals **47**(2):58, 60, 65, 1973.
17. Aydelotte, M. K.: Standard 1—staffing for quality care, Journal of Nursing Administration **3:**33-36, March-April, 1973.
18. Aydelotte, M. K.: Survey of hospital nursing services, New York, 1968, National League for Nursing.
19. Barth, P. S., and Williams, C. A.: Compendium on workmen's compensation, Washington, D.C., 1973, National Commission of State Workmen's Compensation.
20. Behrens, A. D.: The pleasures and problems of the director of nursing in a small hospital, Journal of Nursing Administration Vol. **5**(2):31-34, 1975.
21. Blanchard, R. H.: Liability and compensation insurance, New York, 1917, D. Appleton & Co.
22. Brachman, P. S.: Isolation techniques for use in hospitals, DHEW pub. no. (HSM) 71-8043, Washington, D.C., 1970, United States Government Printing Office.
23. Breiding, R., and Pellegrini, F.: How to comply with OSHA, Hospital Progress **54:**69, June, 1973.
24. Bringman, M.: Safety action sheet keys program, Hospitals **48:**85-88, Jan., 1974.
25. Cantor, M.: Standard 5 — education for quality care, Journal of Nursing Administration **3:**49-54, March-April, 1973.
26. Chavigny, K. H.: Nurse epidemiologist in the hospital, Hospitals **75:**638-641, April, 1975.
27. Console, C. P.: Safety council innovates, Hospitals **48:**88-90, Jan., 1974.
28. Department of Diploma Programs: The changing role of the hospital and implications for nursing education, pub. no. 16-1551, New York, 1974, National League for Nursing. (Papers presented at the Annual Meeting of the Council of Diploma Programs, held at Kansas City, Mo., May 1-3, 1974.)
29. Department of Hospital and Related Insititutional Nursing Services: Four approaches to staff development, pub. no. 20-1578, New York, 1975, National League for Nursing.
30. Division of Community Planning: Quality assessment and patient care, pub. no. 52-1572, New York, 1975, National League for Nursing. (Presentations at the Fall, 1974, forum for nursing service administrators in the West held at San Francisco, California.)
31. Division of Community Planning: The future is now, pub. no. 52-1553, New York, 1974, National League for Nursing. (Presentations at the Conference of the Northeast Regional Assembly of Constituents Leagues for Nursing.)

32. Durbin, R. L., and Springall, W. H.: Organization and administration of health care: theory, practice, environment, ed. 2, St. Louis, 1974, The C. V. Mosby Co.

33. Ellis, B.: Infection control, Hospitals **49:**151-152, April, 1975.

34. Ellis, B.: Frequently occurring accidents can be prevented, Hospitals **50:**86, May, 1976.

35. Etzioni, A.: Modern organization, Englewood Cliffs, N.J., 1964, Prentice-Hall, Inc.

36. Gardner, J. W.: Excellence, New York, 1961, Harper & Brothers.

37. Hamil, E.: Vice-president in charge of nursing. In Roles in today's health team, New York, 1969, National League of Nursing.

38. Hoover, S. A.: Job-related back injuries in a hospital, American Journal of Nursing **73:**2078-2079, Dec., 1973.

39. Joint Commission on Accreditation of Hospitals: Accreditation manual for hospitals, Chicago, 1976, The Commission.

40. Kramer, M.: Nursing care plans . . . power to the patient, Journal of Nursing Administration **2:**29-34, Sept.-Oct., 1972.

41. Langewisch, C. D.: How to establish an infection control program, Hospital Topics pp. 52-53, March, 1974.

42. Levine, E.: Nurse manpower—yesterday, today and tomorrow, American Journal of Nursing **69**(2):290-296, 1969.

43. Levine, H. D., and Phillips, P. J.: Factors affecting staffing levels and patterns of nursing personnel, DHEW pub. no. (HRA) 75-6, United States Department of Health, Education, and Welfare, Bureau of Health Resources Development, Superintendant of Documents, Washington, D.C., 1975, United States Government Printing Office.

44. Little, D., and Carnevali, D.: Nursing care planning system, Nursing Outlook **19:**164-167, March, 1971.

45. Lysaught, J.: Motivation in nursing. In Nursing digest focus on the work environment, Wakefield, Mass., 1975, Contemporary Publishing, pp. 4-13.

46. McGibony, J. R.: Principles of hospital administrations, ed. 2, New York, 1969, G. P. Putnam's Sons.

47. Michaelsen, G. S.: Evaluating the hospital environment, Hospitals **49:**69-72, May, 1975.

48. Miller, A.: Up-up the organization, Fortune **71:**306, May, 1970.

49. Miller, D.: American Nurses' Association nursing service standards viewed as norms, International Journal of Nursing Studies **5:**69-75, 1968.

50. Miller, D. I.: Standard 2—organization is a process, Journal of Nursing Administration **2:**19-24, March-April, 1972.

51. Moore, M. A.: Philosophy, purpose and objectives, why do we need them? Journal of Nursing Administration **1:**9-14, March, 1971.

52. Moore, M. A.: The Joint Commission on Accreditation of Hospital Standards for Nursing Services, Journal of Nursing Administration **2:**12-17, March-April, 1972.

53. National Commission for the Study of Nursing and Nursing Education: an abstract for action, New York, 1970, McGraw-Hill Book Co.

54. National Fire Protection Association: Life-safety code, Boston, 1972, The Association.

55. National League for Nursing: Criteria for evaluating a hospital department of nursing service, New York, 1965, The League.

56. National League for Nursing, Department of Hospital Nursing, in pursuit of quality—hospital nursing services, New York, 1964, The League.

57. News: Controversy flares over baccalaureate as licensure base, American Journal of Nursing **76:**14, Jan., 1976.

58. Peterson, G. G.: Do nursing administrators need advanced clinical preparation? American Journal of Nursing **70:**297-303, 1970.

59. Peterson, G. G.: The director of nursing should be a nurse, American Journal of Nursing **73:**1902-1904. Nov. 1973.

60. Pierik, M.: Joint appointments: collaboration for better patient care, Nursing Outlook **21:**576-579, Sept., 1973.

61. Public Law 91-596, 91st Congress, S. 2193, 1970.

62. Ramey, I. G.: Setting nursing standards and evaluating care, Journal of Nursing Administration, **3:**27-35, May-June, 1973.

63. Report: Proposal of the New York State Nurses' Association to implement the resolution on entry into professional practice, newsletter of N.Y. State Nurses Association No. 9-10, 7(2), 1976, 7(2) 1976. 6(4,5,9,10,12), 1975; 7(2,3), 1976.

64. Rotkovich, R.: The role of the director of nursing in creating an environment for the practice of nursing, Journal of the New York State Nurses' Association, 4(1):20-25, 1973.

65. Ryan, B. J.: Nursing care plans, a systems approach to developing criteria for planning and evaluation. In Planning and evaluating nursing care, Wakefield, Mass., 1974, Contemporary Publishing, Inc., pp. 40-48.

66. Shapiro, A. G., and Kernaghen, S. G.: JCAH standards learn to use tool—new mandates for respiratory care, Hospitals **48:**100-106, May, 1974.

67. Secretary's Committee to Study Extended Roles for Nurses: Extending the scope of nursing practice, Nursing Outlook **20:**46-52, Jan., 1972.

68. Sheahan, D.: Short shrift for hospital nursing . . . the directors' defection, American Journal of Nursing **73:**485-490, March 1973.

69. United States Atomic Energy Commission: Emergency handling of radiation accident cases, Washington, D.C., 1969, United States Government Printing Office.

70. United States Public Health Services: Hospital planning for national disaster, Washington, D.C., 1968, United States Government Printing Office.

71. Young, L.: Room at the top: a place for nurse administrators, Journal of Nursing Administration **2:**81-86, Nov-Dec., 1972.

6 | Management perspectives and principles

Today's hospital can be thought of as a complex of relationships between people, material resources, and work, kept together in an appropriate structure aimed at meeting the health needs of our society. Achievement of hospital goals and objectives depends a great deal on the consumers who use the services offered, the professionals who direct the services, and the individuals who supply the services. Today's hospital must function in a society faced with technological, social, economic, political, and legal forces. The ability of the hospital to cope with these forces will determine how effective its management will be. Hospitals, like other industries, will be pressured to examine their environment and their structure to apply appropriate management concepts and techniques.

IMPACT OF CHANGE IN HOSPITAL MANAGEMENT

The modern organization is the most effective means yet planned to pool members' mental and physical efforts and channel them into productive means of need satisfaction. Management can be a positive or negative force in an organization's progress. Hospitals have many professionals and managers who are delegatd the responsibility and authority to determine and plan the necessary work, staff the operations, organize the jobs and tasks, direct the work, and control and assess the results against the objectives. Management authorities and practitioners now are agreeing that the organization and management appropriate for operating a product, a business service, or a university are not necessarily appropriate for operating a health institution. However, tremendous changes in our society have affected all organizations, including hospitals.

In the past 20 years structural, institutional technological, and social changes have influenced the kinds of patient services and their management.[9] As a result of biomedical breakthroughs, technological innovations, and government funding, the hospital has become a structured complex providing many specialized medical treatments and care in the cure, and to some extent the prevention, of a wide variety of illnesses. One can see the tremendous technological improvements in our health care institutions—specialty care units, surgeries, diagnostic and emergency facilities, an array of mechanical engineering innovations, and information and computer systems. They exemplify a wealth of human and material resources (see Chapter 3).

In our postindustrial society, many management researchers and members of hospitals recognize that the environment of our hospitals has not been integrated conceptually with management practices. In any hospital, members find the environment frustrating and discouraging. They sense changing attitudes, conflicts, and the impersonality of the system. On the other hand, these same individuals desire a more realistic sense of professional achievement and personal satisfaction in helping patients.

As hospitals become larger and more complex, their goals tend to become less clear, and their relationships more formal. Specialization increases the pressures to protect one's status. Note that amid highly technological changes, institutions and indivduals tend strongly toward the status quo. In the years ahead the nursing profession will have more trained educated nurses wanting a stake in goal setting and in planning the management of nursing care services in the hospital and community agencies. The change in the concepts and goals of the "new" nurse will pressure hospital nursing services to develop a more flexible structure and a more appropriate environment and to use the knowledge and skills of professional nurses more effectively to assure quality nursing at a reasonable price. Through the management processes an environment should be created to permit individuals to achieve optimal goals and reap the benefits of technology while on the job.

Drucker[18] points out that the professional manager has not one job, but three. He believes that the major functions focus on using human and material resources economically and providing optimal productivity, getting people to work together to accomplish the desired objectives, and arranging tasks so that individual skills and knowledge are blended together. He stresses that the organizational structure is the mechanism through which human efforts, attitudes, and ideas are maximized for effective productivity. The actions of the administrator or supervisor are always visible to others. They are always on the stage with the spotlight on them.

EMERGING MANAGEMENT AND PERSONAL GOALS

If one accepts the premise that nursing should provide contributory knowledge and skills based on the physical, biological, and psychosocial problems of patient care, it follows that the operational management of nursing services would be science based. Second, if one believes that environmental elements influence performance, it would indicate that the nursing service system, as one of the hospital systems, should be based on new assumptions that correspond to management realities of our time. Some leaders in the field of scientific management predict that the future manager will be involved as much with the values and attitudes of individuals as with the accomplishment of measurable results. If this prediction comes

true, the managers in the patient care system will be concerned with helping patients and workers achieve optimum well-being within their capabilities as much as with making sure that the "sick" services are rendered in an economical, efficient manner and personnel policies are fair and adequate.[17]

Throughout the centuries nursing has endeavored to adjust its role to other health professional and technical roles in the life process of the hospital. Technological advances and socioeconomic and political events of the twentieth century provide opportunities for nursing to become a more dynamic, effective, efficient occupation. To put to use nursing expertise in a modern scientific operational management system, professional nurses will have to gain an understanding of new management theories as they affect objectives, organizational structure and functions, authority relationships, and processes of technical and social change.

It seems evident that in the future organizational behavior and management practices will be important forces affecting the environment of the hospital. The people who have a management role as part of their job will be very much concerned with interrelationships between personnel who have different attitudes, skills, and jobs. Nurses will be concerned with the *blending of management objectives with clinical objectives in the nursing care of patients.* Nursing as part of the hospital organization will be more involved in the science of nursing as well as the "social responsibilities" (human activities) of patient care management.

Perhaps one of the main reasons for nursing service's resistance to "the management," both as a term and as a concept, has been the emphasis on the managerial internal daily tasks as opposed to the innovating functions of nursing care that become stultified by rules, regulations, and rigid work environments.

Recognition of personal goals

Faced with demands for more technically trained nurses, clinical nurse-specialists, and administrators with expertise, nursing service administrators will face a more permanent need to foster personal productivity among those whose work they direct. To a greater degree than ever before, professionals and technical workers will be required to accept change *in order to gain personal achievement* in their own performances within the established system.

CHANGING THE MANAGEMENT APPROACH IN NURSING SERVICES

New management approaches will mean adjustment to new behavioral patterns so that clinical experts, scientific engineers and researchers, and highly trained technical workers can work together effectively in a satisfying environment for objective accomplishment. This will also mean adjustment to new personnel concepts, including a new incentive reward system for nurses' outstanding achievements on the job.

Scientific management techniques and tools are evolving rapidly, borrowing from the systems approach long associated with the physical, social, and behavioral sciences. As we master new management techniques and skills we should improve our art in managing nursing care services. One assumes that as we initiate a more scientific management approach in our jobs, we will create an environment in which people can perform with greater effectiveness and efficiency. We will know how to use the informational system, the computer, and engineering resources for accurate assessment data and for communication purposes.

Nursing service today is becoming increasingly aware of the fact that in our traditional management environment scientific nursing knowledge and skills are not utilized to their highest potential unless there is a blending of organized human energy, defined objectives, and a system through which people can work toward both personal and hospital goals.

It is obvious that managing is essential in all organized participation at all levels of the organization. Every nurse knows that the quality of nursing is influenced by the degree of group effort expended and that the total organized output depends on the contribution of each person in the group. Each nurse

has a management role incorporated in the job, regardless of her position in the hierarchy. *The art of managing cannot be a separate task apart from the art of nursing.* Note that the practice of managing does not mean performing clerical duties. The art of managing things and people is an integrated process through which organizational goals are set and achieved by means of people who work together within the system.

As part of its new role in the total hospital system, nursing service management will become more aware of its responsibility to generate and direct human energies in a more objective manner.

We realize that hospital objectives and management are different from those of a business, even though the tools and techniques are similar. Nursing can no longer accept remaining outside of "management" or even on the peripheral limits of the scientific management approach.

Gardner[28] states: "Professions are subject to the same deadening forces that affect all other human institutions, an attachment to time-honored ways, reverence for established procedures, a preoccupation with one's own vested interests, and an excessively narrow definition of what is relevant and important."

Traditional rigidity and a lack of knowledge, skills, and mutual agreement regarding objectives, as well as the use of crisis-changed models, prevent change or the ability to manage change.

In this postindustrial age, professionals and other members of the hospital staff have a more difficult time in decision-making activities than those in previous generations due to conflicting groups' goals and expectations.[62] Opposition today is frequently viewed as a way of life involving intraorganizational and interorganizational conflicts, and there are few decisions made in departments or at the executive level that receive unanimous support. Regardless of how clearly facts indicate that a particular plan or strategy should be initiated, there are persons who will oppose it.

To feel comfortable and to be an effective and participatory clinical coordinator, clinical specialist, or administrator, an individual should understand the philosophies and values of conflict.[62] Managing organizational conflict will be discussed later in this text (see Chapters 10 and 11).

INTERPRETATIONS OF THE MANAGEMENT PROCESS

Basically, the practice of managing means getting things done by working with people and using physical resources to accomplish the defined objectives of the group in keeping with those of the department and the hospital. To do this the person who is managing—the director, supervisor, or nurse-clinician—coordinates and integrates the activities and work of others rather than performing all tasks alone.[43]

Terminology

The term *management* is applied in different ways. Because management is a complex process, it is often defined in operational terms for those at the lower level of the management hierarchy. Management is process of designing and maintaining the internal environment for organized effort to accomplish group objectives and those of the total hospital system.

A distinction usually is made between the terms *management* and *administration*. Although both have approximately the same meaning, in hospitals administration usually refers to activities of management carried out by those at the higher levels of the hierarchy. Management refers to activities carried out by those at the middle and lower levels of management (Fig. 6-1). Some scholars and leaders in management use the terms administrator, manager, and executive interchangeably and prefer not to distinguish between management and administration. Others make a distinction between administration and management when it is suitable to the situation at hand; however, the actual distinctions are made by people as they accept the positions in the institution. McFarland[51] points out that the term *management* may refer collectively to those persons who manage or to the management process itself.

To some authorities the term *administration* refers to activities associated with guiding, directing, and controlling the actions of other individuals or groups who have delegated responsibilities contributing to achievement of specifically defined goals (Fig. 6-2).

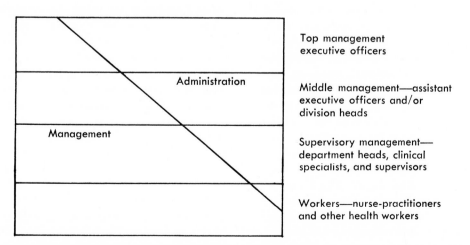

Fig. 6-1. Diagram showing the relationship between management and administrative functions in the organization hierarchy and the distinction that is sometimes made between the two. The functions of the executive officers, the top-level planners, and the lower-level planners must blend together to formulate realistic objectives of programs and policies, implement them, and evaluate the results concerning effective relationships and efficient use of human and material resources.

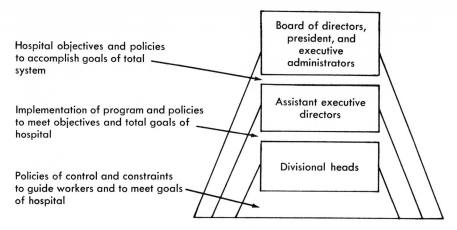

Hospital objectives and policies
to accomplish goals of total
system

Board of directors,
president, and
executive
administrators

Implementation of program and policies
to meet objectives and total goals of
hospital

Assistant executive
directors

Policies of control and constraints
to guide workers and to meet goals
of hospital

Divisional heads

Fig. 6-2. Traditional hospital organizational structure, showing delegation of management functions to those who hold top-level positions in the hierarchy.

Tead[68] clarifies the distinction between administration and management as follows:

Administration is the process and agency which is responsible for the determination of the aims for which an organization and its management are to strive, which establishes the broad policies under which they are to operate, and which gives general oversight to the continuing effectiveness of the total operation in reaching the objectives sought.

Management is the process and agency which directs and guides the operations of an organization in the realizing of established aims.

In the total hospital system the nursing service department is delegated administrative and operational management functions. The nursing service managerial system is influenced by the objectives, policies made by the controlling executive body, span of authority, and organizational structure of the hospital.

Management is a process of organizing and using human and material resources to achieve predetermined objectives. Mary P. Follett,[24] a social worker in the 1920s when highly autocratic practices were the vogue, believed that the manager could get more work done by exercising power *with* people, rather than power *over* people. Follett believed that the human element and the environment of the work situation should be considered for effective achievement of an institution's goals.

THE EVOLUTION OF MANAGEMENT

The various schools of management theories and practices should be considered within the framework of the environments in which they developed. A glimpse at man's past endeavors shows us that management contributed much to successful accomplishments.

It is difficult to classify the different schools of management because they overlap in many instances. Many new concepts are additions to former theories. The evolving field of management may be divided into (1) management concepts in ancient and preindustrial times, (2) the scientific management theory (classical doctrine), (3) the bureaucratic-organizational concept, (4) the human relations theory, (5) the modern management approach emphasizing interdisciplinary, quantitiative and behavioral concepts, (6) the general systems theory, and (7) the contingency management approach.[15,30,48]

Management concepts in ancient and preindustrial age

Management theories and practices date back to antiquity. For example, the building of the pyramids of Egypt with few tools and the labor of 100,000 workers for a 20-year period signifies a tremendous effort on the part of managers and their application of management concepts and techniques of their time.

Like the Egyptians, the emperors in early Chinese history used advisers or staff concepts in planning and operating the government. The Chinese acknowledged the need for an overall system that would blend the required material and human resources in a harmonious fashion to achieve the greatest result for the whole.

Both Plato and Socrates recognized the importance of division of labor.[45] Socrates wrote that there are differences between the functions of a specialized professional and those of so-called management, but that both are needed to attain effective results.

Moses and the Hebrews used the Ten Commandments as guidelines for individual and organizational conduct. It is reported in the book of *Exodus*[21] that Jethro, Moses' father-in-law, counseled Moses on how to reduce his span of control and delegate functions to his subordinates:

. . . Moses sat to judge the people and the people stood about Moses from morning till evening. When Moses' father-in-law saw all that he was doing for the people he said . . . "What you are doing is not good. You and the people with you will wear yourselves out; for the thing is too heavy for you, you are not able to perform it alone". . . . Moses gave heed to the voice of his father-in-law and did all that he said. He chose able men out of all Israel and made them heads over the people, rulers of thousands, of hundreds, of fifties, and of tens. And they judged the people at all times; hard cases they brought to Moses, but any small matter they decided themselves.

This is a good example of delegation of authority, span of control, and a sharing of functions to accomplish objectives.

This first recorded statement on how to design an organization clearly demonstrates how and why middle management positions originate.

The ancient city of Rome expanded to an Empire through the use of the scalar principle of management. The formation of large-scale armies and the bulding of a city did create problems of communication, logistics, organizational structure, and the selection and training of people. History shows us that the path of institutional progress has not been straight but very winding and that

mankind has made many strange compromises, sometimes with deplorable results.

The development of the scalar principle and general staff concepts initiated in military organizations are reflected in many patterns of the traditional management process in our society. Looking back over the long organizational life of the Roman Catholic church, one sees the development of a centralized authority with the specialization of activities along functional lines and the use of staff and line relationships, defined objectives, and establishment of a doctrine and conditions (policies and rules) for membership in the organization.

Feudalism and preindustrial commerce. Feudalism consisted of a tremendous organizational hierarchy headed by a king or emperor, assisted by nobles, lords, subvassals, and laborers.

In the preindustrial age, primarily in England, the guild system regulated economic and employment conditions in the production of the trades. Through the guild system the design, quality, and price of products were determined. This system was the beginning of production controls and the establishment of work loads and wages for the workers. The concepts of the guilds' apprenticeship system were adopted in hospital nursing training schools and, to a great degree, in medicine for beginning physicians.

The Crusades changed the nonmaterialistic life of the Middle Ages with the opening of new trade routes that stimulated interest in commerce. The development of management concepts was influenced by the market ethic, the Protestant ethic, and the liberty (free) ethic.[73,74]

The concept of the division of labor was defined clearly by Adam Smith[64] in the 1700s, with his famous pin example. Smith argued that dexterity and productivity are improved when a worker's task is reduced to a single repetitive operation. This theory introduced the assembly-line production concept.

Early management concepts

The growth of the factory system brought together a relatively large concentration of people, machines, and raw materials in various geographical areas. Some leaders were aware of the need to consider man as well as the machines. In the early 1800's Robert Owen, one of the pioneer industrialists in Scotland, took a genuine interest in the welfare of his workers. In his book, *A New View of Society*, he urged the manufacturer to maximize profits by taking an interest in the workers (human machines). On the other hand, Owens considered the workers as children who must be continually trained and guided by rigid discipline; he still believed that the authority of management was supreme. Today Owens would be called a paternalistic employer. In many hospitals this attitude toward personnel still exists on the part of some supervisors and managers.

In the early 1900s British mathematician Charles Babbage emphasized the application of scientific principles and mathematics in the operation of industries in his book, *On Economy of Machines and Manufactures*. He recommended the formulation of exact measurements and having precise knowledge before reaching decisions. Babbage also desired to see mutuality of interest between employer and employee and opposed labor unions representing the workers. He believed that hard work and high productivity were a source of good wages for the worker and high profits for the employer. Babbage and others helped bring managerial principles into the industrial management process. These concepts had a tremendous influence on the operation of hospitals. In the organizational structure the greatest scope or extent of authority rested at the top, with little or no authority for the workers.

Scientific management theory

Frederick Taylor,[67] a mechanical engineer, is considered the driving force behind the scientific management movement. In 1911 he presented his ideas and concerns about certain conditions that he viewed as problems of industry. His basis for industrial management may be summarized under three major headings: (1) the need for clear concepts of managerial responsibility, (2) the need for measured standards for defining the

worker's task, and (3) the need to remedy the widespread inefficiency of workers in their jobs. It is interesting to note that Henry Gantt and Lillian Gilbreth urged institutions to create an environment with favorable psychological effects on workers.[31,32] In 1887 Gantt, working with executives in a steel company, introduced schedule charts for management planning and control. Today such tasks are part of sophisticated management methodology aided by computers in modern operational management approaches.

Frank Gilbreth also developed work-planning and training concepts for workers.[32] He believed that workers should be trained in the correct methods of work. Although the apprenticeship system of training people has existed for centuries in industry and hospitals, it provided formalized training only for special groups, such as nurses in hospitals. During World War II new principles and techniques in training programs in industry were initiated and have had a great impact on hospital training programs for semiskilled workers. Today hospital managers have learned that workers do not learn new jobs and new skills simply by watching others and by trial and error.

After World War II many studies based on work-simplification methodology, industrial engineering, and human relations concepts were conducted in hospitals to define nursing tasks and functions and interrelationships between nurses and other hospital groups (see Chapter 2). Taylor and later Fayol, Gilbreth,[31] Gilbreth,[32] and others began to experiment in management techniques. They endeavored to conceptualize new principles for a scientific management approach.

One of Taylor's main goals was to determine methods to achieve efficiency of personnel and machines through time and motion studies. He also envisioned new functions for managers focusing on (1) replacement of the rule-of-thumb methods with scientific determination of each element of the job, (2) scientific selection and training of workers for the job, (3) cooperation of management and labor to accomplish work in accordance with scientific methodology, and

(4) a more equal division of responsibility between managers and workers, with the managers delegated to plan and organize the work of others.

Taylor also called attention to the interrelationships that must be considered part of the scientific management approach. He emphasized the value of harmony not discord, cooperation not individualism, maximum output of work rather than restricted output, and the development of each individual to his greatest efficiency and prosperity.

Gantt, a collaborator of Taylor, was one of the early leaders who looked at the psychological factors affecting the worker and took into account the importance of morale and of utilizing nonfinancial rewards to promote efficiency and increase productivity.

Administrative concepts in scientific management theory. Henri Fayol,[22] a French industrialist and former mining engineer, developed a comprehensive theory of organization and management. His monograph "General and Industrial Administration" was published in 1911 and translated into English in 1949. He presents a practical approach to management functions, emphasizing the need to consider the basic physical, mental, moral, educational, and experiential requirements for the job manager.

Fayol, who may be considered the father of the traditional operational school of management, divided the activities of an industry into six major groups: (1) production, (2) commercial, (3) financial, (4) security, (5) accounting, and (6) management. Fayol believed that management courses should be offered in schools and also that management ability should be acquired as technical ability is—through education followed by on-the-job experience.

He listed 14 principles of management, noting that they must be flexible and practical under any conditions. The principles, even today, have general implications for the management process in a hospital department of nursing service.

Fayol[15,22] emphasized the importance of selecting the appropriate principle for a given situation. His principles may be summarized as follows:

1. *Division of work.* There should be specialization of labor such that different people perform different tasks.
2. *Authority and responsibility.* Responsibility should be commensurate with authority.
3. *Discipline.*
4. *Unity of command.* An employee should receive orders from one superior only.
5. *Unity of direction.* There should be only one person in charge of a group of activities having the same objectives.
6. *Subordination of individual interest* to general interest.
7. *Remuneration of personnel.* There should be a system of remuneration which is fair, which rewards well-directed effort, but does not produce unreasonable overpayments.
8. *Centralization.* In each situation an optimal balance exists between centralization and decentralization, and this balance is partly determined by the capabilities of the managers involved. This does not necessarily mean that authority for all decisions be centralized at the top of the organization.
9. *Scalar chain.* There should be a scalar chain of authority and communication ranging from the highest to the lowest position.
10. *Order.* The organization should provide both the material and social order with everything and everyone in the appointed place.
11. *Equity.* Equity in the sense of justice must extend throughout the organization.
12. *Stability of tenure of personnel.*
13. *Initiative.* There should be every opportunity to exercise initiative at all levels in the organization.
14. *Esprit de corps.* There is a need for teamwork and the maintenance of good interpersonal relationships.

Fayol also defined functional processes of management such as planning, organizing, directing, coordinating, and controlling. These functions have general application to administrative and managerial functions in modern organizations (see Chapters 9 and 10 on organizational designs).

Development of management principles based on Fayol's concepts. During the 1920s and 1930s, leaders in management and consultation presented their principles utilizing and broadening Fayol's concepts. Luther Gulick[34] and Lyndall Urwick,[35] British writers, in 1927 presented the *Papers on the Science of Administration.*[35] Gulick used the acronym POSDCORB to represent the functions of management—planning, organizing, staffing, directing, coordinating, reporting, and budgeting.

In the United States, James Mooney and Alan Reilly coauthored a book entitled *Onward Industrial,*[57] based on their experiences in and analyses of government agencies, military organizations, and the Catholic Church. They emphasized four principles: (1) coordination to secure unified action, (2) scalar process to emphasize hierarchial levels, (3) functionalization to establish tasks into departmental units, and (4) staff line to gain advice and information.

Mooney and Reilly[57] viewed the scalar process as the formal mechanism through which coordinating authority can operate by delegation, thus allowing one individual to confer his authority on an individual in a lower position and permitting assignment of functions to units of responsibility by functional definition.

Mooney and Reilly were among the first management writers to recognize man's management problems. Most administrative management theorists did not consider behavioral elements very important to administration. Mooney and Reilly emphasized the structural relations between production, supply, and other units of organization. However, in general, they viewed the organization as a closed system.

Bureaucratic-organizational concept

Max Weber wanted to construct an ideal, formal organization model that would provide maximum rationality in human behavior. He viewed his ideal type of bureaucracy as an efficient form of social organization that could be applied to scientific, religious, business, or government organizations. Weber believed that a bureaucratic form of organization provided greater technical efficiency than any other form.[74]

Weber believed that the ideal model of

bureaucracy, that provided a mechanistic, impersonal form of organization, was necessary to minimize the impact of man's diversities and to support a kind of power legitimized by society. In other words, he thought it would make a man do what he did not want to do. Weber assumed that man was unpredictable, often emotional, not necessarily rational, and would interfere with efficient organizational performance. In the 1940s many sociologists, stimulated by Weber's ideas, began to evaluate the theories of bureaucracy. Merton,[55] in studying the ideal bureaucracy, concluded that bureaucracies have a tendency to produce difficulties in maintaining discipline, and the leadership role tends to be frustrating and repressive. McFarland[51] defined bureaucracy as a "type of organization designed to accomplish large-scale administrative tasks by systematically coordinating the work of many individuals."

Dimock[16] and others[27,38] in their studies viewed the bureaucracy in its specific forms or organizational behavior such as hierarchy, subdivision, specialization, and professionalization, which are similar to those characteristics defined by Weber.

Frequently, people use the term bureaucracy in a denigrating sense to express personal anger and frustration when they encounter inefficiency, red tape, or interference in trying to get something done.

To many executives in our modern hospital industry the bureaucratic approach is a normal, logical developmental process for objective accomplishment of established goals (Fig. 6-3). It institutionalizes and formalizes both the inefficient and the efficient elements of management through control and decision making.

Scalar process in division of work. The scalar process is a division of work into levels providing a scale or grading of managerial functions according to span of authority and responsibilities. Functional definition, plus the scalar principle, is basic to the authority-level principle that is universally applied in all institutions. Fayol[22] and Weber[74] thought of the scalar chain as a "chain of superiors" from the highest to the lowest echelon that,

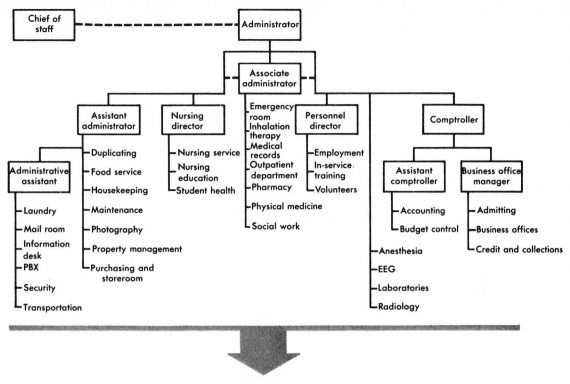

Fig. 6-3. The traditional hospital organization structure of departments and their units reflects the military plan. The management is viewed as one of production of services and a system of authority. (From Taylor, F. W.: Scientific management, New York, 1947, Harper & Brothers.)

although not to be departed from without reason, should be short-circuited when scrupulous following of it would be detrimental to effective management. He also believed that there is a place for everyone and everyone should be kept in his place. This supports a principle of organization in the arrangement of people and things as described by Weber.

The scalar principle refers to a chain of direct authority relationships from superior to subordinate throughout the organization. Fayol described the scale as follows:

. . . the chain of superiors ranging from the ultimate authority to the lowest rank. The line of authority is the route followed—via every link in the chain—by all communications which start from or go to the ultimate authority. This path is dictated both by the need for some transmission and by the principle of unity of command, but it is not always the swiftest. It is even at times disastrously lengthy in large concerns, notably in governmental ones.[22]

According to Weber, a bureaucratic organization would have (1) a well-defined hierarchy of authority, (2) a division of work based on functional specialization, (3) a system of policies and regulations pertaining to the rights and duties of personnel in different positions, (4) a system of procedures that workers must follow in performing their tasks, (5) impersonality of interpersonal relationships, and (6) selection for employment and promotion based on the individual's competence.

Human relations theory

Between the late 1900s and the 1930s events occurred that began to change man's view of himself, his organization, and his environment. Technological factors were primarily the result of the rapid industrialization of the period. Mechanization replaced manpower, and division of work and specialization were emphasized. The population in the United States doubled between 1890 and 1930, with the greatest increase in the cities.

Hawthorne research studies in the human relations movement. In the 1920s and early 1930s the Hawthorne Works of the Western Electric Company in Chicago consisted of a series of experiments and studies conducted by Western Electric investigators and a team from the Harvard Graduate School of Business Administration, led by the behavioral scientist Elton Mayo.[15] These studies endeavored to determine what relationship, if any, existed between environmental factors, such as light intensity, length of workday and workweek, and the introduction of rest periods, and productivity. The analysis of data disclosed that management attitudes toward people often exerted a greater influence on the efficiency of workers and productivity than did physical conditions of work. Prior to this study many management theorists had assumed that the worker was an "inert instrument and the human being a 'simple' machine." As a result of the Hawthorne research the human relations concept began to be recognized in the management approach.

Behavioral organizational theories

Barnard,[8] Gulick,[34] Urwick,[35] and others, members of various scientific management schools, contributed much to the human relations and behavioral models of organizational theory.[46,52]

As a result of the Hawthorne experiments, the depression and high unemployment rate between 1929 and 1933, and decreased incomes, the concepts of individualism and self-help seemed to disappear. The basic premise of the Protestant ethic was challenged.

The behavioral theorists were critical of the concepts of human relations theory that supported the assumption that if management could make employees happy, maximum performance would result. The behavioral theorists believed that providing the workers with money, security, and good working conditions did not begin to solve the human relations problems of organizations. The behavioral authorities moved away from simplistic assumptions toward a broader scientifically based approach, termed *organizational behavior.*

Barnard's contributions. Chester Barnard, a business executive assistant, may be considered the first behaviorally oriented theorist. In the 1930s he supported the theory that an organization is a system and that authority begins at the bottom and moves up (Fig. 6-3). He stressed a cooperative group system and believed that efficiency depends on organizational equilibrium, and effectiveness on the incentives offered by the organization and the contributions offered by the employees.

Barnard recognized that not every order could be analyzed, judged, and either accepted or rejected. Through his analytical approach, Barnard stated that most orders fall in the employees' "zone of indifference." The acceptance or rejection of an order depends on the degree to which the incentives exceed the burdens and sacrifices that employees must make. This concept introduced the exchange theory of organization. In short, the individual will participate in the achievement of an organization's objectives if the personal rewards are greater than the sacrifices.

Barnard proposed the open system of organization, based on the premise that man plays a vital role in the creation and the success of an organization. In the modern organization, Barnard's theory has been refined by means of the systems approach and group and role perspectives.

Simon's decision-making approach. Herbert Simon agreed with Barnard that an organization is not autonomous and that it is dependent on offering sufficient inducements to gain needs contributions from its employees.[63] Simon viewed the open system organization as one composed of employees, executives, managers, board members, community members, and regulatory agencies.

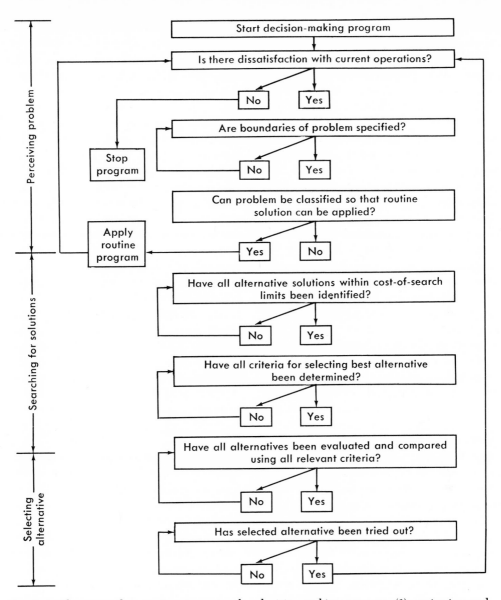

Fig. 6-4. There are four major stages in the decision-making process: (1) reviewing and analyzing the problem; (2) finding or creating solutions based on appraisal of information and known and unknown facts; (3) identifying one or more of the best solutions to cope with the problem after examining the pertinent alternatives, expectations of the results, and objectives in light of established criteria; and (4) formulating a course of action. The flow chart of logical steps that might be involved in the problem-solving process is shown. (From Bass, B. M.: Organizational psychology, Boston, 1965, Allyn & Bacon, Inc.)

Simon believed in the participative approach to decision making. His analysis approach has been refined and broadened by the systems approach to management based on the open sociotechnical concepts (Fig. 6-4). In the decision-making process Simon identified three distinct phases: (1) intelligence activity, (2) design activity, and (3) choice activity.

Likert's contributions. Rensis Likert, former University of Michigan professor, advocated *general* supervision and employee self-direction.[46] He believed that a close, one-to-one supervision tends to promote more conflict among peers than general supervision. He supported the theory that when employees can directly plan and control their own work, structural and authority conflicts are reduced. In the studies conducted in school organizations, Likert's conclusions were not supported, but there tends to be a positive correlation between close supervision and conflict in some situations.

McGregor's assumptions. According to Douglas McGregor, the traditional organization with its highly specialized jobs, centralized decision making, and top-down communications were not the result of economic necessity but portrayed certain basic ideas about human nature.[52] McGregor classified these assumptions as "Theory X," which held that most people dislike work and responsibility, that they prefer to be directed, and that they are motivated to do a good job primarily by financial incentives. Therefore, most people must be closely supervised, directed, and controlled in order to achieve organizational objectives.

In studying these assumptions, McGregor developed an alternate set of assumptions called "Theory Y," which held that people could enjoy work, and if the conditions were favorable, they would exercise sufficient self-control over their performance. He believed that people are motivated by a desire to do a good job and by opportunities to interact with their superiors rather than simply by financial rewards (see Chapter 17 on leadership role using Theory Y).

Application of the bureaucratic concept in the twentieth century

In our society most institutions apply the bureaucratic management concept. Today's organization appears to be the most effective means yet developed to pool members' energies and channel them into productive results to accomplish established objectives.[60] Our modern organization is composed of a highly detailed hierarchy of authority and is supported by an elaborate division of functions, tasks, and decision-making processes (Fig. 6-4). It uses many

different units and departments to accomplish specific tasks and achieve objectives, thus resulting in a horizontal dimensional structure. To coordinate and supervise the work of people in many different jobs, a hierarchy of authority is used, thus creating a vertical dimension to the organizational structure. The combination of depth and breadth gives the organization a triangular shaped appearance when depicted on an organizational chart (Figs. 6-2 and 6-3).

The number of levels in a formal organizational structure, the degree to which personnel are required to follow prescribed channels, and their adherence to all policies and rules have a direct relation to the degree of bureaucracy present. Bureaucracy is felt to a great degree by those individuals in the so-called middle management (Fig. 6-1). In other words, employees between the top level and the rank-and-file workers frequently are frustrated by the constraints and strategies initiated from above and the pressures exerted on them from below.

In the past decade bureaucratic models in hospitals appear to be undergoing substantial modifications. Bureaucratic management principles will no doubt continue to be applied, but in a highly modified form within a more meaningful behavioral environment.

Theories of motivation

It is not my intent to discuss in detail the various theories of motivation and their application to managing people.[23] Because the art and science of nursing involves working with individuals—patients, clients, and personnel—a basic understanding of the values and satisfaction of man's various needs and the motivational process is important for nurses at all levels of the organizational hierarchy.

The theories of Maslow[53] and Herzberg[36] provide the framework for looking at the monetary, security, status, power, competence, and achievement motives of all individuals in a modern organization.

Maslow's contribution. Drawing on personal clinical experience, Abraham Maslow outlined the basic elements of his motivational model in 1943.[54] He believed that a person's motivational needs could be arranged in a hierarchical fashion. When a person's needs at a given level are satisfied, they no longer serve to motivate. The next level of need has to be activated in order to motivate the individual. The progressive terms of Maslow's content are (1) physiological needs, (2) safety needs, (3) love needs, (4) esteem needs, and (5) self-actualization needs. It is interesting to note that Maslow did not attempt to apply his motivational model to individuals in organizations until 20 years later. This need hierarchy has had an impact on the modern approach to motivation. Others have expanded Maslow's theory in their management concepts.[10,55,56]

Herzberg's theory of motivation. In the 1950s Frederick Herzberg conducted motivational studies using the critical incident method of obtaining data analysis.[36] His model became known as "Herzberg's two-factor theory" and is related closely to Maslow's need hierarchy. Herzberg reduced Maslow's five levels to two. Herzberg's two-factor theory was divided into hygiene factors (dissatisfiers) and motivator factors (satisfiers). The hygiene factors represented preventive and environmental aspects such as policies, supervision, salary, and working conditions. He stated that these factors prevent dissatisfaction but do not lead to satisfaction, and do not motivate by themselves. On the other hand, motivating factors such as achievement, recognition, work itself, responsibility, and advancement motivate people on the job. He believed an individual must have a challenging job to be motivated.

Researchers in general have not supported the Maslow and Herzberg approaches to motivation, although these theories have been accepted by practitioners. Studies[4,5,10] indicate that there is not always a clear distinction between factors that lead to satisfaction and those that lead to dissatisfaction.[50] Maslow and Herzberg contributed much to understanding work motivation by drawing attention to the importance of job content factors.

Expectancy models of motivation. The expectancy model approach to work motivation attempts to determine how motivation is translated into action. Victor Vroom[72] in the 1960s, started this approach that has been expanded and refined by recent behavioral theorists Porter,[61] Smith,[65] and others.[76]

Vroom's expectancy model involves the concepts of valence, expectancy, and force (instrumentality).[72] Vroom's concept of force may be viewed as motivation. Valence represents the value or importance that a particular outcome has for an individual and reflects the degree of the individual's desire for or attraction toward the outcomes of a particular course of action. Expectancy refers to the extent that the individual feels his efforts will lead to first level performance outcome.

Luthans,[48,49] in discussing the process and content of motivation, suggests that the Vroom theory could help management. By measuring the worker's output, management could determine how important various personal goals are. Vroom's model can aid in analyzing the worker's motivation and in identifying specific variables.

Smith and Cranny expectancy model. Based on the framework of the 1968 Porter and Lawler[61] motivations model, Smith and Cranny proposed a three-way relationship between effort (motivation), satisfaction, and reward.[65] Rewards affect satisfaction and vice versa, and rewards affect effort and vice versa. However, it is only effort (motivation) that affects performance. The Smith and Cranny model promotes a better understanding of the motivation process for the human behavioral aspects of managing people.

Specific elements in motivation. In our postindustrial society, recent content models have become applicable to the practitioner involved in human resource management.[29,37,39] In this age of specialization and with the larger number of trained, educated individuals working in health care institutions, professional nurses and others should endeavor to improve their understanding and practice in working effectively with individuals in their specific units. The traditional content factors in motivation such as money, security, and status and the more sophisticated factors such as power, competence, and achievement play important roles in work motivation.

Money always will be an important motivation.[10] In today's society, money represents all the things it can bring an individual. Surveys[10] indicate that wages fall in the middle of the list of employment factors. Money is a complex motivator because it can provide power, status, and security and because it can be used to measure achievements. Vroom's model supports the assumption that money has a direct influence on satisfaction. For example, clinical supervisors may be satisfied with their salaries, but that does not mean that salaries are not extremely important. Professional nursing recently has given high priority to enhancing conditions through collective bargaining to provide for quality in nursing care. However, they assume that their salaries will be taken care of by their union or by the labor market (see Chapters 4 and 17).

In our highly technological society, individuals can feel insecure in many areas including graduate education and obtaining and keeping a good job. Job insecurity plays an important part in motivating many employees in our modern complex health institutions.[29] In general, the simple consensus security motive of employees is taken care of to a great degree by insurance, pension, and personal saving plans. The greater complex drive for security is more difficult to understand and has an impact on the behavior of many people.

The status or prestige motive is especially pertinent to a hospital organization. Studies have described the "pecking order" in organizations. The symbols of status, such as the white coat worn by the physician, the stethoscope carried by the nurse, and different uniforms worn by the workers help to identify rank. Cultural roles greatly influence status determination. Physicians, nurses, and workers each have a different status, as do other employees in the administration. As societal values place more emphasis on the health needs of consumers, the status ranking of nursing could be enhanced.

The power motive is recognized by many behavioral scientists as an important motive in organizations. The quest for power is visible in our organizations, but sufficient research is absent to generalize the power motive.

The competence motive has not been considered to any degree in work motivation.[76] Competence is the motive to control one's environment and involves manipulation and activity. In the nursing organization, administrators and supervisors are beginning to realize that if trained professional nurses are not permitted to express their competence motives in the care of patients, the department as a whole will suffer the consequences.

Achievement is a most important factor in work motivation. In 1947, Harvard psychologist David McClelland[50] first presented the aspects of the need for achievement, called n Ach. Gellerman[29] and Luthans[49] summarized the characteristics of the high achiever. As professional nurses become more involved in complex patient care, community health care, and research, an understanding of the achievement motive will be important. The high achiever is one who takes moderate risks, needs immediate feedback, strives to accomplish goals, and is preoccupied with the task.

The behavioral motives of groups are important in systems and contingency management approaches. Interactive effects and dynamics existing in a group make group behavioral motives different from individual behavioral ones (group dynamics in formal communications, informal communications, and team-building in an organization will be discussed in Chapter 8, organizational structures).

Methods for programmed decision making

Due to the escalation of hospital and medical costs during the past 20 years, consumers, the government, and other regulatory bodies have demanded that hospitals be more accountable for their decisions and more efficient in their decision-making processes. Until recently most hospitals did not routinely forecast facility and resources requirements in relation to potential consumer-patient demands or formulate objectives based on determined goals. Today, hospitals must estimate and tabulate their revenues and expenses so that total costs can be controlled. Hospitals are beginning to apply process, quantitative, behavioral, and systems concepts and techniques for maximum goal attainment just as the other business organizations do.

Professional nurses and others who are delegated responsibilities and authority to provide specific services are obliged to forecast, set objectives, make decisions, assess the results in relation to the established goals, and control costs. Professional nurses in administrative and supervisory positions should have insight and an understanding of the decision-making process and techniques used by the organization.

In recent years business and industry, as well as many hospitals, have applied scientific quantitative techniques to managerial problems. The use of management science involves the application of specific techniques and the development of models that usually are computer based. They assist the decision makers in arriving at optimal answers to their problems and permit them to solve the same problems routinely under varying conditions.

Once a problem that considers diverse variables is programmed, such as manhour scheduling, the model permits the supervisory staff to relegate routine decisions to the management information computer system. This can give the staff more time to spend on the planning process in the management of nursing care, on the training of personnel, and in the controlling process of management.

Nonprogrammed decisions

Nonprogrammed decisions in hospitals frequently involve long-range commitments such as providing a new facility, joining with a university medical center, or merging with another hospital. In general, many such decisions were made through following the judgment, intuition, and creativity of an interested group and problem-solving techniques.

Professional nurses use the problem-solving process defined by Dewey some decades ago. This process includes (1) defining the problem, (2) identifying the alternatives, and (3) choosing the best alternative. There are many situations in the management of a service where nonprogrammed decision making is a normal function. Changing conditions and needs of patients consistently give rise to new problems and unforeseen requirements that call for the problem-solving process. The health team in planning the care of the coronary patient now frequently uses the problem-solving process with the aid of a computerized information system.

Hospitals use heuristic (human) programming in management decision making. Heuristic programming actually is an operations-research technique for solving unstructured problems for which precise mathematical models are not feasible. A heuristic program is a rule-of-thumb or computational procedure that directs the computer to limit the number of alternatives to be analyzed. In nonprogrammed decision making some of the alternatives are ignored, and the decision makers select the "right" choice (Fig. 6-4).

Heuristic operational decision making may involve activities that directly support primary operations such as manhour scheduling and inventory systems by means of a subsystem that writes the purchase or requisition orders under computer control.[12,13] The computer presently is used to assist in the decision-making process in programmed and nonprogrammed decisions.[1,3,11]

Operations research (OR) in management

OR is an extension of the scientific method regarding management problems. It originated in Great Britain during World War II to help solve military problems. From 1942 to 1945 the United States used the OR approach to solve complex military planning and control problems. After the war the specialists of the system began to apply its techniques to civilian management problems, focusing on the formulation of goals and objectives and emphasizing interdisciplinary participation.

OR shifted gradually from a broad concept system toward a more circumscribed computerized model (mechanistic) approach.

OR is a method for analysis of specific

types of business and industrial problems by using scientific, mathematical, or logical means to assist the executive staff in making the best decision in dealing with a particular problem. Operations research provides possible outcomes of various available choices. However, the ultimate selection rests with the decision maker.

Tools and techniques. OR models may be physical models. These models may look like the real thing, such as a new facility. They are very useful in discovering errors of equipment placement and work-flow patterns. Other physical models are tangible objects that do not look like the real object but show relationships between objects.

The procedure used by OR and the planning analyst includes these problem-solving actions: (1) formulate the problem, (2) construct a mathematical model, (3) derive a solution from the model, (4) test the model, (5) provide controls for the model and solution, and (6) implement the solution.

Various specific techniques of scientific decision making that make use of models are used. The major models, based on the principles of physical science, include factor analysis (problem solving); linear programming; queuing, or waiting-line, theory; Monte Carlo technique, or probability theory decision theory; game theory; and the Servo theory.

Linear programming. Linear programming is one of a group of similar techniques that are called *mathematical programming.* It is a technique for finding out the best uses of a system's limited resources. Linear programming may be used to solve problems associated with the distribution of personnel assignment patterns. It is used to describe a relationship between two or more variables, a relationship that is directly and precisely proportioned. For example, linear means that a 10% change in the number of work-hours of a certain number of nurses on a night shift (operational input) will cause a 10% change in the nursing care services (output). Linear programming is based on the assumption that a linear or straight line relationship exists between variables and that the limits of variations can be deter-

mined. The technique is useful where input data can be quantified and objectives are subject to definite measurements. It helps the executive make several interrelated decisions that must be made together.

The dynamics of complex nonlinear programming have come into use in making decisions that do not require accuracy on linear relationships.

Queuing, or waiting-line, theory. Queuing theory is a method of decision making under conditions of uncertainty. It applies to those decisions that arise when service must be provided to meet some demand such as the admission of patients, which is neither controllable nor precisely predictable by management. Waiting lines occur when employees or patients must wait for a service because the servicing facility, operating at capacity, is temporarily unable to provide that service. Queuing theory is the application of a collection of methods based on a variety of assumptions and is not a single set of mathematical formulas. The optimal balance between excess capacity and time lost in waiting is an important consideration in the analysis of the problem. For example, the analysis may involve the costs connected with the length of the waiting line in a cafeteria (personnel time lost in waiting vs. the capital and operational costs associated with increasing the capacity of the cafeteria). Queuing theory has its own set of terms such as arrival rate, servicing rate, and rate per unit of time. The queuing theory can be used in determining a system for transporting of people and things from one place to another in the hospital.

This technique is actually an extension of Taylor's scientific management. He endeavored to maximize the output/input ratio through procedures and physical changes. Although queuing models emphasize the output/input ratio, they aim to increase the ratio by having the proper number of servicing units in order to minimize the waiting line. The cost of waiting must be balanced with the cost of adding additional service units. The best solution strikes a balance between these two costs. The queuing model has been applied to the emergency service system. The number of emergency units needed on duty, locating the emergency unit, designing areas of responsibility, and erecting preventive patrol patterns were problems analyzed by a queuing model.

Monte Carlo technique, or the probability theory. This statistical device is based on the inference from experience that certain things are likely to happen in accordance with a predictable pattern. The application of random sampling called the *Monte Carlo technique* is a process for developing data through the use of some random-number generator. For example, management may not know how many personnel are likely to come in at one time to the cafeteria, or patients to the emergency room. It is possible to simulate human behavior in particular situations by developing a device by means of throwing a pair of dice and observing how many times the number two occurs and how often the number two occurs sequentially. This simulation coupled with the queuing theory will lead to a decision on the optimum number of workers the service may need at a particular time.

Actual data from operations may not provide enough information collected over a long period of time. In order to facilitate analysis, the Monte Carlo technique can be used to simulate activity, thus determining approximations that suffice in the decision-making process.

Decision theory. Decision theory is a method of applying certain techniques or statistical analysis to problems involving uncertainty in such a way as to minimize the degree to which the managers are likely to regret the decision they made (Fig. 6-4). Measures of probability are assigned to events, the occurrence of which are uncertain. The various possible payoffs or losses that would occur for each of the possible events are calculated, and statistical manipulations are performed that lead the way to the best decision. Decision theory is a process of analyzing current movement of some variables in an effort to predict the future movment of events. It does not, however, predict whether the event will occur. Decision theory does provide data to help the

executive officer make an optimal decision when taking into consideration the likelihood that certain events will take place. It may be used by hospitals in determining the number of escorts to be scheduled between the units and the radiology department on a particular day.

Game theory. The objective of game theory is similar to that of decision theory: making an optimal decision concerning an uncertain event. This technique involves analysis of the choice of strategies in competitive situations. Brightman[11a] compares the simplest situation to playing a game of gin rummy in which one player makes a good set of decisions to the detriment of the other player, since one player can win only what the other loses. Game theory has contributed to the development of linear programming and a new way of thinking about competitive decisions.

Limitations. OR is only a tool to aid decision makers in the problem-solving process. There are some problems that cannot be solved using quantitative terms. Others are too broad in scope for analytical OR techniques.

In many situations OR techniques are difficult to use because of the time factor requirements. In general, administrators and managers use data only if it is convenient and readily accessible. Moreover, many individuals are not quantitatively oriented.

Network analysis

Many organizations use network analysis techniques for both time and costs. Of the many techniques, one commonly used is the program evaluation and review technique known as PERT.[1,3]

PERT is an excellent aid to facilitate the planning and controlling of a project or program in order to achieve lower costs, reduce project time, and assure effective coordination and utilization of human and material resources.[70] PERT uses three time estimates—optimistic, pessimistic, and most likely—to determine the expected time for each activity.

Major characteristics. Application of the PERT technique involves a graphic detailed presentation of the many tasks to be done within a time schedule that permits the most effective sequence of events in completing the program. The technique is a time-event network analysis designed to watch and evaluate how the parts of a program fit together during the passage of time and events. An event here means a specific definable accomplishment in a program, recognizable at a particular instant in time.

The activities (events) utilize material and human resources such as manpower, equipment, and supplies. All activities have a beginning event and an ending event. PERT expresses the interrelationships and interdependencies of the activities within programs with the use of a device known as a network. The events are usually represented as ovals or circles. The letter "S" indicates that a particular event is the start of the program, and a "C" in the circle or oval (events) indicates that these events are the completion of the activities being programmed. The lines or arrows in PERT networks tell us of the activities themselves as compared to the events of their start or completion (Fig. 6-5).

Values and limitations. Nurse administrators, in-service training staffs, and researchers have found PERT a valuable, effective tool (Fig. 6-5) for planning, programming, and controlling projects. Through the use of this technique, programmers become more aware of the interrelationships and interdependencies in a project.

The four major facets of PERT are (1) goal planning, (2) frequency time planning, (3) scheduling, and (4) control. These techniques help to make systems design and analysis more effective for goal attainment.[75,78]

Computerized PERT control involves simple data manipulations by the computer to produce periodic printed reports on project status. With or without computer assistance, control reports are by no means fixed. New or improved activity estimates, such as those in a budgetary program, may be submitted any time conditions change, or as more is known about the activities to be performed. Activities may be added or deleted if the scope of the project or program changes. Deletion may occur in order to better meet the projected schedule of a specific project.

PERT appears to have limitations, especially in clinical patient service programs, since those programs frequently face uncontrollable events. For example, PERT may help the student understand more about the process of nursing, or the administrative staff more about a project, but PERT will not do the learning or make control automatic.

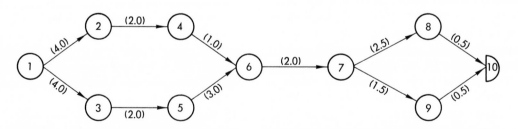

Fig. 6-5. PERT is a type of network analysis involving a sequence of events that are completed to prepare a program or project and the estimated time (Te) in work weeks needed to complete each activity. Encircled numbers *1* through *9* represent the events (completed activities) required in the analysis. Event *10* is the completion of the total planning or factors of the program or project to be implemented. Activities are those things that must occur before the project can go from one event to the next as shown by arrows on the flow chart. The arrows indicate the direction of activity flow. The figures along the arrows designate the estimated time in work weeks that planners agree will be needed to complete the activity. The group must clearly define the objectives of the project, agree on events, make a listing of all activities for each event, time needed to complete each activity, and resources and money required.

However, it is a way to force individuals to undertake detailed planning, and it helps to establish an environment in which sound managerial principles may be applied.

Critical PATH method in network analysis. The PATH method, like PERT, provides a diagrammatical portrayal of the interrelations of all activities in a project. It possesses feed-forward control, focusing on critical inputs so that corrective action may be taken before a major problem develops. The need for network analysis in scheduling project activities depends on having a project of medium size and complexity that is high-time critical.

General systems theory

For the purpose of this book, general systems theory may be viewed as the philosophical and practical supposition of interrelatedness and interdependency of the components (parts) with the whole system.[2,14,25,42]

The general systems theory originated in ancient times and was discussed by Aristotle and Galileo. In 1928, Ludwig von Bertalanffy, a biologist-philosopher considered the founder of the GST, referred to the "system theory of the organism." Following World War II, von Bertalanffy[71] and other well-known management theorists contributed much to the modern systems theory.

General systems movement. In our modern hospitals that focus on specialization, the clinical nurse specialist or supervisor in obstetrical nursing may know very little about the care of the medical patient suffering from a coronary disease, and the specialist in financing may know little about personnel and labor negotiations. Specialists in medicine, nursing, and business have their own jargons and have trouble communicating effectively with one another. This makes coordination and efficiency difficult. Specialization has, to a great degree, created problems in the attainment of overall goals in an institution.

General systems theory identifies and provides common patterns in the opposing philosophies and sciences, but it is not generally concerned with the operational level. A subsystem of GST is concerned with the integration of the parts of an organization from an operational viewpoint.[48] This approach is known as the systems approach to management.

Kenneth Boulding described the hierarchy of the GST in 1956, going from the simplest to the more complex. The hierarchy includes nine systems levels. The most basic level is the status structure such as the anatomy of the universe. That level progresses to the closed system (cybernetics); to the open system level, which is a self-maintaining structure exemplified by the cell; to the genetic-societal level, typified by the plant; to the animal level, identified by increased mobility, teleological behavior, and self-awareness; to the human level or the social and human organizations, which emphasize the organizational role that individuals assume; and to the transcendental systems. Luthans[48] discusses Boulding's concepts and his famous paper General Systems Theory: The Skeleton of Science, published in 1956.

Boulding's writings describe the general nature, purpose, and needs for a systems approach to scientific events. Organizations form in order to gain the efficiency of cooperative endeavor. When an organization becomes too large it may become less efficient. A health care organization does not function in a vacuum, and to be effective in society, it must continually adapt to its environment. A nursing service organization and its environment are interdependent. Nursing service may be perceived as a social and technical system within the total hospital system that copes with constraints from the internal and external environment.[2]

Systems approach to management. In this age of specialization, biomedical and technological research, and the divergence of objectives within the systems of a hospital organization, there is a need to unify philosophic and scientific thought with practical operations. The systems approach to management should be viewed as a subsystem of the general systems theory.[40]

The systems approach is directly concerned with application in management practice in an organization. The modern systems approach integrates former techniques such as quantitative analysis, behavioral concepts, operations research, and decision-making models. Systems approach differs from scientific management. The latter focuses on combining units of work in order to integrate and organize the total system and begins at the bottom levels of the organization; whereas the systems approach begins at the top management level, establishes goals and objectives, and develops work organizational processes downward through the system.

Major characteristics and elements. The basic characteristics of systems approach are central objectives and evaluation of the performance, environment, resources, components, and management. Objectives, decision-making models, and information are key elements in the systems approach to management.

Viewing a hospital as a sociotechnical organization involves people and technology. The inputs into a hospital organization are human resources (patients, personnel, physicians, and others), revenues and funds, materials and equipment, information, research findings, and feedback from the output. Thus, in the systems approach, quality of output is an important variable that affects input in any part of the total hospital system.[66,75]

The hospital, within the framework of the systems approach to management, is considered a structural sociotechnical open system with five major components: (1) goals, (2) concepts (values), (3) managerial processes, (4) conceptual and physical environments, and (5) technology. Both the systems and contingency theorists recognize that the technical aspects of an organization affect the types of inputs and outputs.

The physical environment of a hospital system includes (1) the architectural facilities appropriate for the care of patients with specific health problems, (2) the materials and equipment in the management of patient care and other operations of the hospital, (3) the conference and consultation rooms and visitors' areas, (4) the organizational structure with horizontal and vertical pathways of communication between people, and (5) the distribution and control of equipment and materials from one destination to another.

The conceptual environment of systems approach to management refers to cognitive or mental interpersonal relationships that managers promote in order to create an environment conducive to the practices of health systems. In this environment patients receive optimal care and employees willingly participate to achieve established goals and reap personal satisfaction and rewards from their work. The conceptual or mental environmental factors focus on ways to blend effectively the formal and informal structures of the system.

Administrative roles. In the systems approach, top managers (administrators) guide the organizational processes through (1) planning and evaluation of components and selection of techniques and strategies to attain goals and objectives, (2) development of interfunctional teams and committees that focus on specific objectives, (3) designing a structure for flow of resources and information, (4) development of programs and projects and employment of specialists within the system, (5) implementation of planning-programming budget system, and (6) application of systems analysis techniques for controlling the inputs and outputs to attain goals and objectives.

Meaning of closed and open systems. Systems can be viewed as closed or open. Most of today's management systems are open.

A *closed system* is concerned with cause-and-effect; whereas an open system is viewed as a dynamic system involving resources and change. A closed system, frequently used by the physical sciences, is most applicable to mechanistic systems. As previously noted, in early management theories only the internal operations of the organization were considered without regard to the effect of external forces on the internal environment of the system. In early application, management theory analyzed its problems in terms of internal structure, tasks, and formal relationships. A closed system of management has a tendency toward entropy (measure of chaos, disorganization). It relies on information feedback to achieve control and reach equilibrium.

Cybernetics may be considered a closed system because of its reliance on information feedback.[6] In modern complex organizations, cybernetics may be involved in quality and quantity controls, budgetary control, and inventory control. Cybernetics is applicable when explaining and operating static systems with the aid of electronic computers.

Today, nurses are involved in the use of computer technology in relation to medical records, medication systems, and continuing in-service and educational instruction programs. The introduction of a new automatic system requires critical planning and the development of an effective training program on how to use the computer system to meet the needs of those who will be using it.[3,14] Although mechanistic systems may create negative attitudes or unrealistic expectations from the staff.

An *open system* is one of continuous interaction with its environment. The open system requires information flow, human energy and creativity, and material resources. It depends on strategic considerations such as growth, technological advances, changes in leadership roles, and interaction of components to survive.

An open sociotechnical system such as a hospital must exchange energy and information with its environment. For example, a nursing service system must receive sufficient appropriate input of resources to maintain its operations, thus rendering optimal nursing care to patients and continuing its cycle.

In an open system, hierarchical division results in subsystems that possess some degree of independence. According to Simon and Kast and Rozenzweig, hierarchical structure is based on the concept that a combination of subsystems is needed that merge into a broader system to coordinate activities and processes.[41,42]

Likert[46] states that an important role or function of management is to help link various subsystems to ensure interaction and cooperation between the boundaries of each

system. The role of the nursing service director serves as a pivotal position between the hospital administration and medical staff and the nursing service department.

Boundaries for closed and open systems. A closed system operates within defined precise boundaries, and external environmental factors do not influence its activities.

The open system has unclear boundaries, receives considerable input from the external environment, and transmits outputs back into the environment. In other words, the boundaries of an open system can be penetrated. Fig. 6-6 identifies the boundaries for subsystems, systems, and suprasystems.

The concept of interface in systems approach. The term "interface" refers to the interaction between one system and another. The modern hospital has interfaces with many other systems that are external to the internal organization, such as federal government agencies, manufacturers of equipment and supplies, professional associations, community groups, and labor unions. Within the internal environment of the organization interfaces occur between one system and another where the output of one activity becomes the input for another.

Uncertainties of the systems approach theory. Some theorists wonder if the modern management field may be too complicated to understand and define and if the systems approach to management can be implemented. The systems theory rests on a very broadly based whole with interrelated and interdependent parts. Luthans,[48] Trist,[69] Emery,[19] and others[15] indicate through their research studies that it is useless to search for one best way to manage under all conditions. Complexity, uncertainty, and diversity appear to be important determinants of organizational form.

Von Bertalanffy[71] stated in 1968 that systems science grounded in computer technology, cybernetics, automation, and systems engineering tends to produce another technique than the one originally envisioned. The modern systems approach tends to bring man into a mechanistic system.[79]

The systems approach to management aims to blend behavioral concepts with strictly mechanistic systems and to consider the organization as an integrated whole with objectives to attain overall system effectiveness while reducing conflicting objectives in its components.

The contingency management approach

The contingency approach appears to be an extension of the systems approach.[48] It is based on pragmatic thinking and recognizes the influence of the external environment and the interrelationships between all parts of the whole.[77] Some theorists use the terms *open systems* and *contingency theory* interchangeably and incorporate all schools of thought. Other theorists make a distinction between the contingency approach and systems theory and practice in that the contingency approach aims to develop specific functional relationships between independent environment variables and dependent management variables.

Development. Recent researchers have examined the relationship between the technical and social systems in an organization. A. K. Rice, a member of the research team of the Tavistock Institute of Human Relations in London, states that technological require-ments constrain the type of work organization, but the organization possesses social and psychological elements of its own that function independently of technological advancements.

In 1950 he expanded the Hawthorne findings, emphasizing that technology has an important influence on the organization, equal to if not more than that of its structure and processes.

Gouldner's[33] research supports the contingency framework, indicating that if there is a manufacturing type of technology, a bureaucratic organization structure could be effective. If there are social values of independence and lack of authority acceptance by employees, a more participative style of supervision will help attain goals. In the latter example, social conceptual values become the independent environmental variables, and the type of supervision is the dependent management variable in the contingency approach.

Burns and Stalker[48] classified organization structures and management systems as mechanistic and organic. In general, their research indicates that the most appropriate system depends on the environment. The

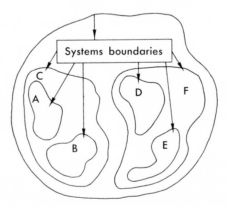

Fig. 6-6. Boundaries for the subsystems, systems, and suprasystem. Hospital organizational systems (open systems) have permeable boundaries. The general and external environment may be considered the suprasystem. *A* and *B* could represent the medical nursing and maternal-newborn subsystems of the nursing service system *C*. *D* and *E* could represent the medicine and obstetrical medical subsystems of the medical system *F*. A more representative suprasystem would be G for nursing service *C* and *F*. The suprasystem for the departments is the hospital organization as a whole, equivalent to the internal environment as shown in Fig. 6-7. (From Introduction to management—a contingency approach by Luthans, F. Copyright 1976, McGraw-Hill Book Company. Used with permission of McGraw-Hill Book Company.)

mechanistic system was found suitable for internal conditions such as specialized tasks control, communications from the top down, and obedience to superiors; whereas the organic system was found to be more applicable to dynamic conditions including horizontal communications, general professional orientation of personnel, unique tasks, nonstructured roles, and counseling rather than direct authority from superiors.

French and Bell,[26] in studying the Burns and Stalker classifications, identify some contingencies concerning mechanistic and organic systems. These assumptions may be provocative in determining transformational structural changes and are clearly summarized by Luthans[48] in his 1976 book *Introduction to Management.*

Theory. The three major components of the contingency approach are (1) the en-

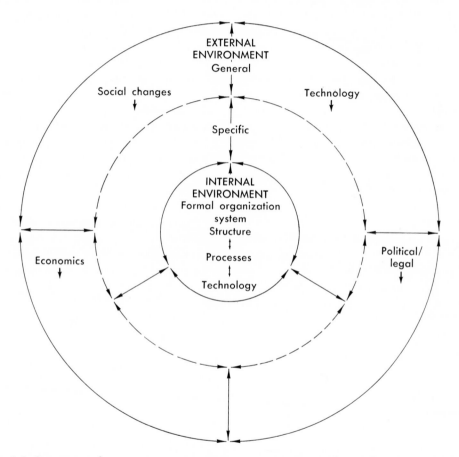

Fig. 6-7. Categories of environment in contingency management in hospital systems. The goal for contingency management of a hospital is to identify relevant environmental factors affecting its management. Administrators of each system must consider the interrelationships between external and internal variables. The external environment is outside of the formal organization system and is divided into general and specific classifications, consisting of social, technological, economic, and political/legal forces that have an impact on the internal formal organization. The subcategories within each of the general environmental forces and the arrowheads in the diagram emphasize that they influence and interact with one another and directly influence the specific environment, such as patients, suppliers, and competitors. The specific environment, like the general variables, interact with the external variables, with each other, and with the internal organization variables. The internal environment makes up the formal organization system. (From Introduction to Management—a contingency approach by Luthans, F. Copyright 1976, McGraw-Hill Book Company. Used with permission of McGraw-Hill Book Company.)

vironment, (2) management concepts and techniques, and (3) interrelations between them. As shown in Luthan's illustration (Fig. 6-7), the external environment is outside of the formal organization system. He divides the general and specific classifications of the external environment and shows the subcategories within each of the general environmental forces, emphasizing that they influence and interact with one another and directly influence the specific environment.

The internal environment consists of the structure, processes, and technology of the formal organization. The organizational structure variables include processes of decision making, communications and control, and the organizational state of technology. In hospital organizations the internal variables frequently depend on the external environment. For example, recent Medicare legislation requires increased measured accountability by the professional staffs and the formation of an accounting system for increased control. In that situation the political variables became the independent variables and the control process of the internal environment became the dependent variables.

The major management concepts and techniques fall within the vertical dimensions of the contingency approach. The major management concepts and techniques may be classified as follows:

- Process variables, which include planning, organizing, directing, communicating, and controlling
- Quantitative variables, which include decision making, linear programming, and operation research models
- Behavioral variables, which include learning, behavioral modifications, motivation, group dynamics, and organizational development
- Systems variables, which include general systems theory, systems design and analysis, and management information systems

The contingency conceptual framework can help professional nurses and others endeavoring to change the existing concepts in the management of patient care services.

The contingency concept attempts to relate the environment to appropriate management concepts and techniques.

MANAGEMENT INFORMATION SYSTEMS

The information system is designed to supply executives with the information they need to make decisions.[40] The information system also must prepare and provide information to outsiders as well as insiders. The kind of information system to be developed in the institution will depend on the type of organizational structure and the kind of information required for planning, control, and decision making by the executives, operational managers, and health professionals and researchers in the various systems (Fig. 6-8). The information system uses data processing that includes several techniques.

The term *data processing* is used in institutions as a means of gathering, sorting, processing, and transmitting information to specified agencies or points. Data processing is part of the information system, but it has no proper decision-making or policy-making functions outside the system itself.

The informational systems may include a subsystem for providing ongoing information by means of data processing, for planning and controlling, and for processing information, material, and manpower resources required for programs, projects and services, and storage of medical and managerial information in the form of records, procedures, manuals, and computer programs[60a] (Fig. 6-9).

Systems analysis

Systems analysis is the process of analyzing and evaluating the various elements of a particular system and the situation in which the system operates. It involves the examination of the inputs into a system and the output requirements. It is designed to achieve the desired outputs in the most effective and economical manner.

Documentation

Documentation is a process of recording every step in a procedure, job, or system in such a way that it can be reproduced in the

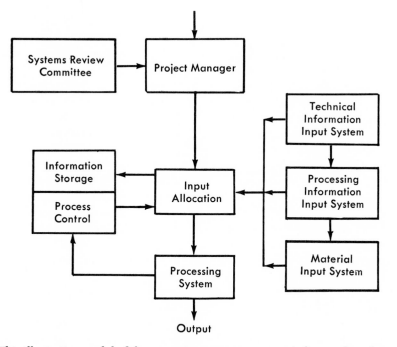

Fig. 6-8. This illustrative model of the operating systems concept indicates the relationship of the functions to be performed and the flow of operating information. In this age of advanced biomedical and business technology, adaptations of the operating systems model have implications for management in the hospital industry. (Reprinted with permission of The Macmillan Company from Wortman, M. S., and Luthans, F.: Emerging concepts in management, New York, copyright © 1969, The Macmillan Co.)

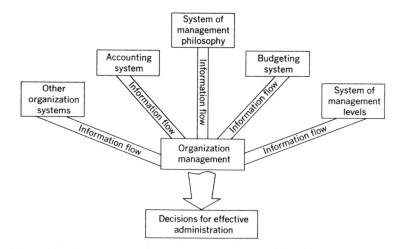

Fig. 6-9. Flow of information in the decision-making process. (From Hodges, B. J., and Johnson, H. J.: Management and organizational behavior, New York, 1970, John Wiley & Sons, Inc.)

future if necessary. Documentation may be used to develop job descriptions and procedures or to document systems activities in the form of flow charts. These documents are one of the basic tools of systems analysis.

Work distribution charts

Distribution charts are used as part of systems analysis in determining what jobs are being done in a particular subsystem, what the interrelationships are with other subsystems, and which individuals working in the subsystem are responsible for the performance of the work. There are many different formats for the preparation of work distribution charts. Work distribution charts are accompanied by detailed forms prepared by the employees on the job. On the individual employee forms each person indicates the percentage of total working time spent in performance of various tasks.[58]

Process flow charts

A procedure analysis work sheet uses symbols (Fig. 6-10) to identify the various operations, thus providing a pictorial description (Fig. 6-11). If it is a new procedure, it can be more effectively evaluated, and if already

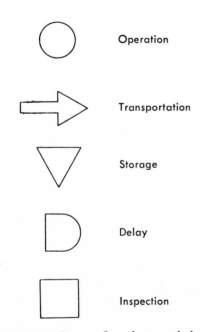

Fig. 6-10. Process flow chart symbols.

Operation

Transportation

Storage

Delay

Inspection

in use, it can be effectively reevaluated.[11a]

Systems flow chart. A systems flow chart is a tool that can be used to document the activities within a subsystem to accomplish specific tasks. Symbols are used in the flow chartings. There are two basic types of flow charts: one concentrates on the flow of forms through a system, the other on chronological steps to be taken in accomplishing a task (Fig. 6-12). The procedure is carried out from the standpoint of finding inefficient activities and developing better ways of doing them. For example, the nursing unit may have difficulty in the processing of a physician's order for laboratory or diagnostic tests such as making out requisitions, preparation of patients, scheduling of patients for tests, completion of tests, and getting test results on the patients' charts. These tasks involve the laboratory, the escort, and the information system. A systems flow chart provides a tool for analyzing all activities within the subsystem involved.

Program flow charts are now being used in businesses and in hospitals for inventory file updating and status reports. The electronic computers do work in response to a set of instructions stored in the computer's memory. This set of instructions is known as a program, and the individuals who write the instructions are known as the programmers. In the writing of a program such as payroll inventory, units of manhours of various categories of workers (input and output) on a floor or service, the clinical status of patients, or the content of a training course plan, the programmer will make use of a fundamental tool of programming, the program flow chart, or block diagram. The form shows the logical sequence of steps that the computer must perform to accomplish the task desired. Documentation in the form of flow charts serves two major purposes in analysis and design. The procedural and forms flow charts serve as tools of analysis and as records to be used in determining how things have been done in the past.

TOOLS FOR HOSPITAL OPERATIONS

The quality control plan for nursing service developed by the Commission for Administrative Services in Hospitals (CASH) has been used as an evaluating instrument. Through the use of this tool, a nursing unit may achieve a systematic, continuous documentation of the relative quality of its service and performance.

A wide variety of tools ranging from pencil and paper to complex electronic computers are available to secure answers to questions and give information. To conserve resources, one should recognize that many national quantitative time-activity studies are available.

The developments in data processing and the use of computers present a new language to nurses working with the devices in the

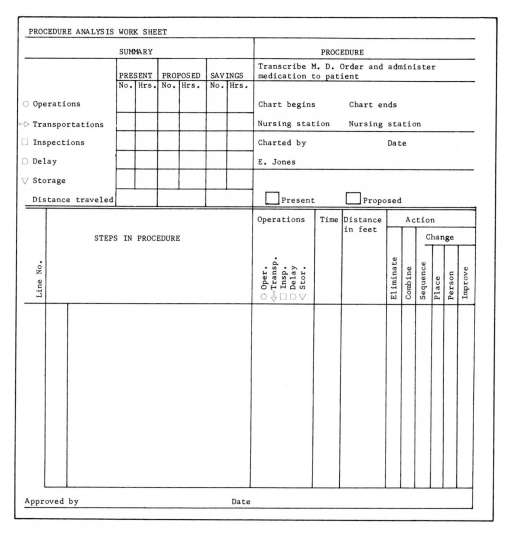

Fig. 6-11. Procedure analysis work sheet. Each of the actions taken in this procedure is listed down the left portion of the form and is identified with a letter indicating which employee performed the particular action. For example, A for the clerk, B for the RN who checked the medication card, C for the nurse who administered the medication and charted it on the patient's chart, D for the patient. Symbols are darkened to show the nature of the activity. The distance traveled and the amount of time required for each activity are recorded at the right of the form. At the top and bottom of the form, space is provided for totals of time and distances, and at the right edge there is a place to indicate what improvements might be made in the procedure.

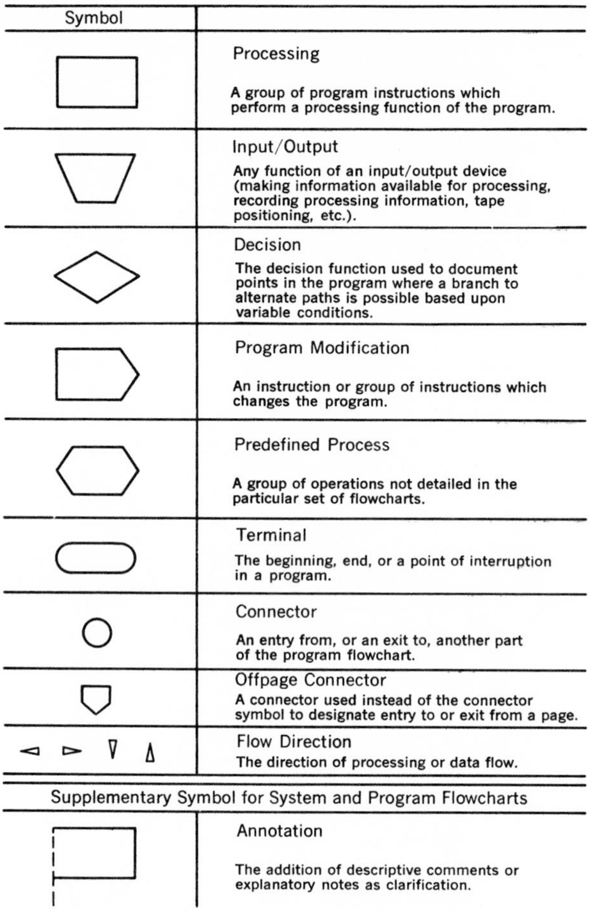

Symbol	
	Processing A group of program instructions which perform a processing function of the program.
	Input/Output Any function of an input/output device (making information available for processing, recording processing information, tape positioning, etc.).
	Decision The decision function used to document points in the program where a branch to alternate paths is possible based upon variable conditions.
	Program Modification An instruction or group of instructions which changes the program.
	Predefined Process A group of operations not detailed in the particular set of flowcharts.
	Terminal The beginning, end, or a point of interruption in a program.
	Connector An entry from, or an exit to, another part of the program flowchart.
	Offpage Connector A connector used instead of the connector symbol to designate entry to or exit from a page.
◁ ▷ ▽ △	**Flow Direction** The direction of processing or data flow.
Supplementary Symbol for System and Program Flowcharts	
	Annotation The addition of descriptive comments or explanatory notes as clarification.

Fig. 6-12. Program flow chart or block diagram symbols typically used in program flow charting. (Reprinted with permission of The Macmillan Company from Brightman, R. W., Luskin, B. J., and Tilton, T.: Data processing for decision-making, New York, copyright © 1968, The Macmillan Co.)

direct care of patients and in the management of nursing service. Nurses and physicians are confronted with such terms as real time, care memory, character set, access speed, and input devices.[75,79] Barker,[7] in her article "The Language of the Computer Age," presents a narrative description of data-processing terms.

Recently, the use of a computer to teach students enrolled in nursing programs has been applied with favorable response from faculty, students, and graduate nurses.[3,14] The computer can provide individualized instruction, immediate feedback, and remedial training. The method of presentation or the type of information can be changed to meet the students' needs. It seems evident that programming with the computer has great potential; however, the manager, teacher, nurse, and physician will have to gain an understanding of the system. Above all, in the operating of hospital systems and their units, the attitudes of the professionals toward roles in handling and using information will require a change toward emphasizing the coordination and analyzing of information.[11,14]

It is important that professional nurses be able to use technological devices based on science to assess clinical needs of patients and to project management inputs and outputs, while keeping in mind that all efforts must benefit the patient. Also, the effective application of scientific knowledge rests on the personnel who are caring for patients and managing the subsystems.

• • •

The PERT, systems, and contingency approaches are perceptive tools developed from a basis of principles on one hand and needs on the other. They are useful theories to be applied in improving the art and practice of management in patient care services. History teaches us that when needs exist and are recognized and when intellectual and cultural levels reach the point of ability to cope with these needs, leadership usually arises to initiate solutions.

REFERENCES

1. Archer, S. E.: PERT: a tool for nurse administrators, Journal of Nursing Administration 4:26-32, Sept.-Oct., 1974.
2. Arndt, C., and Huckabay, L. M. D.: Nursing administration: theory for practice with a systems approach, St. Louis, 1975, The C. V. Mosby Co., chapters 2 and 3.
3. Arnold, M. F., editor: Health program implementation through PERT: administration and educational uses, San Francisco, 1966, Western Regional Office, American Public Health Association.
4. Argyris, C.: Integrating the individual and the organization, New York, 1964, John Wiley & Sons, Inc.
5. Argyris, C.: Management and organizational development, the path from XA to YB, New York, 1971, McGraw-Hill Book Co.
6. Ashby, W. R.: An introduction to cybernetics, New York, 1956, John Wiley & Sons, Inc.
7. Barker, M. R.: The language of the computer age, Chicago, 1970, American Society for Hospital Nursing Service Administrators.
8. Barnard, C. I.: The functions of the executive, Cambridge, Mass., 1962, Harvard University Press. Original copyright 1938 by the President and Fellows of Harvard College.
9. Basil, D. C., and Cook, C. W.: The management of change, New York, 1974, McGraw-Hill Book Co., pp. 2, 182.
10. Beer, M.: Leadership, employees needs, and motivation, Bureau of Business Research, monograph no. 129, College of Commerce and Administration, Ohio University, Columbus, Ohio, 1966.
11. Bitzer, M. D., and Boudreaux, M. C.: Using computer to teach nursing, Nursing Forum 8:234-254, 1969.
11a. Brightman, R. W., Luskin, B. J., and Tilton, T.: Data processing for decision-making, New York, 1968, The Macmillan Publishing Co.

12. Connor, R. J.: A hospital inpatient classification system, Baltimore, 1960, Johns Hopkins University Press.
13. Cook, M., and McDowell, W.: Changing to an automated information system, American Journal of Nursing 75:46-51, Jan., 1975.
14. Daubenmire, M. J., and King, I. M.: Nursing process models: a systems approach, Nursing Outlook 21:512-517, Aug., 1973.
15. Dessler, G.: Organization and management—a contingency approach, 1976, Englewood Cliffs, N.J., Prentice-Hall, Inc., chapters 1 to 3.
16. Dimock, M. E.: The executive in action, New York, 1945, Harper & Brothers.
17. Drucker, P. F.: Management's new role, keynote address, Fifteenth CLOS International Congress, Tokyo, Nov. 5, 1969.
18. Drucker, P. F.: Technology, management and society, New York, 1970, Harper & Row, Publishers, Inc.
19. Emery, J. C.: Organizational planning and control systems, New York, 1960, The Macmillan Publishing Co.
20. Etzioni, A. A.: Comparative analysis of complex organizations, Glencoe, Ill., 1961, The Free Press.
21. Exodus 18:13-26.
22. Fayol, H.: General and industrial administration, London, 1949, Sir Isaac Pitman & Sons, Ltd.
23. Filley, A. C., and House, R. J.: Management process and organizational behavior, Glenview, Ill., 1969, Scott, Foresman and Company, p. 260.
24. Follet, M. P.: Creative experience, London, 1924, Longmans, Green & Co.
25. Fox, D. H.: A contemporary organizational design for maternal and infant care projects, Journal of Nursing Administration 5:26-33, May, 1975.
26. French, W. L., and Bell, C. H.: Organization development, Englewood Cliffs, N.J., 1973, Prentice-Hall, Inc., pp. 188-190.
27. Gardner, A. W.: Patterns of industrial bureaucracy, Glencoe, Ill., 1954, The Free Press.
28. Gardner, J. W.: No easy victories, New York, 1968, Harper & Row, Publishers, Inc.
29. Gellerman, S.: Motivation and productivity, New York, 1963, The American Management Association.
30. George, C. S., Jr.: The history of management thought, ed. 2, Englewood Cliffs, N.J., 1972, Prentice-Hall, Inc.
31. Gilbreth, L.: Bonds of organization, New York, 1950, Harper & Row, Publishers, Inc.
32. Gilbreth, L. N.: The psychology of management, New York, 1914, The Macmillan Publishing Co.
33. Gouldner, A. W.: Patterns of industrial bureaucracy, Glencoe, Ill., 1954, The Free Press, p. 80.
34. Gulick, L.: Notes on the theory of organization. In Gulick L., and Urwick, L., editors: Papers on the science of administration, New York, 1937, Institute of Public Administration, p. 13.

35. Gulick, L., and Urwick, L., editors: Papers on the science of administration, New York, 1937, Institute of Public Administration.
36. Herzberg, F., Mauser, B., and Snyderman, B. B.: The motivation to work, ed. 2, New York, 1959, John Wiley & Sons, Inc.
37. Hodge, B. J., and Johnson, H. J.: Management and organizational behavior (a multidimensional approach), New York, 1970, John Wiley & Sons, Inc.
38. Homans, G. C.: The human group, New York, 1950, Harcourt, Brace, and World.
39. Jehring, J. J.: Motivational problems in the modern hospital, Journal of Nursing Administration 2:35-41, Nov.-Dec., 1972.
40. Johnson, R. A., Kast, F. E., and Rosenzweig, J. E.: Systems theory and management. In Wortman, M. S., and Luthans, F., editors: Emerging concepts in management, New York, 1969, The MacMillan Publishing Co.
41. Kast, F. E., and Rosenzweig, J. E.: Organization and management: a systems approach, New York, 1970, McGraw-Hill Book Co.
42. Kast, F. E., and Rosenzweig, J. E., editors: Organization and management: a systems approach, ed. 2, New York, 1974, McGraw-Hill Book Co.
43. Koontz, H., and O'Donnell, C.: Principles of management, ed. 4, New York, 1968, McGraw-Hill Book Co.
44. Lasca, S. L.: Motivation, evaluation and leadership, Journal of Nursing Administration 2:17-21, Sept.-Oct., 1972.
45. Lepowsky, A.: Administration, New York, 1949, Alfred A. Knopf, Inc.
46. Likert, R.: New patterns of management, New York, 1961, McGraw-Hill Book Co.
47. Luthans, F.: Contingency theory of management: a path out of the jungle, Business Horizons, June, 1973, pp. 67-72.
48. Luthans, F.: Introduction to management: a contingency approach, New York, 1976, McGraw-Hill Book Co.
49. Luthans, F., and Kreitner, R.: Organizational behavior modification, Glenview, Ill., 1975, Scott, Foresman and Company, pp. 140-143.
50. McClelland, D. C.: Achievement motivation can be developed, Harvard Business Review 43:6-25, Nov.-Dec., 1965.
51. McFarland, D. E.: Management: principles and practices, ed. 2., New York, 1964, The Macmillan Publishing Co.
52. McGregor, D.: The human side of enterprise, New York, 1960, McGraw-Hill Book Co.
53. Maslow, A. H.: Eupsychian management, Homewood, Ill., 1965, Richard D. Irwin, Inc.
54. Maslow, A. H.: Motivation and personality, New York, 1954, Harper & Row, Publishers, Inc.
55. Merton, R. K.: Bureaucratic structure and personality, Social Forces 18:560-568, 1940.
56. Merton, R. K.: Social theory and social structure, rev. ed., New York, 1957, The Free Press, pp. 19-24.
57. Mooney, J. D., and Reilly, A. C.: Onward industry, New York, 1931, Harper & Row, Publishers, Inc.
58. O'Malley, C. D.: Application of systems engineering in nursing, American Journal of Nursing 69:2155-2160, Oct., 1969.
59. Perrow, C.: Goals in complex organizations, American Sociology Review 26:855, 1966.
60. Perrow, C.: Organizational view: a sociological view, Belmont, Calif., 1970, Wadsworth Publishing Co., Inc.
60a. Phillips, D. F.: Regulations and data systems questions of demand versus needs, Hospitals 51: 85-90, 202, Oct., 1977.
61. Porter, L. W., and Lawler, E. E.: Managerial attitudes and performance, Homewood, Ill., 1968, Richard D. Irwin, Inc.
62. Robbins, S. P.: Managing organizational conflict, a nontraditional approach, Englewood Cliffs, N.J., Prentice-Hall, Inc.
63. Simon, H.: Administrative behavior, New York, 1959, The Macmillan Publishing Co.
64. Smith, A.: The wealth of nations, edited by E. Cannon, New York, 1937, Modern Library, pp. 4-9.
65. Smith, F. P., and Cranny, C. J.: Psychology of men at work, Annual Review of Psychology 19:469-477, 1968.
66. Somers, J. B.: A computerized nursing care system, Hospitals 45:93, 1971.
67. Taylor, F. W.: The principles of scientific management, New York, 1911, Harper & Brothers.
68. Tead, O.: The art of administration, New York, 1951, McGraw-Hill Book Co.
69. Trist, E. J., and Rice, A. K.: The enterprise and its environment, London, 1963, Tavistock Publications, Ltd.
70. United States Navy Special Projects Office: PERT fundamentals, Washington D.C., 1963, United States Government Printing Office.
71. von Bertalanffy, L.: General systems theory—critical review. In Lutherer, J. A., editor: Organization: systems control and adaptation, New York, 1969, John Wiley & Sons, Inc., pp. 7-31.
72. Vroom, V.: Work and motivation, New York, 1964, John Wiley & Sons, Inc.
73. Weber, M.: The Protestant ethic and spirit of capitalism, translated by T. Parsons, New York, 1958, Charles Scribner's Sons.
74. Weber, M.: The theory of social and economic organization, translated by A. M. Henderson and T. Parsons, New York, 1947, Oxford University Press.
75. Wesseling, E.: Automating the nursing history and care plan, Journal of Nursing Administration 2:34, March, 1972.
76. White, R. W.: Motivation reconsidered: the concept of competence, Psychological Review 9:329, 1959.

77. Woodward, J.: Industrial organization, London, 1965, Oxford University Press, pp. 50-67.

78. Wortman, M. S., and Luthans, F.: Emerging concepts in management, New York, 1969, The Macmillan Publishing Co.

79. Zielstorff, R. D.: The planning and evaluation of automated systems: a nurse's point of view, Journal of Nursing Administration **5:**22-25, July-August, 1975.

7 Purposes, goals, and objectives of individuals and organizations

As health care systems are scrutinized in our society, nurses working in a health system recognize that individual goals and objectives influence those of a nursing department. Nurse administrators realize that compatible, though not necessarily identical, objectives benefit both the employee and the organization.

Today nurses are trying to identify nursing and its objectives to provide optimal quality nursing care to consumers through their professional associations and to participate in the activities of other health groups and agencies on a local, state, and national level.

SETTING PRIORITIES AND DIRECTION

The board of trustees or a similar governing body, assisted by top executives of an organization, define the overall statement of purpose and its goals. Top-level unifying goals and objectives are necessary for operational success.[9,11]

The top-level group of a health system focuses on overall definite goals concerning the financing and management of specific patient services, programs, supportive services, and material and human resources. The executive planning council, including hospital administrators, medical, nursing, and other top-level professionals, should agree upon overall guidelines based on the set of priorities.[13] Such directions are essential to top managers (division or department heads) as they and their staffs determine a set of statements that will contribute to the accomplishment of overall organizational goals.

Factors influencing purpose and goals

Current environmental variables influence the purpose and goals of an institution (see Fig. 6-7). Hospital operations are affected by both the external and specific environments. Environmental elements include potential consumers, social and economic factors, market conditions, health standards, technology and biomedical innovations, and governmental regulations and laws.

The environmental variables of a hospital offer both opportunities and limitations for the attainment of organizational goals. A health system, organized for people and by people, must continually adapt to its environment. Today, the hospital depends on its consumers as well as on the resources and opportunities of its environment for existence (see Chapters 3 and 4).

The principles (philosophy), the values (norms), and the attitudes of consumers and individuals in the organization, as well as their abilities and the quality of their interactions, have an impact on the ongoing goals of an institution and its component parts.[19]

Public expectations of health care. With the public's increased interest in and demands for better health services and the increased participation of private and governmental agencies in health services, all hospitals are becoming more involved in community health problems. For these reasons the controlling officers are faced with making critical decisions regarding the type of services and programs to be offered to the public.

Health, illness, and the treatment of disease have become important parts of the value system of modern society. In our culture the public has come to expect adequate and quality care at reasonable costs as a right, regardless of race, creed, color, religion, or financial status. The public expects to participate in decisions regarding their care and to have the opportunity to benefit from modern scientific medical advances.

It is interesting to note that because health professionals and workers are a subculture of our society, when they enter the health field they bring with them some of the values of the larger society, which are incorporated into the philosophies of patient care.

Biomedical advances. Since the 1950s, health professionals and related businesses, with private and governmental support, have made tremendous strides in relieving human suffering; however, in the process, new health problems have arisen. For instance, hospitals are faced with caring for an increased number of aged people. The combination of a declining death rate and a stable birthrate has produced a population explosion and a great need to provide health care for the young population, and to provide ambulatory services and programs. The ability to decrease the number of patients dying from diseases that used to be swiftly fatal has resulted in more specialization. All these factors have resulted in increased medical costs and the public's demand for more health insurance (Chapter 4).

Specific services and programs. The primary function of a general hospital is to provide diagnostic and therapeutic patient services for a variety of surgical and nonsurgical medical conditions. The primary function of other institutions is to provide treatment and care services for patients who have specific medical and surgical conditions such as psychiatric, orthopedic, or eye and throat problems.

A teaching general hospital situated in a university setting will have a different set of priorities and goals than a general hospital not directly connected with a university or a small general community hospital located

outside the boundaries of a university or a city.

A teaching hospital within a university environment would incorporate into its statement of definition of purpose and goals of patient care services the educational programs conducted in medicine, nursing, and other health science schools of the university. The statement would also give direction concerning its obligations to faculty and students and the expansion of knowledge and skills through refined research. The statement of a hospital organized and supported by a religious order may have slightly different objectives based on its own beliefs, values, attitudes, and intentions.

Hospitals express their system of values and goals in relation to the type of services they will offer the public. Some hospitals offer short-term, specialized services. Others are structured and managed to care for the acutely ill or the chronically ill long-term patients. Moderate- and large-sized private, voluntary, general hospitals have major medical services and many support services. They may have close associations with educational institutions, whereby the faculty and students majoring in health care use the hospital clinical facilities.

The goals of the hospital offering services to chronically ill patients and those requiring rehabilitative care over an extended period of time will focus on a set of relationships between medicine, nursing, and many rehabilitative services such as recreational, physical, and speech therapy and the like.

The statement of an institution should present its primary purpose and goals in the delivery of patient care services, as well as contributory or related goals such as education, research, and community-related programs that enhance and support the patient care system for consumers. The definition of primary purpose of a general hospital may state that the hospital offers optimal quality patient care services to consumers of all ages who have surgical or nonsurgical conditions, regardless of their economic status or other social factors.[9]

Control or ownership of institutions. The ideas and expectations held by the controlling body and the top-level medical and research professionals influence the goals of an institution. The statement of an institution identifies the type of hospital, its ownership, and those with a vested interest who control its operations. For example, the proprietary institution may be financed by "lay" individuals. Such private institutions operate for profit in the delivery of specified patient care services.

A voluntary nonprofit hospital may be considered as a public institution operated under private management and sponsored by a board of trustees composed of representatives of the community who are legally and morally responsible for its professional services and policies.

Institutions registered by the state and the American Hospital Association and accredited by delegated commissions or associations for specific patient care services and programs must meet specific standards. Their goals and objectives are designed to achieve these standards.[9]

PRIMARY AND CONTRIBUTORY GOALS OF AN ORGANIZATION

Both individuals and organizations tend to have many goals. Some are viewed as more important than others. However, individual and organizational goals change as situations change during a period of time. A short-term goal identifies what is to be done in an immediately prescribed future, whereas a long-term goal looks to a plan further in the future and a desired end. Organizational goals change due to advances in biomedical and technological sciences, limiting resources, and rising costs for resources.

The goals of an organization are nonpersonal to most members, but must be compatible with the personal goals of the employees of the institution. If top executives and department heads care to cooperate toward overall organizational goals, it is imperative that they identify in writing and verbally a set of goals that will motivate subordinates, regardless of their areas of indifference, to participate toward the attainment of objectives.[7]

Goals serve as common denominators for all members of the institution. For this reason, goals should be clear and definite. If goals are worded as abstract statements of principles or philosophy, it will be impossible for managers of services to determine objectives for measuring success. For example, an overall organizational goal may state "the entire organization will endeavor to decrease personnel input during the fiscal year, thus reducing rising costs of services." This means that each department head must identify specific concrete objectives to plan to meet this goal, and tangible results to be achieved.

Goals should inform employees on how they should act, as well as explain why they should direct their energies toward accomplishing goals. The assumption is that the system as a whole will suffer if broad goals are not defined. A distinction is made here between goals and objectives. Each department should define a statement of purpose and goals in order to set priorities and objectives as a first step in operational planning.[15]

In defining nursing statements, the nurse administrator and staff members review the purpose and goals of the institution as a whole. They consider the standards of nursing practice and nursing services proposed by professional associations, the current health regulations and laws, and the social factors that influence the management of nursing care and nursing services. The staff recognizes the goals of employees, those of educational training programs, and the physical and conceptual environment required to provide optimal quality care to patients.

For example, the organizational goals of a division or department of nursing in a teaching hospital may be stated as follows:

The division of nursing and its component parts of hospital X recognize that the primary purpose of all members of each department is to provide optimal quality nursing care and treatment to each patient regardless of his economic status and other social factors. Each nursing service department believes that nursing care is a continual process of identifying, assessing, planning, and meeting the physical, social, emotional, and spiritual needs of the patient and that this process requires a collaborative relationship with physicians and other professionals of the health team and with those of supportive services.

Cognizant of the impact that external and internal environmental variables have on patient care services, the division of nursing realizes that its structure, processes, and technology must permit and encourage the staff at the unit level to participate in decision making and to initiate plans of action in the direct management of nursing care (see Chapter 10).

The division of nursing recognizes the need to conserve limited resources and to use the abilities and skills of professional nurses and assistants effectively in providing nursing care needs to patients in each type of facility (see Chapter 9).

The division of nursing in collaboration with hospital administration and medicine supports and encourages the grouping of patients with specific surgical and nonsurgical conditions in appropriate facilities and the formulation of standards and policies that enhance patient care services (see Chapters 5 and 8).

The division of nursing recognizes that competent professional nurses and clinical nurse specialists are required to provide direct nursing care for inpatients, that nurse practitioners are needed to meet the needs of ambulatory patients, and that trained technical nurses can contribute to the quality of nursing care through a defined nursing team management approach (see Chapters 12 and 13).

The division of nursing recognizes that professional nurses are accountable for their nursing practices and are responsible for guiding the performance of those who assist them and for setting and evaluating standards of nursing care services (see Chapters 16 and 17).

The division of nursing recognizes that on employment, an individual requires orientation through a planned program; and that an employee requires instruction and guidance through an appropriate planned in-service training program or staff development program to perform new functions and tasks.

The division of nursing supports and encourages the staff to participate in research programs and projects that will enhance the treatment and care of patients and in educational health programs associated with the institution.

The division of nursing recognizes that professional nurses and technical assistants must assume responsibility for meeting their personal objectives and that each department must provide guidance to assist individuals in meeting their new objectives.

The division of nursing recognizes that all employees should receive financial remuneration and fringe benefits in accordance with the existing competitive market of the community, that employees should be compensated for quality of performance in accordance with established institutional policy, and that collective personnel requests should be communicated to top administrators for review and decision making (see Chapters 4 and 15).

The division of nursing selects employees for promotion based on their knowledge and skills and the requirements of the position, regardless of sex or race.

Each department and its units of the division of nursing is required to determine ongoing objectives and to evaluate them periodically to eliminate deficiencies in the management of direct nursing care and to accomplish the established goals of the hospital (see Chapter 6).

The philosophy and goals of each unit of a nursing department focus on two major goals: (1) contributing to the therapeutic plan of care for each patient and (2) contributing to the hospital management plan for patient services through an effective, efficient organized system for provision of high quality nursing care services to accomplish the objectives established by the governing board of the hospital. A discussion of the philosophy and goals of a specialty unit follows.

Purpose and goals of nursing in intensive care units

Nurse-leaders in each department of nursing service, with the assistance of staff nurses, should identify goals for nursing units to assure quality of nursing care for patients, using the most effective, efficient, and economical system possible and to attain the goals of the division of nursing.

The intensive care unit is designed and organized to assist critically or seriously ill patients who are unable to communicate their daily needs and who require concentrated, expert medical and nursing treatment at frequent scheduled intervals and in emergencies, with the aid of special equipment to meet their changing biomedical needs.[9]

The aims of the health team, composed of the physician and nurse teams and their supportive professional and technical associates, in the treatment and care of the critically ill patients in this unit are (1) preservation of life, (2) restoration of the patient's functional capacity to a safe or maximal level, and (3) reduction of the morbidity rate through direct, rapid, and deliberate intervention.

With the physician as the leader of the health team, the team members develop a system of relationships that will contribute toward effective functioning of the unit. Health teams must recognize and accept the interdependent and dependent responsibilities and duties of each member of the team. In addition, coordination of activities from nursing service and hospital administrators and from supportive hospital services is required.

A safe, clean physical environment and privacy as needed are required for patients and personnel through a systematic, planned regimen carried out by the environmental service departments. The materials-management department will provide the area with supplies and equipment, linens, and other items to meet daily requirements.

The testing and control of all electrical equipment and other apparatus, ventilation, air conditioning, flooring, and materials will be carried out by supportive services, in coordination with the nursing unit.

The professional staff nurses, the clinical supervisor of the unit, the clinical nurse-specialist, and physicians must have a clear understanding of their respective responsibilities and duties and of the medical and nursing objectives for each patient. The nursing staff on each shift accept the responsibility for an effective nursing care plan system and for their nursing practices. Periodic data collecting of present nursing practices and the nursing system will be used to revise the practices and the system in keeping with changing medical, nursing, and technological advances and will help in decision making concerning the functions and duties of the unit personnel and those of other groups who render services to the unit.

The nursing service leaders and nurses of the unit direct their efforts to meet the standards set forth by the hospital and by the Joint Commission on Accreditation of Hospitals for the intensive care unit. Nurses are delegated to assist others in formulation of policies and procedures and to articulate and interpret the goals and policies of the nursing department and those of the hospital as a whole.

The functions and duties of the professional nurses and others who assist them will be stated in the job description for each position. The functional duties of the staff nurse will include nursing diagnosis and assessment of the patients' physical, emotional, and spiritual needs; performing treatments; communicating the essence of the plan to the patient and family and motivating them to help implement it; making judgmental nursing decisions; and communicating them verbally and in writing to the appropriate physician and superiors in nursing.

The physician, nurse, and clinical specialists of the unit accept their clinical responsibilities for conducting planned patient care conferences with other members of the health team so that each person can share his knowledge, clinical observations, and evaluation of equipment and techniques with the others, thereby giving each other guidance in achieving excellence in patient care.

The staff nurses and the nurse-supervisor accept as part of the nursing care system meeting together for planning, organizing, and informing each other of the medical therapeutic plan and nursing care plan for each patient during each 24-hour period and keeping other hospital groups informed to resolve immediate problems and to prevent others from occurring.

Both physicians and nurses agree that continuous staff development is basic to the health team approach in providing patient-centered care, especially in an environment in which guidelines change rapidly and procedures and treatments become outmoded and require frequent revisions. For this reason, the nursing department initiates appropriate programs to meet the educational needs of the staff members in this specialty unit.

The division of nursing recognizes the

importance of having a long-term plan to provide opportunities for qualified, experienced nurses in the general areas to be assigned to the intensive care unit and to receive training and experience in the care of the critically ill patient.

Through the health team approach, implementation of nursing service principles of management, understanding and acceptance of the contribution of all personnel, creation of an environment conducive to personal satisfaction of each worker and high morale of the staff, the philosophy and goals of nursing care of critically ill patients in the intensive care unit can be achieved.

INDIVIDUAL OBJECTIVES IN AN ORGANIZATION

Experience indicates that unless an organization makes a sincere effort to help its employees satisfy their objectives, they will not give the organization their full efforts and may eventually resign. Nurse administrators recognize that today's nurses tend to work toward the attainment of nursing goals and objectives because of what they expect the department will do for them or because of what it has done for them.

The theories of motivation contributed by Maslow, Herzberg, Vroom,[19] Smith, and others,[14] and the specific elements in motivation have been summarized in Chapter 6. In our society, money, status, power, competence, and achievement are major factors in the work motivation of many individuals.[12]

Interactions of personal objectives in an organization

In many situations an employee may give up a personal objective to attain an organizational objective if the loss or compromise is not too great. Both personal and organizational objectives change in relation to past experiences and present and future circumstances over periods of time. Professional nurses and other employee groups with similar backgrounds tend to have similar objectives, although most employees want opportunities to satisfy their needs through an organization.

As nurses and others work to accomplish their objectives and those of the department itself, the interactions between these individuals usually influence their future objectives. For example, a team leader who has high standards in the care of patients, and a keen desire to understand the objectives of team members can usually pull the members in the direction of providing quality nursing care with more compatible objectives.

The basic goal of an organization is to have its employees' objectives coincide with its own so that both can benefit from subsequent actions. Today nurse administrators and personnel managers are more attentive to an applicant's objectives, values, and attitudes and endeavor to determine if the applicant's objectives and organizational objectives are compatible. This is imperative because of rising costs of recruitment, orientation of new employees, and the influence individuals have on the conceptual environment of a unit.

An objective of a department and that of a group of nurses may be to establish primary nursing in a unit. In the work environment the interactions between these nurses and with others can alter the direction of their own objectives, those of other employees, and those of other departments so that new organizational objectives may result. These may include the revision of job descriptions, staffings, and budgetary measures, as well as the allocation of some supportive duties to other departments. Nurse administrators provide direction and support to the group as it reaches out to attain new objectives.

Nurse administrators' awareness of relationships

A department may show compatible individual and organizational objectives, but nurse administrators and assistants should realize that there is no assurance objectives will remain compatible unless appropriate actions are taken by the superiors of the organization. The interactions between nurses and other employees, between the department and individuals, and between the department and others in the institution may divide rather than correlate personal and organizational objectives.[4,6,19]

Hicks[7] provides effective illustrations of totally opposing, partially opposing, neutral, and compatible individual objectives with organizational objectives (see Chapter 9). For example, a clinical nurse specialist in cardiovascular nursing may have an objective to meet the nursing care needs of patients with complex conditions, in collaboration with physicians and other professionals, without becoming a physician's assistant or a clinical coordinator. If nurses cannot work toward meeting personal objectives they will become frustrated. They may be forced to change their objectives, compromise to prevent frustration, or even resign, unless the organizational objective for this position is reviewed, clarified, and made more compatible with their personal objectives.

In some situations individuals may be compromised partially by department objectives. In other instances, individuals' objectives may be totally opposed to department objectives, creating a so-called subversive group within the department.[1,7] In the latter case the influence of the group must be nullified, or their objectives or those of the department must be changed. If interactions of totally opposing individuals and those of the organization continue, conflict will result.

Some nurses may oppose several organizational objectives while wholeheartedly supporting others and thus do not actively hamper the direction of the department toward the attainment of overall organizational objectives. For example, the experienced instructor of long standing in the orientation program for technical assistants in surgery may oppose the organizational objective for the employment of clinical nurse-specialists in the surgical care of patients.

When employees' objectives are neither opposed nor compatible with those of the department, these individuals should be considered nominal members of the staff. In short, these individuals and the organization do not need each other because these employees do not function as a part of the department.

Compatibility of objectives without uniformity

It should be emphasized that not every staff member is expected to have the same objectives as those of the organization. In the past, many nurses allowed themselves to be subordinated to the will of the organization. Some researchers viewed nurses as puppets controlled by their superiors. In such cases the objectives of nurses were often subjugated to those of medical and hospital administrators. Even in today's health system we may find this feeling expressed in such statements as "Nurses are not as dedicated as they used to be," and "Nurses are not interested in the organization as a whole; they only work toward nursing." Nurse-administrators should not expect staff nurses to identify with the organization in the same way that they do.

The personal objectives of the nurse-administrator and those of the hospital administrator should be compatible, not completely identical, just as the objectives of physicians and a nursing unit should be compatible but not identical.

In an institution that accomplishes its goals and objectives the members of each department recognize that they have opportunities to satisfy personal objectives and to voice their opinions and ideas and that the institution as a whole must set the overall direction and priorities of the organization. In such an environment the staff members of each department move in the same direction to attain both personal and organizational objectives, resulting in relationships that will contribute to effective productivity and necessary organizational changes.

ORGANIZATIONAL OBJECTIVES

The objectives of any organization are distinct from those of its members even though they are determined by the members. The setting of organizational objectives to meet determined goals is a critical first step in managing any type of organization. The plans flow from the determined objectives of each department in the institution.[2,5]

Objectives in management of nursing services

It is the responsibility of nurse-administrators to collaborate with staff members to determine what nursing service is doing, where it wants to go, and the direction it should take to attain objectives.

Nurse-administrators should communicate their own organizational objectives to the staff, seek their ideas, and be able to answer such questions as, What are the objectives? What areas in nursing services should be involved? How are the objectives to be determined and measured by the department heads and their staff? Who will participate in setting the objective of a unit and evaluating the results? What are the relationships between personal and organizational goals and the objectives?[5]

Objectives should establish the results administrators and staff members expect to accomplish and provide precise guidelines for what must be done to accomplishing those results.

Kurt Lewin points out that an objective is not achieved until the steps required to accomplish it are completed, regardless of how much an individual or an organization wants to achieve it. Peter Drucker[5] first advocated management by objectives (MBO) in his book *The Practice of Management*, emphasizing the motivational and self-control aspects that emerge from within rather than outside of the system. George Odiorne,[16] John Humble,[8] and Palmer[17] supported and encouraged the MBO approach.

Management by objectives, also known as the hierarchy of objectives, is a systematized technique for joint participation by staff members at all levels of the hierarchy in decision making. This technique aims to increase the vitality and personal involvement of all the employees in managing nursing services. Objective setting may be viewed as the yardstick of effectiveness for each department and its subsystems.

Objectives define expected results clearly and imply that the organization has committed itself to these results in the sense that it is prepared to use the necessary human and material resources to achieve them.

Developing organizational objectives

Nurse administrators and staff members review and analyze those areas of performance that are most critical and identify the primary objective of the division of nursing. The so-called critical objectives are the results departments must achieve to ensure the outstanding performance that results in the accomplishment of the primary objective. The most important needs and deficiencies of nursing services are determined to accomplish the critical objectives. Following the needs analyses, the staff determines specific objectives that are results they must achieve to satisfy determined needs and to overcome identified deficiencies.

An objective will not be of value unless there is acceptable evidence that it has been accomplished. Nurse-administrators should establish standards to serve as constant guides for themselves and for their staffs who are working toward the objectives. The statement of organizational objectives specifies continual results in specific areas of performance that the staff must achieve to accomplish the key objective.[1] For example, a key objective of the nurse-administrator may be to develop, establish, and maintain a logical, efficient, collaborative system of planning, including 1- and 3-year forecasts, and objectives, programs, schedules of staffing, and budgets to be reviewed monthly and quarterly and revised if necessary with supporting standards, policies, and procedures. To meet these standards of performance, each month the nurse-administrator discusses nursing care forecasts, and economic and technological conditions influencing nursing with all personnel, secures their understanding and acceptance of plans, and initiates and revises plans based on their contributions and data.

Hierarchy of objectives

In the hierarchy of objectives the objectives (ends) of each subsystem become the means by which broader objectives are achieved. For example, in a complex hospital structure composed of divisions, departments, units, and work groups, each division's broad objectives, based on hospital goals, are converted to objectives for each of its departments. A department's objectives serve as a basis for determining the objectives of each of its units. Each unit's objectives are converted to objectives for its work groups. Thus, the objectives of each level of the division of nursing are developed in sequence, starting with the highest level.

Each level in the hierarchy of the division of nursing contributes differently because of its critical performance objectives and its direct concern with daily operational inputs and outputs. To develop and maintain organizational objectives, nurse-administrators and immediate assistants must continually motivate the staff to participate in the attainment of the overall objectives of nursing.

Organizational objectives give direction to staff members and serve as guidelines to channel interests into joint efforts. Broad objectives with subobjectives for the entire division of nursing are vital to determine specific short-term targets. Objectives for a division of nursing are defined based on the determined goals. For example, viewing the goals previously described, the key objective for the division of nursing may be stated as follows:

• Develop and maintain an organizational structure, managing processes, and technology that will permit the nursing staff at all levels of the hierarchy to contribute effectively and efficiently in meeting the physical, socioeconomic, and spiritual needs of each patient.

• A subobjective or intermediate objective may state: delegate and support decision making at the level the action takes place.

• An objective of an intensive care unit of the surgical department will convert the department's objectives into realistic attainable objectives. For example, an objective may state: maintain an adequate ratio of at least one competent experienced professional nurse to every two patients that require continual complex nursing care and probable emergency treatments that must be performed accurately and quickly as lifesaving innovations.

Developing operational (specific) objectives

A statement of an operational objective specifies the measurable, time-limited results that must be accomplished to achieve the critical or subobjectives of a department.

Specific objectives should be realistic, obtainable, and within the power of the staff. The objective must identify expected results, specify quantities (preferably in numbers) necessary to establish meaningful programs, schedules, and budgets, and develop appropriate controls. The more tangible an objective, the more direct and specific the effort to achieve it tends to be.[11] Thus, intangible ideas must be converted into statements related to material things. For example, an objective—maximize personnel resources in the direct care of patients—is useful only when it is related to concrete facts such as decreased nursing aide positions during each quarter, totaling ten positions during the fiscal year amounting to x number of dollars, due to limiting financial input and rising costs of care. To meet this objective, a systematized plan is required to reduce such resources in specified units. It may be necessary to review the management processes of the units and redefine job descriptions of particular positions to provide optimal care to patients. It is imperative that all staff members understand the targets for their own work and how their objectives relate to the broader objectives of the division and to the institution as a whole.

Only immediate and attainable objectives can be related to a standard unit of time, and the characteristics of a nursing care system make it difficult to measure results. Results (indicators) can be made more tangible by using ratios, percentages, or scales for the measurement and the evaluation of results. For example, the objective may state: "Decrease personnel turnover by 5% within a 6-month period using the personnel records of each employee to determine the percentage of objective achieved."

Another objective may state: "Operating personnel manpower costs will be kept at the same level as the past year and based on an average patient occupancy rate of 85%. This objective will be measured by accounting and admission records and requires commitment to analysis of related budgetary factors."

Selecting objectives and evaluating progress

In searching for sound objectives, the nurse-administrator and staff endeavor to select specific objectives from several sources.[18] Analyzing recent facts and experiences and reviewing the strengths and weaknesses of nursing services in relation to key objectives should be undertaken. Standards proposed by commissions and professional associations should be reviewed and updated. Objectives may be based on new documented research information such as the direct care of 30 patients given only by professional nurses that would be x number of units, x number of dollars in savings, and x amount of cost. This information would be converted to a unit for an objective such as, "Develop and initiate primary nursing management in x units to provide optimal quality nursing care and improve productivity of professional nurses for nursing care without increasing input costs during the fiscal year."

An objective may be based on an average of similar operations by other organizations. For example, effective actions taken by other organizations to reduce absenteeism or decrease personnel accidents may be considered by the department heads and their staff. The implementation of management by objectives is not easy to accomplish, but attempts to identify results through performance is superior to evaluating nursing department heads by measures such as the number and cost of nursing personnel input, the maintenance of general policies, or whether the individual is cooperative and pleasant.

Every department head and unit supervisor should be accountable for securing staff participation in a goal and objective setting.

All staff members must be kept apprised of their progress toward objectives. Personnel should know where they stand. Each department head and unit supervisor should know when deficiencies occur and have the information to analyze the progress made toward objectives. They should be responsible for taking corrective action as indicated. Effective objectives may be summarized as follows:

1. Objectives should lead to definite, meaningful performance. They must be meaningful to the workers who are delegated to execute the plan.
2. Objectives must enhance and advance the basic goals of the hospital.
3. Objectives may provide answers to the questions concerning the what, how, and who of the plan. Objectives must state, whenever possible, what is the measurable end result to be accomplished and how it should be done, by what means the objective should be achieved, when it should be started and completed, what material and human resources would be required and their costs, and the individuals or groups who should be involved in accomplishing the objective.
4. Objectives should be described in terms of what the planners desire to initiate. As previously mentioned, objectives must be feasible.
5. Objectives are best described by use of verbs subject to few interpretations. Terms such as *to believe, to feel, to know, to be aware of*, which denote an internal state of mind, should be avoided because such words cannot be evaluated except as they are manifested in observable behavior. Action verbs subject to few interpretations are *identify, list, compare, contrast, interpret, apply, classify, predict, determine, state, differentiate, relocate, develop*, or *reduce*. A plan may state "Reduce the severity and frequency of accidents," or "Revise the appraisal performance system," or "Introduce a nursing audit program."
6. Objectives should be specific and indicate their linkage to the group on which their execution depends and interrelationships with other departments or groups.
7. Objectives should emphasize the uniqueness of the plan in achievement of hospital goals. An objective should be important to the hospital employees, serve a community health need, or create interrelationships with local and state social and educational agencies or institutions.
8. Objectives may be described in terms of a main objective with specifically stated subobjec-

tives. This type of objective may be used in describing an in-service supervisory program or for inpatient teaching. For example, a plan to train team leaders may have a subobjective of developing skills in conducting nursing team conferences on the care of patients who are acutely ill or of training team leaders to make out team members' assignments based on complexity of patients' needs, workers' skill, and job descriptions.

9. Objectives may be described precisely in their meaning by stating the important conditions under which action is expected to occur and by specifying the criteria of acceptable performance. A plan to render care for detoxification of drug addicts may state "Allocate facilities for men and women drug addicts in a methadone maintenance program, employ trained professional and technical workers, and coordinate activities with related community agencies." Objectives that require planning under specific conditions should state the minimum acceptable performance and the time limit for accomplishing the objective.

10. An objective must be reasonably attainable by the lower-level plannners and in manpower resources.

Developing programs and schedules

A department head should develop a program for each specific objective. This means writing out an abbreviated statement of all steps to be undertaken to accomplish the objective. Each step of a program should be accompanied by a schedule including starting and completion times. The steps of a program using the PERT approach have been described in Chapter 6.

The key points to programming and scheduling include (1) providing improvement through continual study of new methods such as peer review and auditing, research findings, and other data that focus on new thinking and innovations, (2) coordinating programs and schedules at each level and securing approval by supervisors, and (3) ensuring confident action from the staff members, and keeping a high degree of stability to withstand daily operational pressures. Vital changes should be made only if necessary to the success of the objective.

The particular mix of broad attainable and immediate objectives is associated with various levels of the hierarchy. The higher the organizational level, the more focus on broader objectives, and the lower the organizational level, the keener the focus on more precise immediate objectives.

The development and communication of organizational and individual objectives are important because they provide the framework for coordinated effort.[10,12] Organizational objectives give purpose and meaning to all personnel.

Planned and managed change is the present method administrators should use to move the staff toward a specific predetermined objective. The steps in the planned and managed change process include the following: (1) the staff evaluates the situations that create dissatisfaction with present conditions; (2) the staff establishes new objectives; (3) the staff develops a plan to research objective; (4) the department head and staff implement the plan using resources of the organization; (5) the department head and staff get feedback on results achieved; and (6) the department head and staff reevaluate and adjust the objectives or the plan.

As Lewis Carroll[3] so aptly put it:

Alice said, "Would you tell me, please, which way I ought to go from here?" "That depends a good deal on where you want to get to," said the Cat. "I don't know where," said Alice. "Then it doesn't matter which way you go," said the Cat.

REFERENCES

1. Allen, L. A.: Professional management—new concepts and proven practices, New York, 1973, McGraw-Hill Book Co., chapters 5 and 6.
2. Cantor, M.: Philosophy, purpose and objectives: why do we have them? Journal of Nursing Administration 3:21-25, July-Aug., 1973.
3. Carroll, L.: The annotated Alice—Alice's adventures in wonderland, New York, 1960, Clarkson N. Potter, Inc., p. 89.
4. Chapra, A.: Motivation in task-oriented groups, Journal of Nursing Administration 3:55-60, Jan.-Feb., 1973.
5. Drucker, P. F.: The practice of management, New York, 1954, Harper & Row, Publishers, Inc.
6. Etzioni, A.: The semiprofessions and their organization, New York, 1969, The Free Press.
7. Hicks, H. G.: The management of organizations: a system and human resources approach, ed. 3, New York, 1976, McGraw-Hill Book Co., chapters 3, 4, and 5.
8. Humble, J.: Management by objectives, New York, 1971, McGraw-Hill Book Co.

9. Joint Commission on Accreditation of Hospitals: Accreditation manual for hospitals, Chicago, 1976, The Commission.

10. Kalab, D. A., and Bayatzis, R. E.: Goal setting and self-directed behavior change. In Kalab, D.A.: Organizational psychology, Englewood Cliffs, N.J., 1971, Prentice-Hall, Inc.

11. Koontz, H., and O'Donnell, C.: Principles of management, ed. 5, New York, 1975, McGraw-Hill Book Co.

12. Lawrence, P. R., and Lorsch, J. W.: The relationship between organizations and their environment are examined. In Irwin, R. D.: Organization and environment, Homewood, Ill., 1969, Richard D. Irwin, Inc.

13. Luthans, F.: Introduction to management—a contingency approach, New York, 1975, McGraw-Hill Book Co., p. 50.

14. McClelland, D. C.: An introduction to motivation, Princeton, N. J., 1964, The Van Nostrand Publishing Co.

15. Masssee, J. L., and Douglas, L.: Managing—a contemporary introduction, Englewood Cliffs, N.J., 1973, Prentice-Hall, Inc.

16. Odiorne, G. S.: Management by objectives, New York, 1972, Pitman Pubishing Corp.

17. Palmer, J.: Management by objectives, Journal of Nursing Administration 3:59, March, 1973.

18. Schlolfeldt, R.: Planning for progress, Nursing Outlook 21(12):766-769, 1973.

19. Vroom, V. H.: Work and motivation, New York, 1964, John Wiley & Sons, Inc.

8 Planning, policies, and procedures

Effective planning for a department, a division, or for an entire institution involves four major aspects of planning that contribute to organizational purposes, goals, managerial operations, guides for decision making, and standards of control. Planning always precedes the execution of any managerial function or course of action.

The efficiency of a plan must be measured by the degree to which it contributes to goals and objectives, offset by the costs in human and material resources and other actions required to formulate and activate the plan.

All plans derive from organizational goals and encompass courses of future action. In general, plans may be classified as purposes or missions, objectives, strategies, policies, rules procedures, programs, projects, and budgets.

PLANNING

Planning is one of the most basic managerial functions of the systems approach for accomplishment of the goals of departments, their subparts, and the hospital system as a whole.

Definition and role

Planning may be defined in broad or explicit terms. In general, it is selecting the best course of action when alternative courses of action are discovered that may resolve a problem. *Planning is deciding in advance what to do, how to do it, when to do it, and who is to do it.* In other words, planning is a cognitive process for decision making. If we accept the definition given by Kast and Rosenzweig,[7] nursing services'

planning function is an integrative, evolving activity that seeks to maximize the total effectiveness of the department as a subsystem of the patient care system in accordance with the goals and objectives of the department that enhance those of the total system. The management planning function emphasizes the planning process in terms of systems relationships. For example, the personnel budget plan for nursing services is the input contributed by team leaders, supervisors, and department heads to meet specific nursing objectives and by the executive planning staff of the hospital, who are linked to the plan through the organizational structure and the goals of the total system.

Thus a plan has three characteristics: (1) it must involve the future, (2) it must involve actions, and (3) there is an organizational identification of the future course of action that will be taken by a particular planner or someone designated by him or for him within the organization. The planning process should generate multidisciplinary goals within the systems of the institution. A plan is a description of actions and anticipated results.

According to Goetz,[4] planning activities are of many different types. In the hospital system, management planning function includes the design of the total organizational structure and its goals, the design for the subsystems and their parts, selection of human and material resources, specification of policies and procedures, budgeting, allocation and scheduling of human and material productive designs, educational and training programs, and revision of structures and objectives to meet new needs and goals.

In the hospital, all the varied activities of all the departments together make up the planning network by which the people in the organization govern themselves to meet the established goals. Thus a plan is created from any planning process. Organizational goals, policies, procedures, budgets, staffing, rules, in-service training and research programs, community care programs, facility projects, and strategies are the output of the planning process.

Johnson, Kast, and Rosenzweig[6] state that "Under the systems concept the planning process can be considered as a vehicle for accomplishment of system change." From a practical planning viewpoint, the hospital is a social organization composed of three basic resources: (1) physical, in the form of plant, equipment, supplies, machinery, and inventory; (2) human, in the form of physicians, nurses, technicians, administrators, supervisors, engineers, social workers, accountants, and many other workers; and (3) financial resources, in the form of money, securities, borrowing power, and other assets. Thus the principal function of the total hospital industry is to convert these resources into services that will accomplish the objectives of the total hospital system. In short, in each hospital the executive officers are obliged to optimize the hospital's total resource conversion efficiency. This means to organize, to control costs, to produce, to develop management lines, and to offer patients services in such a way as to get the greatest performance possible out of its materials and personnel manpower hours in the daily operation of the system. Prior to executing these administrative activities, the staff must participate in planning them.

Because of the application of scientific medical advances in patient care, the demand for complex expensive equipment, machinery, and highly skilled workers brings up the relevancy of the hospital's present ability to initiate new patient care services and programs. The planning groups will need to find answers in relation to how they are making use of their present human and material resources for particular services and programs. The planners may ask themselves, "Would it be more profitable and beneficial to the consumer of health care to combine certain resources for specific services or programs?" Should the organizational structure of the hospital system be reorganized so that several services and programs can be combined under one system? Should the hospital continue to use resources for particular services or other outputs such as education of personnel, students, and medical workers? Would it be more profitable to patients and the community to combine certain resources for a specified service or program? In other words, through the planning process the hospital's resources are allocated to those subsystems that offer the greatest potential return and meet established goals and objectives.

The systems concept of planning for services and programs charges all administrators of each system such as the medical, nursing, materials-management, financial and business, informational, and personnel and eduation systems to work together within the multidimensional framework of the total hospital system. Under this concept, nursing service, as any other subsystem of patient care services, is no longer required to adapt to changing requirements in isolation.

Purpose of the planning process

The purpose of a plan is to bring about behavior that leads to desired actions and outcomes. The planning function aims to provide a framework for integrated decision making that is vital to every individual who works in the hospital. Plans are the guides by which people in the various organizational subsystems interact with each other. Planning provides the primary source of coordination toward defined and mutual goals in each system and in the hospital system as a whole.

Decision making and planning are closely intertwined; however, a decision is not a plan but basically a resolution of alternative choices. Decisions are necessary at every stage in the planning process and therefore are closely linked to planning (Figs. 6-4 and 8-2).

Long- and short-term planning

It is true that current actions greatly influence the potential range of future actions, and planners must work within the latitude required for future action. For example, recent legislative acts support consumer demands for a more definite role in health care planning and in evaluating its quality. Supported by the Patients' Bill of Rights, patients who enter the hospital are aware of their health needs and demand that these needs be met (see Chapter 4). This means nursing administration must change its attitudes toward patients and review its existing policies for the future.

A long-term plan looks ahead as far as possible and visualizes a desired need result. When this desired result is clarified and approved by the superior body, the intermediate steps of planning are developed. The number of years an institution will look ahead depends on what decisions are made, the anticipated environmental assumptions (premises), and the anticipated resource expenditures involved over a period of time to accomplish the desired results. Some decisions will influence the goals and objectives of nursing services in the institution. Nursing administrators must be aware of the nursing implications of such long-term decisions as they determine plans for the immediate future. Management researchers emphasize that planning should always be formulated from the distant year to the present. What is done the first year should provide the foundation and the direction for movement through each successive year. Thus, there is an integral relationship between short- and long-range plans to attain specific goals[1,3] (Fig. 8-1).

The selection of short-term plans proceeds from an evaluation of priorities related to long-range plans. Long-term planning frequently places a different perspective on short-term plans. For example, an institution may decide to build a new medical and surgical inpatient facility or an ambulatory facility 4 years hence to meet potential consumer demands within the areawide regional planning standards assisted by governmental funding. The priorities of a short-term plan to improve existing surgeries and intensive care facilities change in relation to the long-range plans.

Such changes in planning influence the long- and short-range plans for nursing in relation to organizational structure and leadership, as well as influencing personal and material resources. An institution may decide to close its school of nursing 5 years hence and become associated with a community college offering technical health programs. The nurse-administrator responsible for planning will develop short-term plans to meet this long-range plan.

A short-term plan determines what to do in the immediate prescribed future. Planning for 1 year differs in many respects from

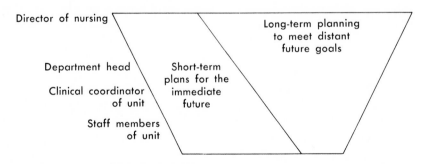

Fig. 8-1. Planning at different levels of the organizational structure and the time mix on planning activities by individuals in various positions in the organization. (From The management of organizations; a systems and human resources approach by Hicks, H. G. Copyright 1976, McGraw-Hill Book Company. Used with permission of McGraw-Hill Book Company.)

planning for 3- or 5-year periods. Short-term plans involve the immediate commitment of resources and must be clearly understood by the individuals who will be involved in carrying them out. A short-term plan must be precise and relatively inflexible.[2,13] For once it is initiated it may be expensive to change. For example, the type and ability of the personnel employed today will largely determine the quality of manpower input in a department in the next 3 years. Thus, current decisions tend to affect future actions.

The changing complexity of inpatient care, the upgrading of the standards of nursing practices, the increased costs of health care, and the implementation of management research techniques all influence long- and short-term plans for nursing services. A nursing service long-term plan may be to increase the professional nurse input by 50%, decrease the nonprofessional input by 60%, and reallocate supportive nonnursing duties to other hospital departments to provide optimal quality of nursing care services wthout increasing overall costs. This 4-year long-term plan would involve planning changes in the organizational structure and managerial processes of nursing services and other departments. The nursing service short-term plans, based on important priorities, would be developed to meet specific objectives for each year and to attain the long-term plan.

Short-range objectives help to achieve intermediate and long-range plans. It is necessary to draw a plan for accomplishing each objective and to combine them into a master plan for logical, consistent, and pragmatic evaluation.

Planning at different levels

The logical approach to the planning processes is determined by top executive officers and communicated to all interested groups. For instance, the director of nursing is the individual delegated to determine plans directly associated with nursing services such as in-service training and staff development, staffing and standards, and the input needed from other professional colleagues. The plans submitted by nursing

service are fed into the total managerial planning structure for decision making.

Administrative guides for planning have advantages in that they provide (1) a basis for unified and integrated planning, (2) the direction that detailed planning should take, (3) a basis for the performance of the control function and at the same time encouragement to accomplish known plans, (4) a basis for well-defined delegation of responsibility and authority to lower-level planners, and (5) a basis for coordination of activities between linked subunits and between diverse and functional units at the lower levels of management within the organization. Each subgoal generated by this process gives rise to lower-level planning, which in turn may generate still lower-level subgoals as a means of achieving goals.

Higher-level officers refers to executive administrative officers or department heads of medical, nursing, and other services. Lower-level officers refers to those who belong to the lower echelon of top management and middle management in the organization. The term *planner* will be used to describe the person having decision-making authority for planning at a given level in the organization.

Hierarchy of planning process for integrated decision making

A plan serves as a formal vehicle for communication throughout the organization. Thus the administrative officer's act of choosing and approving a plan submitted by a lower-level unit of management constitutes one of the most important functions of management. On approval, a plan becomes part of a network of plans that serves as the basis for execution, coordination, evaluation, and modification, if necessary.[9,18] The plans of the hospital only become operational after they become the plans of its subsystems and units of the total system (Fig. 8-1).

Description of plans

A plan may continue in effect until it is formally rescinded or modified by a higher-level plan or by higher levels in the organization that govern lower-level performance. Nursing objectives and procedures may be modified in keeping with changing medical/nursing practices, or ad hoc plans such as periodic budgets and schedules may be devised to describe behavior over a specified time period.

Some plans may be expressed in a functional form in which the values of certain variables in the beginning are not specified. For instance, a "variable" manpower budget might describe a resource input such as cost of four clinical specialists or 15 staff nurses as a function of output or the quality and quantity of manhours for patient service. The functional, organizational relationships must be established and a specific plan determined. The plan must be evaluated to discover the unspecified variables.

A plan may be explicit, leaving little discretion to those responsible for its execution. A plan may also constrain or require only certain actions as in the case of a wage salary policy that requires the nursing service division to pay individuals specific wages in certain positions. However, the supervisory staff may have opportunities to recommend merit increases to individuals based on performance in accordance with established salary ranges.[14]

Any significant additions, deletions, or modifications of an approved plan should be effected only through the same official approval mechanism that first authorized the plan. This type of control system is essential to assure the original planner that objectives will not be thwarted. In other words, a control system aims to "close the loop." Planners at all levels in the organization can view the latest plan network as a reliable source of information for execution and further planning.

The hierarchial nature of planning is manifested in three primary ways: (1) the scope of planning, (2) degree of aggregation of planning variables, and (3) the time sequence in which the planning occurs.

High-level planners concern themselves with broad issues of organizational activity and time, thus providing for more precise accomplishment of the total objectives of the organization as a whole. The high-level "stra-

tegic" plan may describe behavior for the entire organization or for a major portion of it. High-level planners use aggregate data for such dimensions as time, manpower, operational units, functions, and cost classifications. In the process of elaborating high-level plans, each level in the planning hierarchy continues to add information to the description of intended behavior.

The planner is responsible for achieving the transition of the approved plan into lower-level plans in a manner that maintains consistency and coordination between levels. A complete set of plans throughout the organization constitutes a precise hierarchical description of intended actions. The plans at all levels describe portions of the same total behavior.

The lower-level planners deal with detailed disaggregated data; however, at the lowest planning level, plans normally do not describe every detail. Because of the resource constraints set by high-level planners, the lower-level planners must recognize the availability of such resources as managerial talents, manpower, and materials. Lower-level planning pertains to limited activities and extends over a relatively short span of time. The higher-level plan affects the actual behavior of staff members and things only indirectly through lower-level planning.

The organizational system must rely on hierarchial consistency of coordination to achieve productive behavior that is directed to the accomplishment of its overall objectives.[17] Realistic planning requires that high-level planners assess the detailed implications of different alternatives. To achieve this, planners can no longer rely on information about past performance. They must have access to a much larger source of information to determine the probable consequences of nontested plans. If information is not available to planners, they must choose a plan without detailed consideration of the lower-level plans used to implement it.

To develop efficient, purposeful plans it is the major responsibility of the chief executive officers to develop and maintain a proper planning system that is appropriate to the organization. In a large hospital, the department heads in the division of nursing service are delegated responsibilities for evaluating the alternatives. Planners at the various levels of the hierarchy must be sure of their delegated responsibilities. Clarification of the roles of participants in the planning process is important.

Central control constraints

The range of acceptable plans presented by lower-level managers may be restricted by constraints imposed by the hierarchy of standing plans, policies, or a lack of precise information. Thus the lower-level planners may interpret constraints as a guide to assure that all phases of the plans of each subsystem conform to the overall goals of the hospital and provide explicit criteria with which the planner and assistants can assess the relative merits of alternatives open to them. Centralization of planning restricts lower-level actions. It is important that constraints imposed by high-level planners do not restrict the motivation and creativity of lower-level planners.

Higher-level planners may not be able to determine all important interactions; however, lower-level planners should still have some guides to the expected behavior of closely related units. The lower-level planners must know the general schedule before they can establish their own schedule. Thus lower-level planners should at least be able to formulate their own schedules with some knowledge about the changes through which they interact with other units. For instance, the weekly staffing schedules may constrain actual management of nursing care. Guided by the staffing schedules, each supervisor must transform manpower input into units of patient care. This requires breaking down the weekly staffing input into detailed plans. Staffing information is reported to the high-level planners responsible for the overall staffing plan. If deviations become significant, replanning may be required to alter the staffing plan in light of current variables such as an increase or decrease in the number of patients or their requirements for nursing care.

Each planning process is subject to con-

straints of some kind. Each subsystem can improve its performance by making appropriate adjustments to constraint through a continual process of hierarchial adaptation. Whenever possible, the organization should identify the effects of change and make those adjustments that bring improvements. Thus adaptation is a continuous search process.[15] If nursing service desires to exert a fundamental influence on the behavior of the organizational system, it must do so primarily through improvements in the planning process. It is the process that generates the plans. Adaptation takes place through changes in the planning process of the total system. Nursing leaders should be alert to the causes of inadequate planning, not its symptoms.

Control process

Control of the approved plan compares the actual performance against the plan. The planning system should determine and report significant deviations that require management attention. The high-level planners establish control tolerances for each relevant variable. For instance, deviations in budgeting of manhours, materials, and policies are reported.

Information feedback to management serves three important functions. It encourages more realistic planning, closer adherence to approved plans, and a control system that guards against excessive deviations from current plans and reduces the amount of coordinative activities.

The information feedback also provides a hierarchy of responses to reported deviations and provides information for adaptation. The identification and correction of deficiencies in the planning process provide a method for the organization to achieve basic improvements through adaptation.

Information technology has advanced to the point where large man-machine planning systems are technically and economically feasible in the hospital industry. The planning process largely governs performance; thus basic improvements in patient services must become a reality through better planning.

Developing and implementing plans results from using the talents of people, as well as the data-handling capacity of the computer. Man's ability to reason, improve, innovate, make judgments, and recognize complex patterns makes him an essential contributor to high-level planning.

Interrelationships

In each of the different types of plans there is a wide variety of detailed plans ranging from broad high-level goals and objectives covering the operations of the entire organization to detailed plans for activities of each subsystem in the hospital system. In the systems concept of planning one must recognize that *interrelationships of all planning activities are vital for the accomplishment of any plan and goals of the hospital.*

The administrative officer of the division of nursing is a member of the hospital management team. The nursing department heads, clinical specialists, and supervisors serve on hospital committees that are composed of representatives of related subsystems of the total hospital system. The organizational structure of nursing service, including committee participation, is discussed in Chapter 9. In this structure individuals with particular specialized skills have an opportunity to contribute to the improvement of patient care. The planning system offers opportunities to nursing service to feed into the total hospital system. This concept helps nursing service to remove traditional walls and to work with other administrators and managers of other services. The systems concept should enhance the health team concept in the clinical care of patients, as previously discussed in this chapter.

The higher the position individuals hold in the organization, the farther into the future they must plan. For example, directors of nursing may spend a majority of their planning activities on broad nursing service goals and objectives, orienting staff and others to the plans and evaluating short-term plans (Fig. 8-1).

Department heads will spend considerable time planning activities that are expected to be attained within the year and in evaluating the results of programs, policies, and procedures in accordance with established objectives.

The clinical coordinators and senior staff nurses of each subunit will be concerned with immediate short-term plans and their results. They will develop and evaluate monthly staffing inputs and schedules of their unit and policies and procedures that influence staff and department goals and performance.

Strategies

Strategy sets long-range and broad plans, and associated tactics define the many short-range maneuvers required to implement the strategic plan. Strategies are overall plans of the higher management system to achieve objectives. Tactical strategy may be used by employees in middle or lower management to meet individual plans that contribute toward desired results. For example, a nurse administrator may decide to implement a plan to employ nurse-clinical specialists for inpatient nursing services and nurse-practitioners in ambulatory services in next year's program without increasing the costs of manpower resources or decreasing the quality of nursing care.

This administrator is willing to risk hiring this type of nurse to improve nursing care. To make this plan succeed the administrator must initiate tactical strategic decisions, explaining and describing each position's qualifications and salary, and the interorganizational and intraorganizational relationships these nurses will have with other professional nurses and related health professionals as they assist in providing direct nursing care to patients. In long-term plans that introduce individuals in new nursing positions, the nurse administrator works with department heads, who in turn secure opinions from clinical coordinators and team leaders of the units. The nurse administrator secures the ideas and support of the top executive administrator and medical representatives using analytical facts and possible tactical strategies.

Strategy, although a subjective planning process, should be viewed as a decision on how to use resources to attain desired goals when dealing with difficult conditions, individuals' attitudes and opinions, and other possible barriers. Planners are most attentive to forecasting the future behavior of specific environmental factors and in formulating alternative courses of action regarding expected events. Tactical plans are rather narrow and flexible in scope, focusing more on details (see Fig. 8-2).

Strategies result from the process of deciding on organizational objectives or changing them to implement desired programs and policies. Strategies may be classified under the following three major types: (1) external social strategies, (2) external economic strategies, and (3) internal organizational strategies.[20,21]

Strategies adopted to reduce conflicts. In all institutions various kinds of strategies are adopted by management to control the conflict between groups and reduce the tension and stresses between people. Nurses should realize that the degree of conflict existing among professional and technical workers outside the hospital per se greatly influences the tensions within. For instance, physicians' lack of understanding of nursing practice and vice versa and the desire of groups to control the boundaries of nursing practice cause conflicts and tensions between health workers in providing efficient economical services

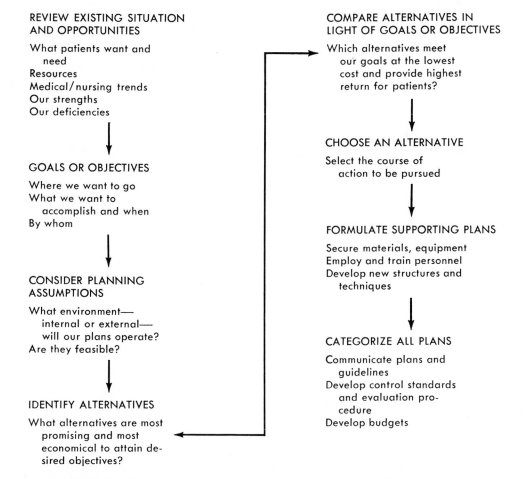

Fig. 8-2. Steps of the planning process. (From Principles of management, ed. 6, by Koontz, H., and O'Donnell, C. Copyright 1976, McGraw-Hill Book Company. Used with permission of McGraw-Hill Book Company.)

to patients. Labor organizations may create pressures on hospital leaders and conflicts among the personnel.[2]

What is an acceptable range of conflict and tension that can be tolerated at various levels in the hospital strategy? The controlling officers may accept one of several strategies. For instance, through verbal and written communications, the controlling officers may make every effort to resist all professional and technical group campaigning for collective bargaining and for particular agreements concerning their role in decision making in the hospital system. Or the controlling officers may apply the fragmentation process by which particularly complex activities are assigned to people in several subunits. The application of this type of strategy means that no one group has controlling operational jurisdiction over any one function. This type of so-called game strategy has many implications for nursing service because of its pivotal location in patient care services.

Qualitative and quantitative goals

The hospital as a social open system has primary basic functions assigned to it by society. The nursing services, as an integral system of the institution, develops primary purposes and goals that support the institution's overall goals. In developing goals, the nurse administrator and staff view and evaluate the existing system and concentrate on the desired direction of movement of the nursing organization.[16] The purpose, organizational goals, and objectives of nursing services have been discussed in Chapter 7.

Planning establishes the objectives necessary for group effort. Plans are the foundation of management,[11] and the actions of staff members are aimed toward goals or objectives. The goals of nursing service constitute the basic plan of the division and its departments.

The nature of overall objectives and management by nursing objectives have been discussed in Chapter 7. Most qualitative goals cannot be reasonably quantified.[5] In the management of nursing care of patients the administrators should not depend too

heavily on staffing numbers since their pleasing accuracy can be misleading in relation to the quality of care. However, many qualitative goals of nursing can be verified, although not with the accuracy possible in quantitatively stated objectives. For example, the in-service training department's goal may be to develop and implement a new program for clinical coordinators with specified characteristics by a certain date. Qualitative goals can be verified by stating precisely the nature of the elements of the program, the objectives to be attained and evaluated, and the date of accomplishment.

The objective may intend to make more effective use of clinical coordinators' knowledge and skills in providing optimal nursing care to patients. In some situations qualitative objectives are evaluated by the standard of "how well" the individual performs.

Quantitative objective usually are gauged by "how much," but without a workable coordinated set of plans and objectives, budget figures become a planner's desires and guesses. Budget figures are results of plans and expected performance. A budget reflects joint planning of all components of the division of nursing with assistance and input from accounting, personnel, and other sources. Budgeting techniques are discussed in Chapter 15.

POLICIES

All hospitals have policies—written, unwritten, or implied, sound or unsound, understood or not understood, complete or incomplete, and followed or not followed. One should consider the sources of policy decision making in the organization.[14] Policies are referred to as standing plans and are used repeatedly.

Purposes and values

Top management originates policies for the express purpose of guiding managers and other workers in the daily operations of the organization. Policies are guides that stem from the goals of the hospital, whether they are defined by the board of trustees or the executive officers. Policies originating from the controlling body may be broad in scope or may be defined in precise terms having little need for interpretation.

It would be almost impossible for an executive officer or a supervisor to share authority with others in an institution without policies. Without policies to guide the managerial staff in the daily activities of patient care services, they are unaware of the appropriate, desired, and correct decisions intended by the controlling officers. Policies should express the attitudes and opinions of the executive officers about the range of behavior within which they will permit or desire others to act. Policies that reflect the thinking of executive officers and management staff serve as a point around which the all efforts can be coordinated to meet the objectives of the subunits and those of the hospital as a whole.

Policies should be considered a part of the hospital's planning process. Frequently, the traditional bureaucratic structure of the hospital prevents coordination of policy planning because of the compartmentalization, fragmentation, and isolationism of departments. Planning by objectives and policies pressures medicine, nursing, and managers of hospital support services to coordinate their goals for the improvement of the patient care system.

Well-defined policies give potential employees and other interested groups information that reflects the philosophy and objectives of the hospital's systems. The policies inform the employees of how satisfied and secure they can expect to be in their jobs. To professionals and highly trained technical workers, the written hospital management, clinical, medical, and nursing policies assure them of how they may work with others in carrying out nursing practices and activities in the care of patients. Policies serve as guides in the workers' appraisal of the hospital's intended, as well as its present, behavior in achievement of objectives.

The formation of written policies can actually be a labor-saving device that curtails innumerable written and verbal communications concerning problems demanding daily attention. Policies provide guides to assure safe patient care. They give the direction

that all people require to do their jobs efficiently and with personal satisfaction. Written policies emphasize that the hospital is a social organization managed by people for people.

When executive officers approve an objective to train professional nurses to perform specific procedures requiring medical judgmental assessment, it becomes a policy; thus policies give direction and authority to those responsible for achieving objectives. The input in formulating policies should come from professionals who have responsibilities associated with the policy. For instance, the policy for licensed practical nurses to administer certain medications requires input from the pharmacy/therapeutic committee, in-service training director, personnel department, and medical committee of the hospital, as well as the administrative nursing service council.

Policy decision making is a superior order of activity in executive responsibility that leads to the establishment of appropriate procedures. It is important that those who set policies and those who engage in developing crucial procedures work together within the structured system. Both a policy and its procedures must fit together and contribute to the major objectives of the hospital. Once a policy decision has been issued, it serves as a guideline to supervisory staff as they establish derivative policies for those in the lower levels of the system.

Policy aims to create uniformity of operations throughout the organization and provide similarity of actions in resolving similar problems. Clear, written policy statements assure patients and employees of uniform decisions.

Characteristics and outcomes

There are many different types of policy considerations associated with the hospital industry. As in all businesses, there are policies connected with providing patient services; purchasing drugs, equipment, and supplies; type and volume of services; inventory of resources; and controlling financial inputs and outputs. There are policies dealing with cash, working capital, investments, capital procurement, depreciation allowances, hospital personnel, and public relations.

In most hospitals the largest group of policies is concerned with personnel and other supporting services such as nursing, dietary, maintenance, engineering, and public relations. The nursing service management group should have a good understanding and keen awareness of the business policies of the hospital to interpret them to others and to use them effectively.

The degree of centralization or decentralization of authority within the organizational structure will determine how policies are formulated and initiated. Frequently, regardless of the structural organization, the managers of subsystems are charged with originating policies for approval by the executive officer. In some situations the executive planning group decides how policy is to be initiated.

Policies may stem from a pressing problem concerning conflicting behavior of people in a particular situation. As incidents are taken up for decisions, certain actions take precedence over all others and become policies for future managerial actions. Policy decisions arising from urgent appeals of managers and supervisors may be incomplete, uncoordinated, and confusing. Frequently such policies are made on the basis of a given set of facts, without evaluating the possible effects on other aspects of the operation. When unidentified derivatives develop from a policy, it may not guide the thinking and actions of subordinates as really desired by the top executive officers. To provide for effective coordination of all policies to achieve the hospital's objectives and goals, top executives should be made aware of any policy that is formulated and dispersed to any level in the organization.

The so-called implied policy may arise from instances where the stated policy is not enforced. In such situations the organization may desire a certain kind of *image policy* but is unable or unwilling to enforce it. Or an implied policy may develop when there is no stated policy. When policies are not available, supervisors and others tend to adopt their own unwritten guidelines. Those individuals who promote unwritten policies, consciously or unconsciously, usually believe they are helping to achieve the goals of the hospital. For instance, a hospital may have a stated policy of promoting from within; but if the workers see available positions filled with outsiders or the absence of development programs to qualify insiders for promotion, the implied policy will be understood to be different from the stated policy. In a complex situation the top executive may not develop a written policy. Difficulties also arise when those who submit ideas are never informed of what action is to be taken to meet the objectives or resolve the problem.

Nonconformity of action may occur when a policy is quickly revised and initiated to fit a new plan. A policy should be developed in advance when there are indications that many questions will be asked concerning a proposed plan. For instance, when the executives agree to revise the salary structure or the patient admission and discharge policy, time is needed to orient those individuals who will be interpreting the policies and revising procedures to fit the written policies (see Chapters 11 and 12).

A policy involving different groups of people with different values, attitudes, and desires should be stated in terms of the hospital's needs, with due consideration for compromise.

In some cases, department heads should not forget the concept of management by exception, used as far back as Jethro's advice to Moses in the Bible, that only exceptional matters should be brought to Moses' attention. Frederick Taylor advocated management by exception (see Chapters 6 and 11).

Policies require that people use a high level of reasoning and judgment in the interpretation and implementation of a particular policy. For example, nursing service may have a policy that states "To assure optimal patient care and to give all personnel holiday time and days off together during the period between Christmas and New Years, employees are advised not to request vacation during this period, except those who are assigned to areas where patient care services are greatly reduced." This kind of derivative policy gives guidelines to division heads and supervisors and should be written in advance. Each supervisor should make sure that all coworkers understand the policy. Such policies should be carefully reviewed with new employees during their orientation to their role and job in the hospital. The management function of motivating and directing personnel is important for effective results and good human relations.

Every action requires thinking through each problem, evaluating the alternatives, and making a correct decision that follows both the policies of the hospital and, if possible, the desires of the employees. The supervisor who is delegated to take appropriate action concerning policies may have difficulty in applying management by exception, preferring to consider the policy as a rule with no exceptions. It may be correct for the supervisor to make an exception to the policy and give a vacation during the Christmas season to an employee who has an urgent request. Policies that do not specify action or stipulate penalties require that the department head or the supervisor exercise initiative as well as direction.

Policies range from broad major policies covering major departments to minor or derivative policies applicable to the subunits of the total system. For instance, the hospitals' written personnel policies state the working hours of employees, vacation allowances for all categories of workers, compensation, health, and pension benefits for all employees, and the like. Each subsystem may find it necessary to have derivative policies to meet the objectives of the system. The nursing service may have a written derivative guide concerning the number of evening and night shift employees who may be required to work during each fiscal year if they are employed on a rotation plan (Chapter 9). As situations change, the nursing service executive staff should study the desires of the employees and the anticipated nursing service demands and revise the policy within the boundaries of the hospital's overall objectives and policies. All derivative policies should have the support and approval of the executive officer of the system.

Policies, as descriptions of actions, provide a plan representing "messages" through which supervisors may communicate to their staff members and provide guidance and a feeling of assurance to all in the system.

Policies affecting nursing practice

Today many professional registered nurses carry out complex procedures requiring careful assessment that were formerly done by physicians. Physicians' assistants, physicians' nurse-associates, and nurse-practitioners are also performing tasks formerly considered medical procedures. In the face of malpractice suits, hospital and professional liability costs, and the need to clarify the functions of various employees in the institution, nursing service policy involving an area in nursing practice should be clearly defined in accordance with the nursing practice state law and the standards recommended by official accreditating agencies and professional health associations.

For example, the program and procedural plan for closed chest cardiac resuscitation, emergency cardiopulmonary resuscitation, and other complex procedures should include the tasks that may be performed by the trained professional nurse, the qualifications, experience, and the kind of training program required for this nurse, and evaluation measures to assure competence prior to acceptance of the responsibilities stipulated in the policy. The plan should provide for period review of the policy as the practice of nursing and medicine changes to meet patients' needs.

Policy procedure for the assessment of the quality of nursing care being provided to patients is now being defined. This tool should be reasonably objective, reliable, easy to use, accurate, and closely associated with a description of procedures and methods used[19,22,23] (see Chapters 16 and 17).

RULES

Rules issued by the executive officers, department heads, and supervisors of each subsystem should specifically state what must be done or what may not be done. Like policies, rules are designed to influence the conduct of patients, workers, and others in the hospital. Rules are plans in that they are courses of required actions that, like objectives, are chosen from many alternatives. They describe specific, definite actions to be taken or not taken with respect to a situation. Rules do not allow for deviations from a required course of action and in no way interfere with procedure for handling orders. For instance, "No Smoking" is a rule.

PROGRAMS

The term *programs* represents policies, procedures, projects, and other elements required to carry out a given course of action. Based on the demands of the systems, such as patient care, ambulatory care, education and in-service training, diagnostic and laboratory systems, and others, hospital resources are coordinated and utilized by means of programs.

Resources for programs to meet goals. Resources must be utilized to fit the program's needs and designed to accomplish the objectives of the total hospital system. To assist planners and others to meet the goals of the total hospital system objectives, policies and procedures are fomulated and initiated with inputs from the subsystems.

Through programs, internal processes can be matched with external goals and with marketing research orientation. The modern decision-making techniques for both programmed and nonprogrammed decisions suggest major changes with processes as compared with the traditional methods of planning. The scientific operations research approach, composed of mathematical analysis, computer simulation, and electronic data processing, is used in programming decisions (Chapter 6). For nonprogramming decisions heuristic problem-solving techniques may be applied.

One of the primary purposes of integrated programming processes is to provide a hierarchy of objectives, based on predetermined premises about the external and internal resources and the environmental behavioral processes necessary to achieve desired actions. As each department becomes more specialized and the activities to be done more complex, the planning and controlling become more complex, requiring expertise.

Programs interlocking within the systems

Programs may be classified as major or minor. A major program may consist of objectives and derivative objectives, policies and procedures stemming from those in different subsystems that are linked together by particular interfaces. For instance, a major objective may be to build a 30-bed specialty unit. Derivative objectives and policies are formulated by people in the various subsystems who will have interrelated input into the operations of the unit. Medicine, nursing, dietary, engineering, personnel, business and finance, and education and training systems will help formulate specific objectives and policies to utilize their resources effectively and efficiently for the accomplishment of the overall objectives of the program and hospital as a whole. High-level planners must see that the resources and programs mesh within the total system.

Thus building and operating a 30-bed patient unit involves physicians, nurses, administrators, engineers, architects, director of materials-management, educational and training representatives, and others in related subsystems (see Fig. 8-2).

Minor programs are those that do not involve many different subsystems. The business and finance system develops a budgetary mechanism so that the budget programs, cost accounting, and performance classifications become integrated into a plan. The budget usually implements a program through the development of objectives, policies, and procedures. These elements of the budgetary program of each system are closely interfaced with elements such as the measurements of manhour productivity and costs of the quality control system. Nursing service budgeting objectives are important to the financial business program. One of the important aspects of program budgeting of the cost and income control program is the input of those at the operational level. This is discussed in Chapters 11 and 15.

Nursing service departments may develop a nursing audit program. This program involves graduates in the various levels of the organization. However, the findings of this program may involve other related subsystems to accomplish the goals of the program and the patient care system (see Fig. 8-2).

To make certain that programs function effectively, policy and procedure guides are necessary, as are coordination of efforts and proper scheduling and timing. The failure of any part of the network of derivative objectives may mean delays in the accomplishment of the total program (see Fig. 6-5).

The subunits of each system and the programs tend to lend themselves to linear programming of resources for patient care and support services, teaching, and research purposes. The application of linear programming techniques, as described in Chapter 6, forces a clear-cut statement of goals and the kind of programs and resources required to meet these goals. Linear programming pressures people to state how limited resources are to be used to accomplish a particular objective at the lowest cost and highest productivity, at least when those resources have alternative uses. Through this type of programming the flow of resources for specific purposes is introduced into the management unit to accomplish the interrelated activities of the program.[8,11]

Any program should be significant enough to stand by itself in the system. However, many programs are part of a complex structure of programming dependent on several groups and affecting several systems. There is always interdependence, which at times makes planning and initiating programs difficult.

Constraints

Programs may be subject to constraints imposed by the existing structure, limitations of human and physical resources, inadequate information, or poor coordination. It is important to be aware of constraints because they will influence lower-level planners in the implementation of the programs. Constraint may be interpreted as guiding lower-level planners in a way to assure that all plans of each subsystem conform to the overall goals of the hospital. The constraints imposed by the executive planning group should provide explicit criteria so that lower-level planners can assess the relative merits of alternatives open to them. Constraints may be imposed by the hierarchy of standing programs, policies, or lack of informational data (see Chapter 12).

Centralization may restrict the activities of middle- and lower-level planners. For this reason restrictions should only be used to assure effective overall organizational behavior. In this age of specialization there are often pressures from several different departments or committees to initiate particular programs, policies, or objectives as they wish them to be. The planners are responsible for determining the priorities, using management research techniques.

Scheduling

A schedule can be defined as the time sequence necessary to carry out the steps of a program. Although a schedule is determined by program planners, it is independent of the program in that it can be changed without altering the program.[1]

In carrying out a schedule, planners should (1) develop the best way to do it by reviewing new innovations that will improve the operation; (2) develop a schedule at each level and coordinate it with the first level; (3) refrain from changing schedules unless absolutely necessary to provide stability and ensure effective, confident action from those who work together; (4) avoid overestimating time requirements for self-protection and insist on honest, realistic commitments so that superiors will stand by them; and (5) secure approval from superiors to implement the schedule.

Scheduling techniques used range from appointment books, patient reservations for the use of facilities, personnel staffing, and schedules for complex mathematical programming.

The Gantt chart,[9] a general purpose tool for scheduling, consists of a bar chart with time or dates on the horizontal axis and the factor to be scheduled on the vertical axis. Specific adaptation of Gantt charts can be used to show personnel assigned to specific nursing units, for equipment inventory control, or to show budgetary position vacancies.

Critical path analysis uses networks for scheduling program inputs or constructing facility projects and in research and development activities of a program that require time and performance estimates when it is important to identify the sequence of activities of the program.[9] PERT (program evaluation and review technique) is an accepted network technique for planning all links in a program. PERT and other scheduling and analysis techniques are discussed and illustrated in Chapter 6.

PROCEDURE

A procedure is considered a standing plan since it may be used more than once. A procedure provides a more specific guide to action than a policy. Nursing procedures in the care of patients aim to achieve a high degree of regularity and competent performance, support preventive maintenance of equipment and materials, and establish safety measures to protect individuals from bodily harm and potential hazards.[21a]

The steps of nursing care and managerial procedures are arranged in a logical predetermined order of actions to be taken. When a procedure is carefully planned and followed, labor and time are saved. An effective procedure includes the objective and the steps of the plan.

Managerial procedures help staff members and top-level administrators. For example, a personnel hiring procedure aims to ensure that the interviewer will cover all points in the selection of an applicant. This procedure includes past training and education, experience, previous work records, health, present job, test results, individual objectives, and the results of the interview. Each step in the sequence may eliminate some applicants, and the individual responsible for hiring is only required to interview several applicants instead of the entire group who originally applied for the position (see Chapter 17).

An example of a procedure policy that should be a part of the nursing service management manual is as follows:

Subject: Rotation policy for nursing service personnel

Objectives: To provide an appropriate and equitable distribution of man-hours for all categories of personnel for direct care of patients during the day, evening, and night shifts

To consider each individual's shift preference without jeopardizing the quality of nursing care services

To utilize in the most effective and economical way the manhours of various categories of workers, considering their job descriptions and competencies and patients' needs

To ensure implementation of fair labor standards as stated in the hospital personnel manual

Policy: In general, registered graduate nurses, supervisors (head nurses), licensed practical nurses, and auxiliary workers on a full-time status shall be required to work on two different shifts—the day shift and either the evening or night shift—during any given period, except during a permanent or long-range change of shift assignment.

An individual worker may work on a permanent basis during the evening or night shift, except during the orientation period or when it is necessary to attend a special in-service program conducted only during day hours.

Each individual who is working the evening or night shift by personal preference may request to work on a rotation shift plan by presenting a request in writing to his or her immediate superior at least 6 weeks in advance of scheduled rotation dates.

Each individual who is on the scheduled rotation system must work more manhours on a preference shift than on other shifts.

Each individual shall have at least 8 hours and preferably 12 hours between the time of completing one shift and beginning the next shift, except in cases of emergency.

The system of rotation chosen in consultation with the staff members shall be consistent.

The department heads, under the guidance of the director, and in accordance with the overall departmental staffing plan, shall have rotation schedules posted several weeks prior to the scheduled effective date, except in cases of emergency.

The regular part-time staff members shall be required to work an appropriate number of manhours, or two shifts, based on the total number of manhours worked each month, and their scheduled assignment shall be posted as for the full-time personnel.

Full- and part-time staff members who work in a unit where evening and night coverage is usually not required shall work those shifts when it is necessary or on a planned scheduled "on-call" system.

A desired number of full- and part-time staff members shall be assigned to work as the complementary (float) staff on the day, evening, and night shifts, according to variance in patient needs, turnover rate, and absentee rates for an established number of weeks during each year.

The occasional and regular part-time staff members who work 1 to 2 days a week shall be assigned to the complementary staff for a section or to units to which they have been oriented.

All personnel shall be informed in detail verbally and in writing of the rotation scheduling nursing service policy during their initial orientation, with follow-up by their immediate supervisors.

Nursing service procedural manuals

The nursing service procedural manual provides guidelines to ensure adherence to consistent recognized standards of nursing practice. Procedures should be developed on the basis of current scientific knowledge and the use of new equipment and current practices. Each procedure should be designed so that all aspects of its performance are clearly explained.

The nursing procedure manual provides a tool for training programs to enable new nursing service personnel to become acquainted with the standards of care to be followed. It provides a ready reference for the staff in each nursing care unit and service area, as well as other services and departments of the hospital. The procedure manual assists in the standardization of procedures and equipment and serves as a basis for evaluation and study to assure continued improvements in techniques. The procedure guides also are used in conducting the auditing of nursing care of patients.

The chief criteria for the policy and procedure format of nursing service manuals are simplicity and practicality. There is no one best format, but a manual must not be difficult to follow[10] (see Chapters 11 and 12 on communications). A few criteria may be considered:

1. A code system should be used to enable the reader to find the related policy and procedural statement.
2. All policies, procedures, and directives should be dated and signed by the executive officer.
3. The most common terminology used in the institution and the department should be included.
4. The purpose for the policy or procedure and a brief description of the directive should appear at the top of the document and be followed by actions to be taken.
5. Manuals can be divided into definite sections and subsections, each having its own number of pages that appear in the outline of contents of the manual. A cross-indexing system facilitates location of material. Nursing procedures may be organized under major headings such as the care of patients with circulatory, gastrointestinal, neurological, cardiopulmonary, cardiovascular, eye, throat, and orthopedic conditions.
6. Manuals should use loose-leaf notebooks so that policies can be readily removed or added to the section.
7. A plan should be developed and maintained for periodic review of policies and updating of the contents of each manual.

STEPS OF THE PLANNING PROCESS

Planning is accomplished through a sequence of steps, each dependent on the others to attain expected results and desired goals.

Influence of external and specific environmental factors

Planning assumptions may be thought of as arising from forces outside of the institution and from within (see Chapter 6).

Consider the patients, consumers, vendors, government agencies, and labor unions as external forces and the board of trustees, physicians, researchers, administrators, nurses, and other staff members as specific factors. The external forces influencing the institution generally are beyond the control of the nursing service administrators, even though such forces must be considered in planning for the future (see Fig. 6-7).

Koontz and O'Donnell[9] emphasize the importance of following a systematic planning approach (Fig. 8-2). The nursing service administrator is responsible for planning nursing services for the present and future, for examining existing strengths, deficiencies, and opportunities, and for initiating changes to improve the quality of nursing care. The administrator and the immediate assistants should discuss trends in nursing practices, new management techniques, and methodologies that might be innovated. Today nursing service administrators are obliged to consider changing concepts of patients toward their care needs, new legislative acts in health care planning, quality controls, changing collective bargaining laws for personnel, and conflicting groups' actions (see Chapter 4). Nursing service administrators should recognize the trends of specialization and the upgrading of the status of professional nurses, and the current standards of nursing practices and nursing services (see Chapter 5). An understanding of these forces and their implications for the future planning of the existing nursing service organization should be carefully considered.

Establishing organizational goals and objectives

The primary step in planning is to establish planning goals for the entire division of nursing and then for each department and its subunits.[12] The hierarchy of planning within an institution has been previously discussed in this chapter. The statement of goals and objectives for nursing services specify the expected results and emphasize the important actions to be undertaken by means of programs, procedures, and projects. Goals and objectives throughout the planning process have been discussed in Chapter 7.

Assessing strengths, deficiencies, and capabilities

Some management consultants prefer to call this process one of premising.[9] For effectiveness, top planners should establish and agree to use and disseminate critical planning assumptions (premises). They should agree to use specific forecast data of existing plans concerning programs, policies, and projects.

Coordinated actions will not take place when the administrator and the department heads use different factual data and the administrator does not provide specific and realistic guidelines to be followed. For example, nurse administrator, believing that planning should begin at the bottom, asked department heads to develop and submit their own manpower and equipment budgets. The administrator faced a dilemma on receiving a collection of inconsistent, unrealistic budgets that did not fit together to accomplish the goals for the entire division of nursing.

One must take into account the limitations as well as the resources of each situation when setting realistic priorities in planning. A plan will be useless if resources are not available to implement it. As previously mentioned, assessment involves answers to such questions as, Where are we at the present time? Where do we want to go? How do we get there? When do we do what? Who is to do it?

Planners may find general answers to important aspects of planning, such as, What changes should be made in the organizational structure and management processes to initiate effective team nursing? What kind of a program is needed to improve the existing nursing audit plan? What quality measurement techniques should be used to evaluate performance of personnel? What quantitative techniques should be used to attain better standards of control? What kind of a program should be implemented to reduce personnel turnover? (See Fig. 8-2.)

Alternative courses of action

In reviewing and evaluating the environment of the organization, anticipating costs to implement a plan, and determining priorities, it may be necessary to examine alternatives and choose the best course of action to achieve long-term goals or objectives. As previously mentioned, planners should be aware of the effect of short-term plans on the primary long-term plan.

Alternative courses of action are evaluated for their feasibility and their impact on both the quality of care and organizational objectives. For example, a plan may be to employ clinical nurse-specialists in inpatient services and nurse-practitioners in ambulatory services to upgrade the quality of nursing care. Another plan may assign only professional nurses for the direct nursing care of patients, supported by clerical and unit management personnel to perform indirect services to patients and the unit to utilize the knowledge and skills of personnel more effectively and economically in providing optimal care to each patient.

After examining a plan and reviewing the available resources and the existing conceptual environment, planners may agree this goal cannot be achieved within 2 years. Thus, alternative courses of action are determined to direct action toward the first goal. An alternative plan may be to initiate a project on one unit using the basic objectives of the first plan and to provide for the examination and evaluation of the results for future planning.

Selecting a plan of action

Selecting a plan of action requires decision making by the executive staff with assistance from the staff members of the units.

Formulating supportive plans

Formulating supportive plans may involve purchasing equipment and materials, securing personnel, setting up in-service training programs, and making organizational structure changes. Secondary plans may be required to support the basic plan.

The implementation of a plan requires many decision-making activities affecting the organization as a whole, and thus actions to be taken require clear, detailed directives from the nursing service administrator or the department heads to those individuals who will carry out the plan. Here, the questions of what, when, how, and where must be spelled out in simple language.

Evaluating the planning process

Every plan should provide a methodology to measure outcomes against objectives. Periodic progress checks shoud be built into the planning process as a means for modification prior to the planned evaluation period. Records must be kept to provide the data necessary for appraisal at definite times. Statistical data compiled by accounting, personnel, and administration staffs are needed to check quantitative phases of the plans. Review and assessment of patient care plans, observations of personnel performance in the direct care of patients, and conferences with supervisory and team leaders are needed to evaluate qualitative phases of actions.

Results from the total evaluation and standards of control must be fed back to department heads and staff members so that they can be considered in future planning. The criteria for formulating objectives have been discussed in Chapter 7, and the standards of control in Chapter 16.

BASIC MANAGERIAL CRITERIA IN PLANNING

Even though researchers cannot give us one perfect technique for planning, there are some basic managerial criteria that nurse service administrators and members of the planning team should consider. They may be summarized as follows:

• The nursing service administrator should decentralize planning, but recognize that staff members cannot be allowed to do precisely what they want. Effective leadership provides realistic guidelines and controls for others to safely carry out their own course of action.

• The nursing service administrator should recognize that a systematic planning approach provides an opportunity to ascertain the abilities and skills of staff members, to utilize resources effectively to attain desired results, and to provide staff members with opportunities to be creative, innovative, and gain achievement or personal satisfaction from their successful effects.

• The nursing service administrator and department heads, in facing emergency changes in the direction of a plan, must give priority to the objective of the plan and secondary concern to the objectives of the group and all others involved.

• A coordinated plan between involved departments in an institution tends to bring a more general agreement concerning the desired direction of movement of the separate department toward the overall goal.

• The nursing service administrator recognizes that a plan is only as good as the ability and motivation of the staff to carry it out. Staff on the units are closer to the real problems and thus understand them better.

• In a changing hospital environment the plan of action must be flexible enough to make necessary changes in the groups' direction. On the other hand, the plan must possess enough stability to generate confidence in the group.

• The plan should be based on clearly defined goals or objectives and should itself be clear and simple.

• The plan should be economical in terms of the resources required to implement it.

• The plan should provide for a thorough analysis of the various activities and determine the criteria for evaluation. A plan's efficiency must be measured by the degree to which it contributes to goals and objectives, offset by costs and other actions required to formulate and put it into effect.

Nursing service administrators cannot control the actions of staff members without realistic plans. Through the planning process, both administrators and staff discover where they want to go, and through the controlling process, they know if they are going in the desired direction.

REFERENCES

1. Allen, L. A.: Professional management, New York, 1973, McGraw-Hill Book Co., chapters 2 and 6.
2. Arndt, C., and Huckabay, L. M.: Nursing administration—theory for practice with a systems approach, St. Louis, 1975, The C. V. Mosby Co., chapters 3 and 4.
3. Chandler, A. D., Jr.: Strategy and structure, Cambridge, Mass., 1962, The M.I.T. Press.
4. Goetz, B. E.: Management planning and control, New York, 1949, McGraw-Hill Book Co.
5. Hicks, H. G.: The management of organization: a systems and human resources approach, ed. 3, New York, 1976, McGraw-Hill Book Co., chapters 4 and 16.
6. Johnson, R. A., Kast, F. E., and Rosenzweig, J. E: The theory and management systems, New York, 1963, McGraw-Hill Book Co.
7. Kast, F. E., and Rosenzweig, J. E.: Planning for an integrated decision system, Washington Business Review, p. 39, April, 1960.
8. Kazmier, J. L.: Principles of management—a programmed instructional approach, ed. 3, New York, 1974, McGraw-Hill Book Co.
9. Koontz, H., and O'Donnell, C.: Principles of management, ed. 6, New York, 1976, McGraw-Hill Book Co.
10. Lawson, J. W.: How to develop a company personnel policy manual, Chicago, 1967, The Dartnell Corp.
11. Luthans, F.: Introduction to management: a contingency approach, New York, 1976, McGraw-Hill Book Co.
12. Mali, P.: Managing by objectives, New York, 1972, John Wiley & Sons, Inc.
13. Massie, J. L., and Douglas, J.: Managing—a contemporary introduction, Englewood Cliffs, N.J., 1973, Prentice-Hall, Inc., chapters 11, 12, and 16.
14. McFarland, D. E.: Management: principles and practices, ed. 2. New York, 1964, The Macmillan Publishing Co.
15. Morris, W. T.: Decentralization in management systems, Columbus, Ohio, 1968, Ohio State University Press.
16. Palmer, J.: Management by objectives, Journal of Nursing Administration 3(5):59, 1973.
17. Perrow, C.: Complex organizations, Glenview, Ill., 1972, Scott, Foresman and Company.
18. Plachy, R.: Delegation and decision-making, Modern Hospital 120(2), 1973. In Stone, S., Berger, M. S., Elhart, D., Firsich, S. C., and Jordan, S. B.: Management for Nurses, St. Louis, 1976, The C. V. Mosby Co., pp. 58-65.
19. Ramey, I. G.: Setting nursing standards and evaluating care. In Planning and evaluating care, Wakefield, Mass., 1974, Contemporary Publishing, Inc., pp. 17-25.
20. Salacik, G. R., and Pfeffer, J.: The bases and use of power in organizational decision-making, Administrative Science 19(4):453-473, 1974.
21. Simon, H. A.: Administrative behavior, ed. 3, New York, 1976, The Free Press.
21a. Tucker, S. M., Breeding, M. A., Canobbio, M. M., Jacquet, G. D., Paquette, E. H., Wells, M. E., and Willmann, M. E.: Patient care standards, St. Louis, 1975, The C. V. Mosby Co.
22. Wandelt, M., and Ager, J.: Quality patient care scale, New York, 1974, Appleton-Century-Crofts, Inc.
23. Weinstein, E. L.: Developing a measure of the quality of nursing care, Journal of Nursing Administration 6(6), 1976.

9 | Organizing–role structure

The function of organizing is an important aspect of the total management process in providing nursing care services to clients. It coordinates these services within the nursing service system itself, and with other systems in the institution. Designers determine a role structure within the division of labor, and an organization structure through which all personnel may perform their jobs effectively and efficiently to achieve goals and objectives. Formal and informal organization structure is discussed in Chapter 10.

MEANING OF ROLE AND POSITION DESCRIPTION

The meaning of role structure as used in this book should be clarified. In our modern society, we progress as individuals through a succession of roles. A role is a position that an individual can act out. The content of a given role is prescribed by the prevailing norms of a society. Norms are social or institutional in nature.[34] Physicians, nurses, administrators, and secretaries are occupational roles. Each of these roles has widely accepted expectations of how a person should perform in a given position. Both the individual occupying a position and those outside it are familiar with the role expectations.

Some researchers believe that the organization, to some extent, changes the individual and that the individual, to some extent, restructures the organization. In this context personalizing and socializing processes are kept together through functional specifications, the status system, the communication system, the reward-and-penalty system, and the organization structure.[4] The specification of behavior that an organization requires of its members is spelled out in its policies, procedures, and rules (see Chapter 8).

In this book the prescribed nursing service roles take the form of job descriptions to attain organizational goals. The roles are based on the division of nursing service responsibilities and hierarchy of authority that must exist within the system.[14]

The activities of each professional nurse include such functions as organizing, planning, communicating, motivating, creating, and controlling, whether caring for patients or supervising subordinates. Nurses in any position set examples for others to follow. They represent nursing to outsiders when talking with visitors, participating in community projects, or settling differences among personnel, patients, and others (Fig. 9-1).

EXTERNAL INFLUENCES ON GOALS

Defining the goals and objectives of a nursing service system has been presented in Chapter 7. The long- and short-term plans that involve the practice of nursing, policies, standards, and management processes are discussed in Chapters 5 and 8.

The goals of an organization and its plans of action result from its interactions with the environment of the total system. The environmental variables of a health care system influence the role and organization structure by means of goal setting (see Chapter 6).

Several environmental factors influence changes in the role of nursing in the delivery of health care to clients. Among external environmental variables are federal governmental regulations, research, the introduction of technical health care workers and physicians' assistants, revised licensure stat-

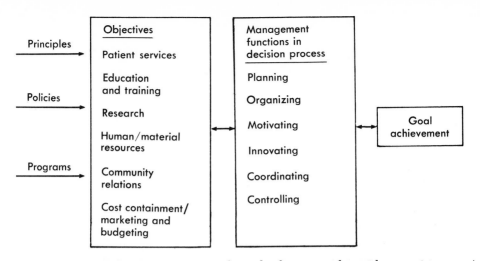

Fig. 9-1. A statement of management principles and policies provides guides to assist nurses in carrying out their daily activities. To accomplish the objectives of nursing and initiate programs, nurses at all levels of the hierarchy carry out management functions. It should be noted that the traditional management operation concept does not consider the environmental and human variables that are so important in the scientific management approach. (Adapted from Wortman, M. S., and Luthans, F.: Emerging concepts in management, New York, 1969, The Macmillan Co.)

utes for technicians and nurses, and consumer demands for better and more health care services at a reasonable price. With the introduction of scientific technologies in management, the growing complexity of health care in institutions and agencies is forcing nursing leaders and others to examine and rearrange levels and types of positions in the system.

Short,[44] in discussing planned organizational change, defines it as any planned program that results in significant alterations of the behavior of individuals or groups within the organization in a direction desired by management. A health care organization can be viewed as a system composed of subsystems consisting of four basic interacting variables—tasks, structure, technology, and the human element.

PURPOSE AND NATURE OF ORGANIZING

Organizing is the establishment of relationships between tasks to be performed, individuals to perform them, and necessary physical elements. To coordinate nursing service resources, nursing service administrators and their professional staffs design a formal structure of jobs and authority re-

lationships that will allow them to attain their goals. *The major challenge in organizing nursing services in a changing health care environment is to determine the grouping of nursing care and management functions and establish a graduation of authority. Top nursing service administrators must empower professional nurses in the middle and lower levels with the means to achieve the objectives of their positions.*

Sociotechnical system concept in organization structures

As we view nursing care services within the sociotechnical framework, any task requires both technical organization—equipment, processes, and skills—and social organization to relate staff members who perform necessary tasks. To a great extent, these two forms of organization determine each other, even if viewed independently.[39]

Professional nurses want to experience gratification in meeting the total nursing needs of their patients, feel some control over their own activities in the practice of nursing and experience satisfactory relationships with those persons performing related activities in the care of patients and in the management of the health care system. The gratification of autonomy in the control of a professional nurse's activities is closely related to the need for self-expression and self-determination.[7,18,37]

In our scientific medical and management health care system, this need is becoming the basis of nurses' identification with their jobs; that is, the need for satisfactions that derive directly from the performance of job functions at any level of the structure.[10,22,35] In some institutions our sociotechnical system has not been properly organized. The nursing teams composed of a variety of workers with different goals, values, and skills have promoted poor relationships, the formation of cliques, and difficulties between subordinates and peers.

Grouping of resources

The organizing functions performed by individuals at various levels of the organization involve grouping various inputs—human, technological, and social—and combining and interrelating them to each other, to result in organization outputs for the purpose of attaining desired outcomes.

As previously mentioned, the human element consists of the individuals in the system. Each member comes with individual knowledge, skills, values, expectations, and personal behavior.[20] Personal goals have been mentioned in Chapter 7.

The technological element consists of the technical skills of individuals, their practices, and the standards, materials, and equipment required to produce a work flow pattern of activities necessary to attain objectives. The impact of technology on nursing and its organization structure will be discussed later in this chapter.

The social element of organizing refers to the informal organization that influences the behavior of individuals within the units.

IMPACT OF TECHNOLOGY ON NURSING SERVICE

Throughout the ages each society has created a technological system, however simple, to use the physical and biological environments of man to solve critical problems of human survival and to attain material comforts and well-being for its people.

Advances in scientific and medical knowledge, more sophisticated techniques, and the increasing use of electronic equipment are affecting the medical and nursing management of patient care, as well as the operational processes of the institution.

Meaning of technology

Charles Perrow[38] viewed organizational technology as the activities that various individuals perform on objects, with or without the aid of equipment or materials, for the purpose of making definite changes in that object. The object may be a living being, human or otherwise.

Luthans and others[27] view technology as having three separate but related elements: (1) the job design promoting increased professionalization, specialization, and institutionalization of technical and complex tasks, (2) the introduction of new relationships between technology and science based on more systematic research and innovative managerial concepts, and (3) the adoption of the systems approach.

As previously mentioned, professional nurses in any type of health institution or agency should be more aware of external and internal environmental variables such as sociopolitical values of consumers and groups and governmental financial support for health services that influence the profession of nursing in our modern technological society. Increased specialization will continue to make organizing the role structure of nursing service more difficult.

Technology and interdependency

Technologies have become the primary determiners of the nature and locus of interdependence.[21,51] How professional nurses at all levels of the structure become embedded in the network of interdependence is a major factor in their identification with the total patient care system.

Using Thompson's classification of technologies,[50] the hospital care system is using more and more intensive technology. Intensive technology influences the ways that groups' activities relate to each other, thus creating intensive interdependence.

For example, in the surgeries, the emergency room, or the specialty patient care units, as well as in the research programs, physicians and nurses perform their portion of a task in diagnosing and treating each patient without precisely following a standardized routine. They perform their activities in accordance with the dictates of patients' particular situations that may require adjustments of their tasks to those of others as they receive feedback of the results from ongoing activities. Intensive interdependence involves the development of knowledge and skills and the selection and application of appropriate actions for a particular purpose at particular times and places.

Interdependence tends to strain relationships between members of the organization, especially where one role serves a number of other roles. When high specialization exists there are many steps involved in a management procedure or the treatment of a client. Several different categories of workers may be involved in one procedure. For example, the physician writes an order for a GI series for his patient (output) that becomes the input of nursing in the preparation of the patient. The nursing service output becomes the input of the x-ray technician. Finally, the total staff and equipment of the hospital (input) is used by the physician to make his diagnosis (output) of the patient's problem.

In this type of interdependence no one unit of work can proceed until it receives its input, and coordination becomes an important function when an organization turns highly specialized. Koontz and O'Donnell[25] remind us that occupational specialization is based on an economic, not on a management, principle. Recent use of computers has reduced paper work and employee worktime, thus improving the feedback of information.[15,19,53]

Technology and role structure

New lifesaving techniques that involve complex equipment and require on-the-spot judgmental assessment of the patient's condition at any time have resulted in the expansion of professional nurses' responsibilities.[5,9] In the past decade the number of various specialty patient care units has increased because of their effectiveness in the treatment of acutely ill patients. These units are staffed by professional nurses who have clinical expertise in their particular specialty such as coronary, respiratory, pediatric, or postoperative surgical care, burn trauma, or psychiatric emergency care. Nursing service administrators should focus on determining dependent responsibility with authority and accountability as well as interdependent relationships for nursing roles.

Researchers[27] studying unit production technology found that it requires a relatively high level of skills in terms of technical knowledge of the job method, equipment, knowledge about operation errors, evaluation of skills, and control. Research indicates that highly skilled workers are more likely to perform effectively when they are given freedom on the job and require less supervision than those performing repetitive tasks.

Skilled and professional workers feel more involved with their jobs and more eager for an opportunity to participate in making job-related decisions. In a work environment such as modern nursing, nurse administrators should exercise a more democratic supervisory approach within all levels of the nursing service system. Democratic supervision is effective where the nature of the tasks permits individuals to enjoy autonomy. Researchers of technology provide important information for nursing service leaders in the rearrangement of role structure.[13,15]

Cognizant of the influence of technologies on nursing service both clinically and administratively, nursing service administrators are being forced to analyze the effects of innovations on the role and organization structures of nursing service and to make appropriate adjustments that could influence the total health system of an institution.[1,2,24]

Technology and hospital supportive and management operations

With the introduction of unit management and materials management-system, informational systems aided by computers have had a tremendous influence on the nursing role structure and the work flow patterns of nursing service units.

Supportive and management operations should be designed to assist the health staff in providing quality care to their clients and result in the economic use of hospital resources. Unfortunately, nurses in some hospitals permit these innovations to constrain their primary role in the practice of nursing. Nurses at the first managerial level should participate in decision-making processes concerned with hotel-ancillary and auxiliary activities that are rendered to their clients and affect their nursing services activities. The role structure should not be fragmented, and it must be designed for the achievement of nursing service objectives.

With the advent of technological changes, too frequently nurses continue to become absorbed as the primary managerial coordinators of hotel, ancillary and supportive services involving activities of the pharmacy, laboratories, admissions, materials management, x-ray, and housekeeping. In general, the formal structure of the hospital has not focused on the coordination process of management but has depended on the informal organization and communication network. Technology demands that nurses and others commit themselves to determining realistic objectives and their attainment. In other words, shall the first line managerial nursing service role be one of organizing nursing care services for clients or one of coordinating all hospital services for clients on a unit or a floor?

Informational systems have been particularly effective in providing clinical and operational management data on past activities. Analyses of quantitative and qualitative nursing services through quality control records, budget, standard costs information, and personnel turnover statistics are essential to determine ongoing results.[16,19,47] By carefully analyzing the information, nursing service administrators are aided in assessing current deficiencies and in determining an alternative course of action (see Chapters 6 and 8). This type of technology provides for more accurate decision making. It also creates greater interdependence between adminis-trative groups and increases the need to define more clearly interrelated activities in the planning, organizing, and controlling processes of the system.

Technology and organization structure

Researchers of organization have demonstrated that there is a correlation between technology and organization structure. The implementation of technologies makes it necessary to develop a strong coordinative and control network laterally rather than primarily vertically within the system.

Technical expertise and knowledge tend to influence the dispersal of power as opposed to individuals' hierarchical rank in the structure. It is through the organization structure that the activities of many different groups are coordinated and controlled. With rapid changes in medical approaches and the introduction of technologies, there is a continual shifting of coalitions between top administrators, physicians, and top nursing service administrators.[45] The power distribution between the top controlling groups of an institution influence the organization structure of nursing service, its objectives, and the role of professional nurses.

CONCEPTUAL ENVIRONMENTAL CHANGES AFFECTING NURSING SERVICES

Throughout hospital history, physicians have been the primary users and controllers of new medical technology. With a tremendous increase in the use of advanced technology and an increase in clients through health insurance, the influence of the medical staff in health institutions has widened in scope and power (see Chapter 3).

Changing role concepts

In recent decades, more physicians are full-time employees of the hospital. Others are paid for specific functions such as teaching, administering inpatient medical services, or treating clients in ambulatory and outpatient clinics. This shift in the division of labor concepts has increased the power of physicians in the major decision-making processes in the patient care system.

Traditionally, nursing has accepted coordination activities of the "care" functions of the hospital with little defined authority, whereas medicine accepted the "cure" functions of patient care.[8] For this reason nursing services' coordination activities are based on illusive authority relationships between nursing and other departments.

Nursing has been viewed as the doctors' helper and the patients' and hospital administrators' representative, and is closely associated with the patients' care and cure activities. With the expansion of professional nursing roles, based on intensive training and specialization, the expertise of nurses in their specialized area has resulted in moving the role structure of nursing away from that of the physicians' and administrators' helpers. A colleagueship rather than a superior-subordinate relationship is occurring between professional nurses, physicians, and administrators to meet the health care demands of clients, but although the role of the nursing service administrator is gaining in status as a member of the top executive team, traditional expectations of physicians, administrators, and clients still exist.

Sills[45] in discussing the hospital organization triad—hospital administrator, physician, and nurse—deplores the fact that existing organizations do not rearrange the structure to give nursing more power. However, in some cases, one sees a greater equalization of power between medicine, nursing, and hospital administration.

With increased professionalization in hospital administration, administrators are gaining professional status and more power in the hospital care systems. There is more movement toward power with equalization between the top executives, the board of trustees, and the medical staff. To meet the primary mission of the hospital—quality health care to clients—nurses should focus on strategies to further equalize power between medicine, nursing, and administration.

A rearrangement of the role structure could help to reduce the self-interests of administrators, physicians, and nurses within the total system. The controlling officers recognize that crucial problems of the hospital can no longer be resolved effectively and efficiently by one individual or one or two groups. Consumers and administrators of health services now recognize input of nursing services to clients, as well as the input of nursing in the in-service training and education of professional and technical groups.

The "new" professional nurses are willing to improve their skills in a nursing specialty.[11,29,52] They want a stake in determining nursing service objectives and in rearranging the organization structure to use their skills more effectively for the nursing care of their clients. According to the 1972 HEW studies on the present and future supply of registered nurses, the projection indicates that graduations from baccalaureate and associate degree programs will show considerable increase. At 5 years after graduation almost 47% of the baccalaureate program graduates reported full-time employment in nursing.[23]

Some health leaders emphasize the need to completely differentiate between clinical nursing roles and those of the management of nursing services. In this postindustrial age, this book emphasizes that it no longer benefits clients or nursing to separate nursing functions into two distinct categories of professional nursing service workers. Such an approach fragments the management process at all levels and reduces the nursing autonomy and unity needed to attain goals.

The design of a role structure must blend nursing practices in clinical aspects of care with the management of resources, the assessment of performance, and the control of operations to attain nursing service objectives. The job design must promote expertise in both clinical specialization and the administration of nursing care services.[16,18,37]

It is imperative that professional nurses at all levels in the structure differentiate between nursing service management functions and nonmanagement and clerical activities. Repetitive managerial tasks should be delegated to others in the hospital system. For example, with the informational system and new techniques, nurses should develop and evaluate a staffing scheduling plan but delegate its operation to trained secretaries. Administrators should do the same concerning budgets and other control devices, using the resources of accounting and other business personnel. In other words, if nurses wish to have a stake in providing better nursing at a reasonable price to their clients, they must use their energy and imagination confidently to eliminate wasting resources in nursing service and must participate more actively with other disciplines in and out of the system (see Fig. 6-7).

Widening status of professional nursing

For many years, nurses have been considered paramedical workers, rather than professionals, in the division of labor. In recent years, nursing as an occupation has taken on more and more of the ideal characteristics of a profession. One of the deficiencies experienced by designers of nursing service has been the lack of sufficient professionalism. In recent years there has been a tremendous increase in the number of nurses who can be ranked high on the continuum occupation scale and who possess all the characteristics of a professional.

Professional nurses promote professionalism through their efforts in their professional associations and through their work with related health, community, and educational associatons, consumer groups, and government representatives (see Chapters 4 and 5). Nurses recently initiated the revision of their state licensure statutes to permit the expansion of the professional nursing role and to differentiate between the roles of professional registered nurses and registered technical nurses[30,42] (see Chapter 4).

In 1975 the credentialing mechanism was introduced in an effort to identify competence and excellence in nursing practice, as was the assessment system to determine the quality of nursing service (see Chapters 4 and 16).

Through the collective bargaining process professional nurses emphasize the difference between the roles of nursing and those of industrial workers and supervisors (see Chapter 4). In recent years in the hospital industry, which employs about 70% of working professional nurses, nurses appear to have more choice about working in their specialty. Rising salaries for nurses, reduced vacancy rates for hospital nurses, the closing of hospital-operated diploma nursing programs because they were no longer profitable, and an increase in the number of nurses with advanced degrees have affected the division of labor and nursing positions.

In recent decades more universities have begun to offer graduate programs in advanced clinical and administrative nursing. Medical centers are providing specialty training for nurses who wish to move into an expanded role such as nurse-practitioner in ambulatory health care or clinical nurse specialist in an acute hospital setting.

Blair,[6] in describing a new nursing service administration program at the University of Colorado School of Nursing, a project sponsored by the W. K. Kellogg Foundation, emphasizes the need to synthesize clinical nursing knowledge with management skills.

The Women's Liberation movement has promoted professionalism in nursing. As nurses become more autonomous in their practice of nursing care and its management, they will be more confident with greater responsibilities in decision making affecting their clients' services and in helping to create colleagueships with other health professionals in and out of their health care system.

ROLE STRUCTURE OF NURSING SERVICES

The general hospital has become a center of extensive differentiation and specialization of activities performed by a very large division of labor (see Chapter 3). The nursing service system has the largest manpower budget in the hospital because of its delegated responsibilities in the delivery of health care services. The organizing process of hospitals, including the nursing service department, is frequently not relevant in the need to coordinate interdependent activities between medicine and nursing and between nursing services and the supportive services. As previously mentioned, at this stage of hospital specialization and technologies the design of the nursing role structure is an important aspect of management (see Fig. 9-1).

Purpose of role structure

A role structure finds ways to develop a purposeful division of labor in the subunits of an organization and ways to provide appropriate authority and relationships for all individuals to work effectively toward defined objectives. A role structure, frequently referred to as job design, should encourage individuals and groups to meet their own goals within a logical system.

A logical, carefully structured work pattern efficiently performed provides for individuals' security and personal material rewards.[41] Professional positions should encompass important activities that require an individual's best knowledge and skills; providing each with the opportunity to satisfy personal goals and the highest monetary returns for individual efforts. Positions must clearly define responsibility, authority, and territorial boundaries to satisfy security and encourage creativity and freedom in areas where it can be most effective.

A role structure design considers the staff's limitations toward meeting the objectives of each position as well as the values and behavior of individuals. Designers should recognize that they cannot modify personal behavior while making changes in the tasks to be done, although both must be considered in relation to the requirements of the situation. The process of organizing a role structure in nursing service is not mechanistic or static, but dynamic. It requires continual evaluation and logical restructuring due to environmental and technological changes.[28]

Constraints and implications in role structure

The freedom of nursing service administrators and professional nurses to design a role structure is constrained to some extent by the conceptual environment of the patient units and the organization structure of the hospital. The degree of constraint nurses feel depends on the amount of agreement that exists between their concepts and the policies of job design, as well as those underlying the general direction taken by the nursing service organization structure. According to Miles,[34] designers should recognize that the types of job design reflect, as do the forms of organization structure, both environmental and technological variables, and real or perceived human attributes of individual nurses and others in the total organization.

Technological advances and intensive role programming

The impact of technology on the practice and management of nursing has been discussed previously in this chapter. Intensive programming can relieve individuals, including nurses in middle and top positions, of their former activities. A large portion of supervisory tasks can be programmed and computerized. The informational system provides statistical data on personnel input and output and turnover data concerning budgetary control and material inventory control. The use of the information feedback system in the assessment of patients' physical conditions influences the nurses' activities and initiates changes in the charting and communicating of physicians' orders.

Will the positions of supervisors in middle management consist of routine technical tasks, or will these positions be eliminated or rearranged to focus on creative, judgmental tasks directed toward the attainment of defined objectives? Will upper level positions be delegated tasks in programming and projects to resolve major problems affecting the patient care system? Technology will probably force those in upper level positions to perform tasks involving planning for introduction of innovations, and decision making to determine realistic objectives for resolving problems. *Technology is forcing a shift from the activities-oriented approach to the result-oriented systems approach.*[19]

It has been predicated that as we move toward a so-called postindustrial economy, there will be a decline in semiskilled routine technical tasks in nursing services and a movement toward more sophisticated specialization within a functional system.[15]

The quality of life at work currently receives a great deal of attention from management, workers, union leaders, government officials, professors, and the press. The successful application of job enrichment greatly depends on the nature of the job itself.

Reduction in nursing and hospital costs may be realized when the enriched professional nurse takes over more quality control responsibilities in the care of patients.[32,33]

One factor that appears to affect career planning by nurses is the structure of nursing and their personal needs.[23]

Trend toward job enrichment

Dickson,[15] in discussing the coming revolution in jobs, focuses on job redesign for motivation, applying principles of participative management, group goal setting, and decision making to reduce costs and improve outputs in business and industrial enterprises. In 1971 the Quality of Working Life Program in Los Angeles was founded by L. E. Davis, a professor at the UCLA School of Management and a well-known expert in the field of job redesign. In late 1974 this program became the Institute for the Quality of Working Life, providing indicators to measure the effectiveness of change, and to test new concepts.

Also in 1974, T. Mills formed the second organization—the Quality of Work Center; it was established in conjunction with the University of Michigan's Institute for Social Research as a nonprofit institute. Its new premises are not radical but based on common sense, flexibility, humanism, and enlightened self-interest. There must be a proper mix of what is good for the institution as a whole with what is good for the personnel toward the attainment of goals.[41]

Position description

A good position description for professional nurses informs them and others about what they are supposed to do, clearly states the objectives of the position, and identifies lines of authority required to perform the job. The description states the basic functions, major duties, and interdepartmental and intradepartmental relationships to be observed.

The degree of institutionalization in positions is a relative concept involving the establishment of standard roles, tasks, and behavior.[26] A small degree of institutionalization exists when the objective of each position is clearly defined. A high degree of institutionalization is present when rules and procedures for each position are defined.

A job description should be broad enough to permit changes when necessary. As a means of control, position descriptions serve as a standard guide against which to judge whether each position is necessary and, if so, its organization level and exact location in the structure.

JOB ANALYSIS

Personnel literature provides information and methods for defining, grading, and classifying jobs within a total system. Job analysis is defined by the United States Department of Labor as the process of determining the nature of a specific job by observation and study and reporting pertinent related information.

The personnel and industrial relations hospital committee may be responsible for job descriptions for all positions. A job design program aims to describe all jobs, analyze their relationships to each other, and describe those jobs that have to be created or eliminated. The wage administrative program becomes closely associated with the job analysis program.

Job analysis plays an important role in manpower, organizing, planning, employee recruitment, placement, performance appraisal, and training programs. The literature on job analysis and work improvement methods should be studied by nurses to gain a better understanding of the program and its influence on the practice of nursing and nursing service classification of positions or jobs within the hospital system.

The job analysis program is a mechanism for determination of equitable rates of pay *for the duties done by each employee*, not those duties that may be done occasionally or what the nurses have written on a piece of paper as the job description of each position. The method of analyzing jobs consists of gathering information by means of observation, questionnaires, and interviews. All personnel have a part in the formulation of the job descriptions based on the data collected.

New position descriptions are introduced by the job design committee to the nursing council for review. The nurse-executive presents the recommendations for the new position for executive approval.

Implications for nursing service positions

Frequently, nurses are unaware of the power of control that the job analysis program has over nursing practice concepts and the grading of nursing positions within the total hospital personnel system. Job evaluators may not recognize the activities of the nursing director, department heads, clinical coordinators, and staff nurses as autonomous functions, but rather view them as performing highly skilled activities under the direction and judgment of a physician or executive. The overlapping concept of duties is not considered. The value or worth of the nurse's cognitive thinking and skills in applying social and scientific information in developing and initiating a plan of care for patients is not clearly identified in the grading system.[32]

For instance, nurses may state that the nursing care plan is the most important duty of professional nurses. But the observations of the job analyst and the professional nurse's listing of activities done indicate that activities of nursing care plans were done infrequently or not at all during the actual study. The frequency of planning, organizing, and coordinating activities of clinical care and the managements of nursing that require cognitive thinking influences the grade of the position (see Chapters 12 and 13).

On the other hand, nurse-specialists with several years' experience and a master's degree in a nursing specialty usually hold a lower position than other professional specialists, although over 70% of their duties require application of knowledge and skills in handling and resolving complex patient care and human relations problems. To remedy this confusion, nurse-administrators and staff should examine the functions and scope of authority in such positions.

In the traditional organization, determination of the relative worth of a job within the hospital system is decided by the executive officers.

The executive staff evaluate and compare wages paid in the organization with those paid for similar jobs in other institutions.

Nurses should review current national, state, and regional wage surveys and through peer review and ongoing appraisal evaluation compensate individuals for competent performance (see Chapters 16 and 17).

Job titles

Position titles in most hospitals cause problems and confusion in that there is little standardization in their use. The title of director may refer to a position at a high level in the structure. In another hospital the same title may refer to a lower, subordinate position. The position of director of the division of nursing may appear at a high level in the structure, whereas in other hospitals it may appear on the operational level along with other department heads under an associate or assistant executive director.

In some nursing services, position titles are both misleading and unrealistic. For instance, the title of head nurse may refer to supervisory duties in a 30-bed unit. In other hospitals the title of head nurse refers to a team leader position with the rate of pay of a head nurse.

In some situations, much of the confusion stems from the fact that the executives and some nurses believe titles make little difference in the nature and characteristics of a position. However, there is much evidence to confirm that position titles greatly influence both the nature and performance of a job.

It is important to accept the fact that many people identify strongly with the title of their position and that subordinates also identify with the title of their superior. Titles are closely bound to our status concepts and desire to be recognized for reaching the top of the ladder.

Position titles should be clear, brief, and as descriptive as possible. General conformity to usage assists in better interdepartmental communications. Titles should be chosen carefully, taking into consideration the probable consequences within the various levels of the structure and the innovations contemplated in the near future.

APPROACH IN JOB DESIGN

In study and redesign of professional nursing service positions, the bottom-up approach rather than the top-down classic approach should be used. The pivotal point of nursing care and coordination of care to patients begins with those individuals who actually render the care and manage their activities toward the attainment of objectives.[10,12,18]

The job design of positions at the middle and higher levels depends on the job design of those at the bottom level of the organization. Job design should be based on a rational systematic plan, involving analysis of nursing activities, research data, and computer and modern informational systems input. Due to increased demands for more health care, nursing service frequently creates new positions without considering their effect on existing positions. This adds to more fragmentation, confusion, and overlapping of activities and increases in manpower costs.

The nursing service administrator, as a member of the hospital top management team, can have a vital influence in redesigning positions to attain a better quality of health care for clients and in conserving manpower resources.

Designers should review the long- and short-term plans and objectives of the nursing service system (see Chapters 7 and 8). They should seek instruction from researchers who understand nursing practices in the various specialties and the role of the nursing service system.

As previously mentioned, the job design of professional nurses in all patient areas must indicate their scope of authority and accountability for the clinical nursing care of their clients. They need to know their dependent functions and interdependent relationships with subordinates and peers. For several decades, many nurses have been interested in patient care in the hospitals but have become frustrated and dissatisfied with their powerlessness to effect needed changes in client care or feel a sense of accomplishment. With increased health care costs, the fragmented and precarious design of bedside nursing must change (see Chapters 13 and 14).

Nursing care design

In our technological health system clinical nursing care can no longer be accomplished by semiskilled workers and technicians. Beginning registered and technical nurses need to work with the help of competent clinical nurses.

Designers, including representatives of the nurse-practitioners and clinical specialists groups, should seek answers to several questions in developing the nurse-clinician positions. For example, what is the objective of the experienced nurse-practitioner in charge of a group of patients? In reviewing the responsibilities of this position, designers must decide how nursing care will be managed for a group of patients. Will the team or primary nurse care approach be used?

Moreover, who will perform, supervise, and coordinate the hospital-hotel and supportive services for patients in the units or for those in the clinics, surgeries, and other areas? Depending on the availability of electronic informational systems, what are the nursing service clerical tasks, and who will perform them every 24 hours, 7 days a week? These and many more questions must be answered to design a smooth work-flow pattern for clinicians and others to meet the changing clinical and supportive needs of patients.

Another reason for using the bottom-up approach in position design is that professional nurses' autonomy begins with the nurse-client at the lowest level of the organization chart. It is there that effective nurse-client relationships are established and continued throughout the client's hospitalization. This is also true in the care of clients in clinics.

The position design of the professional nurse who provides nursing care should allow for creativity to initiate nursing innovations within prescribed standards of nursing practices and in accordance with legal authority given her through a nursing practice act. The job description of practicing nurses should provide opportunities for them to satisfy personal goals while working toward the attainment of nursing service goals (see Chapter 7). To eliminate confusion and uncertainty, professional nurses at the bottom level should know who is to do certain activities and who is responsible for certain results.

The professional nurse role at the bottom level should help strengthen the dependent and interdependent functions of nursing, as well as attempt to create effective colleagueships with other professionals.

With increased nursing professionalism, specialization, the adoption of sophisticated management systems, and new patterns in the health care delivery system, it is evident that the traditional position of the staff nurse must change in order to provide a better quality of nursing care to clients. Secondly, research data indicates that the knowledge and skills of the nurse must be utilized more effectively to decrease costs.[1,15,17] The job design of professional nurses at the lower level must give them a feeling of status and more satisfaction in rendering nursing care to clients.

Position design for first-line managing role

For many years there has been a registered graduate nurse "in charge" of the activities of workers and the care of patients in an area or floor. This first-level managing position of nursing care services is often called the "head nurse" position.[48] It has always been an ambiguous and conflicting role because of the many inconsistencies in its responsibilities, its scope of authority, and its relationships with superiors in decision-making processes.

Development of the head nurse role. In the past, when selecting nurses for this first-line supervisory position, nurse administrators chose good bedside staff nurses who gave evidence that they could run the ward in an efficient manner. Frequently, these nurses accepted the position since it was the only avenue open to advancement, better pay, and better working hours. These nurses then carved out their own territorial authority relationships through the informal system as they worked with subordinates, peers, and others.

Administrators and many nurses have viewed the head nurse position in the context of the foreman's job in industry, not as a first-line supervisory position at the bottom level. The functions of the job have focused primarily on personnel, policies, and procedures rather than on the outcome results of nursing practice in the care of patients. The major clinical and management decisions are made by superiors. This position does not permit the head nurse to participate with the nursing service team in making crucial decisions.

Efforts to change traditional head nurse role. In the 1950s, with advances in medical care and more hospital supportive services, the head nurse's management activities were increased. Nurse administrators endeavored to upgrade the position, increase the rate of pay, and provide clerical assistance and more staff personnel. In some hospitals, hospital management took over some of the hotel duties of the unit, and team nursing was introduced. The title was changed to "assistant supervisor," or "supervisor." However, in many situations the head nurse's scope of authority was not widened or considered a first-line nursing service supervisory position.

In the early 1970s, because of the confusion of nursing job designs in health institutions and agencies, the proliferation of different titles, and the increased hospital and supportive duties performed by nurses, nurse administrators and nurse educators advocated that the primary role of professional nurses focus on nursing management of the clinical aspects of patient care and not on the functions of a hospital manager role.

In 1972 the New York State Nurses' Association presented New Positions Descriptions in Nursing. This document emphasizes that the responsibilities and authority given to professional nurses must stem from their position as practicing nursing professionals and not from their managerial positions in the organization. The NYSNA also recommended that titles of nursing service positions be changed. For example, the title of head nurse should be replaced by that of associate clinical coordinator. Although job descriptions and titles proposed by the NYSNA emphasized the role of nurses in the practice of nursing, they were too vague in defining major tasks and scope of authority.

Recently, some administrators have advocated a distinct separation between clinical and management positions. Others have advocated that all services be coordinated by a unit director. The literature indicates that the later approaches have not proven successful either administratively or economically. There are indications that the coordination of nursing services requires an equalization and synthesis of both clinical and managing tasks in the care of patients in a given unit.

In many hospitals the head nurse or nurse care coordinator shares responsibilities with the evening and night supervisors or assistant directors of these tours, who may participate in the nursing service decision-making process. This fragments the position and creates conflicts.

With advances in medical technologies, the automation of health care activities, the use of computers to facilitate charting, care planning, patient monitoring, and scheduling personnel assignments, and the use of management informational systems in reporting data, there is a need to clearly define the functions and scope of authority of the first-line position of managing nursing services at the bottom level.

This position is crucial in coordinating, transacting, and integrating the practices of nursing toward the attainment of the primary goal of nursing service—that of rendering a high level of nursing care to each patient in each unit (see Chapters 11 and 17).

The nurse in the first-line supervisory position first needs a clinical background and experience as a team leader or primary care nurse and then a knowledge of management practices and skills. This book views the first line managing position like that of any nursing service administrator, except that it is narrower in scope and complexity, and the scope of authority in decision making focuses on a smaller area.

The functions of the first-line supervisory position must provide an interface between clinical nursing and nursing service administration. Blair,[6] in a recent article "Needed: Nursing Administration Leaders," emphasizes the need for a master's program that synthesizes clinical nursing knowledge with management theory and skills. With increased numbers of recent graaduates who have advanced clinical preparation, the use of an all R.N. nursing staff to deliver nursing care, and increased medical and nursing specialization, there is an urgent need to design a first-line supervisory position at the bottom level of the organization. It is a vital role in strengthening nursing autonomy toward a better quality of care at a reasonable price.

Nursing leadership must reorient itself and restructure the bottom level of nursing service, remembering that nursing education, nursing practice, and nursing service are inseparable. Present head nurses should be given the opportunity to improve their knowledge of nursing practices and gain an understanding of modern management process and skills through advanced education and in-service training.[35,36a]

The new council of nursing service facilitators should consider the first-line supervisory position as a member of nursing service administrative team, making the head nurse eligible for membership in the council.

The position design may be wrong, but usually it is the overall management concept of nursing service that needs to be changed. The nursing service facilitators should attend to planned organizational change programs directed toward intervention strategies designed to change the human element and structure in nursing services.

Position design at the middle level

As previously mentioned, this book stresses the need for a strong, effective, competent role structure at the bottom level of the nursing service system, regardless of its type, size, and complexity, to deliver to patients the quality of care that is now possible. This procedure also supports the assumption that hotel-housekeeping activities will be assigned to hospital aides and other workers.

With a competent nursing staff for clinical nursing care services and a well-coordinated work pattern in each unit, designers must decide what supervisory positions are needed at the middle level to coordinate, integrate, and evaluate nursing activities at the first level with those at the top level. The kind of job description and the number of positions will depend on the number of units, the type and complexity of specialization and services, and the objectives of the nursing service system and the institution.

It should be mentioned that creating a middle supervisory role structure to satisfy a span of control has been proven unproductive, resulting in more conflicts and problems at the bottom level, or in going downward from the top level. Span of control is discussed in Chapter 10.

Constraints and problems of traditional supervisory positions. In this age of advanced medical and nursing practices and specialization, health care workers and the head nurse in a unit often view the supervisor as an "outsider." The physicians and nurses caring for a group of patients work toward the attainment of their objectives; however, the supervisor is expected to be on the units and to perform specific tasks.

The traditional supervisor spends considerable time writing concise reports, investigating staffing resources and needs, and evaluating ongoing patient, personnel, and equipment problems. At the end of the tour supervisors frequently feel their accomplishments have not amounted to anything toward the attainment of objectives.[7,49]

Because the professional nurses and the supervisor in the unit have more clinical competence than the supervisor at the middle level, feelings of uncertainty and conflict occur on the part of both the superior and the subordinates.

Traditionally, much of the time spent by the supervisor at the middle level, especially those on the evening and night tours, concerns material resources, secretarial and interdepartmental activities, and business office activities. During evening and night tours the supervisors perform activities for such hospital departments as pharmacy, dietary, housekeeping, and admitting office. Little time is spent on integrating, coordinating, and evaluating the clinical and management performance of subordinates toward the attainment of nursing service objectives.

In some nursing service organizations, management processes have been decentralized and management technological innovations initiated. This has eliminated the traditional tasks of supervisors. With intensive in-service training and advanced education courses the traditional supervisor has functioned effectively in a restructured position, focusing on clinical aspects of patient care—planning programs and projects toward providing quality patient care.

Future role of middle management in nursing care services. In our sophisticated and technological hospital delivery system, designers should define the purpose and objective of each supervisory position. The position design should be based on a scientific rationale. What kind of organizing, planning, directing, and controlling activities must be done by nurses in the middle level to maintain a productive, cohesive staff at the bottom level and to assist administrators in the attainment of goals? What are the activities concerning quality assurance, peer review, budgeting, and controlling resources?

Some nursing service administrators have initiated changes in the role structure of supervisors. They are responsible for the quality of nursing care delivered to patients. They act as nursing coordinators for several

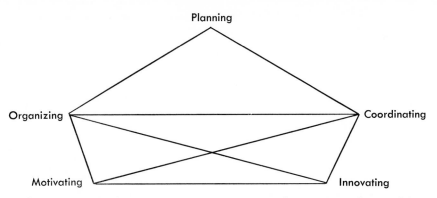

Fig. 9-2. The management function is not a separate entity but an integral part of the entire process of decision making and accomplishment of goals. A realistic image of the management process is shown in the diagram. The management process involves a set of relations among the various units of the system to assure that the activities of the constituent units accomplish the desired objectives.

components of the nursing units in their specialty and assist administrators in developing standards, quality assurance, budgeting, and peer review programs. This type of clinical supervisor has a master's degree in a clinical specialty and preparation in management systems and skills. This individual has competencies and knowledge that help those at the bottom level (Fig. 9-2).

Stevens,[49] in discussing supervisory functions, suggests dividing the functions into several positions—one supervisor to coordinate patient care services, a second supervisor to coordinate nursing personnel and staffing, and a third supervisor to coordinate nursing systems. In this environment the first line supervisor would be obliged to work with each of the others in relation to a particular category of need. This concept does not encourage the group participative approach in planning, organizing, and controlling nursing care services.

To reduce fragmentation and the overlapping of functions, designers should transfer as much paper management work as possible to the computer and use informational systems. Nurses in supervisory positions must be able to develop and use informational systems in the management of nursing services.

To be able to work effectively with the staff at the lower level and evaluate patient care, supervisors need to have interpersonal and clinical competencies and practical skills in interviewing and guiding others. They must be able to set up effective mechanisms of feedback to understand the "social" environment in which they work.[9]

It is imperative that nursing service system provide for the maintenance of the clinical competence of supervisors as well as other personnel. This can be accomplished through in-service training and education programs. Nurses on evening and night tours should be assigned to day tours and appropriate programs periodically during the year. In addition, the position design of the supervisor in the middle level must be different from those of first line supervisory positions and their superiors.

Position design of clinical specialists. In recent years the position of the clinical specialist has been created to upgrade the level of nursing care in the delivery of patient care.[5,11,24]

In many institutions, clinical nurse-specialists have been most effective in providing quality care in coronary, cardiovascular, surgical, and pediatric specialty units.

Frequently the position design for clinical nurse-specialists does not clearly define the scope of authority and accountability or the relationships with nurses in line positions. Difficulties arise between the health care group, head nurse, and the specialists because of unclear communication relationships and authority. Nurses may function in a staff role even though they perform direct nursing care for patients. Conflict and confusion may arise as nurse-specialists endeavor to change patients' nursing care plans. Guiding and teaching other nurses in the unit is principally accomplished by example and persuasion.[4,9]

Nursing service administrators should try to use knowledge and expertise of nurse specialists to raise the general level of nursing practice in the care of patients with acute or chronic health problems. In some hospitals clinical nurse-specialists are responsible for special programs offered to professional nurses and act as consultants to nurses in the care of patients with complex nursing care problems, functioning as staff consultants and teachers (see Chapter 10).

When clinical specialists are employed as members of a nursing team, head nurses or supervisors are usually unable to use their expertise in planning, assessing, and evaluating care. The results of such outcomes have proven expensive and unproductive in upgrading general nursing.

It has been found that clinical nurse-specialists who have completed a master's program may not have sufficient experience in nursing practice. Frequently these nurses do not have basic knowledge in management services and skills. Many seem frustrated in their jobs due to vague position descriptions or the assignment of some management tasks in the unit.

Both specialization and generalization in nursing should be considered when designing the position of the clinical specialists. Nurse-administrators must find an effective and economical way to use the expertise of nurse-specialists to improve the quality of nursing, either through a better understanding of line-staff concepts or by restructuring the supervisory position using the expertise of clinical nurse-specialists.

In our age of technological sophistication and demands, to provide a better quality of care at a reasonable price, nursing service should design the clinical supervisory position with the objective of improving the quality of nursing care. Clinical specialist

supervisors would have the authority role in creating change. They could be assessor-evaluators, innovators, participant-consultants, and informal teachers. Nursing service administrations should support research programs to determine the future role of the clinical supervisor with specialized expertise in clinical nursing.

Position design for administration role structure

The role of the nurse-executive of the nursing service system has been defined by the American Nurses' Association and the American Hospital Association as presented in Chapter 4.

Top level leaders in nursing service perform four major functions—planning, organizing, implementing, and evaluating activities toward the attainment of the goals of nursing service and those of the total system (Figs. 9-1 and 9-2). Decision making occurs throughout the entire management process (see Chapters 6 and 8).

In the role structure of top-level positions, functions should focus on nursing, input and output, administrative processes, and research. Nurse administrators and their immediate assistants must be able to analyze their health care system in relation to external environmental variables.

Productive leadership patterns. Shelty emphasizes that the leadership pattern of an individual in a supervisory or administrative position depends on many forces that act and interact. These forces shape the pattern of authority and control in a system. Thus, the leadership pattern is a result of many forces—those in the individual, in subordinates, in the organizational system, and in the type of situation that requires immediate action.[43]

Our modern health delivery system requires sophisticated competence in each member of the administrative team. There is a need for colleagueships between specialists and administrators (see Chapter 11).

A successful nurse-administrator is neither an autocrat nor a democrat, but tries to integrate the forces operating in relation to specific situations. The leadership appropriate in one organization may not apply to another, and a productive leadership pattern depends on what is most consistent with other elements in a particular system.

Using modern management systems. Top administrators of the nursing service system should have modern management techniques and skills in patient classification systems, cost analyses of resources, staffing, budgeting, evaluating, and controlling. Top nurse administrators must continually evaluate the existing system and recommend necessary actions from staff members, physicians, and others to improve the system or change objectives (the role of the nurse in administration in collective bargaining is discussed in Chapter 4; planning in Chapter 8; budgeting and controlling in Chapter 15; and evaluation in Chapter 17). Nurse-administrators are the leaders in innovating changes based on facts and data, and in coordinating programs within nursing, with other leaders within the health system, and with health and educational groups in the community.

Research has demonstrated that computers, hospitals' information systems, and input from accounting and personnel departments have changed the activities of central nursing administrations.

Power of nurse-administrators. Historically, the director and the department heads of nursing service have struggled for title and power commensurate with their functions as administrators of the largest division in the total health care delivery system.

Today the nursing service administrator reports to the president and associate director of the institution. Some nurse executives hold the titles of associate administrator or vice-president. The nurse-executive is a member of the top executive administration staff and attends the board of trustees meetings.

The nurse-executive and the department heads of the division of nursing should be included in the informal organization structure. This is vital since the attitudes and direction of a system stem from informal power groups, rather than from formal conferences.[20] A nurse-executive should be part of the power groups that influence organiza-

tional direction. These groups include executive officers, the board of trustees, and chief physicians of services. It is usually difficult for the nurse-executive to gain access to such informal committee groups, regardless of title.

With the rapidly changing patterns in the delivery of care, the nurse-administrator should try to develop colleagueships with physicians who have equivalent organization positions. The influence of nursing service depends to a great degree on the development of these colleagueships.

Nurse administrators are primarily responsible for promoting quality nursing care to all clients in accordance with the practices of nursing and health care standards, for designing a structure of organization to use human resources effectively and economically, for initiating a process of management through which personal satisfaction is gained in the accomplishment of goals of the nursing service system, and for supporting the overall goals of the enterprise.

Philosophy of nursing service administrators' positions. In the past few decades the criteria of nursing service administration have not changed drastically, but the way it is accomplished has changed. The decisions now must be based on verifiable facts; the administrator must appropriate the necessary degree of responsibility to those in lower levels, and the nurse administrator must achieve a conceptual and physical environment, an ongoing communication network flowing vertically and laterally, and a flexible structure to meet and adapt to changing needs in the system and the external environment.

STRUCTURAL AND POSITION DESIGN FOR IN-SERVICE DEPARTMENTS

External pressures for high quality of care services, the application of new scientific technological advances, and emphasis on continued learning through education and training have made administrators and professional nurses more aware of the need for competent performance and the development of individuals' capabilities in the care of patients.

The ANA's Standards of Nursing Practice and Standards of Nursing Services aim to fulfill the profession's obligation to provide quality of nursing care to consumers (see Chapter 5). The JCAH's Nursing Service Standard V requires a nursing service department to provide a program for staff education and training composed of orientation, in-service education, and continuing education.

Assumptions of in-service education

One assumes that education and training activities will assist workers to acquire, maintain, or gain new knowledge and skills to produce the desired outcomes in the clinical care of patients and the management of nursing services. To achieve the primary mission of the hospital and that of nursing services, nurses must be given the opportunity to acquire the necessary knowledge and skills for their jobs. To provide an acceptable quality of patient care to consumers at a reasonable price, the human, material, and financial resources for in-service programs must be identified in relation to the learning needs of personnel, so that employees can perform their activities effectively and efficiently. The objective of the in-service programs is not to provide education for the sake of the staff's personal interests, but to help them provide better care to consumers.

Structure and position design of in-service programs

The type of positions and the number of nurses required for in-service education and training will depend on the kinds of programs required to ensure good performance from personnel. Orientation, induction training, reinforcement, and the maintenance of nursing practices will depend on the job descriptions of various categories of workers in the organization.

Does the organization employ nursing aides, recent graduate nurses with an associate or a baccalaureate degree, or licensed practical nurses? If so, these new employees will need intensive induction training to learn the hospital's and the nursing service's objectives, policies, and regulations as well as the nature of their activities and communication feedback with others. Will practical nurses require training in the administration of medications? The nurse-executive and director of the in-service department can plan such programs in advance during the fiscal year, based on statistical manpower data from recent years. In some situations a part-time experienced professional nurse may be available for projects such as the administration of medications or the training of nursing aides.

Another factor influencing the activities of in-service education will be the structure of nursing service positions. Does nursing service differentiate between levels of responsibility with concepts of staff nurse, clinical nurse, and master clinician? Are the levels designed according to the content of the position and the clinical proficiency required for competent performance? Is promotion granted on the basis of possession of knowledge and demonstrated competence to perform a given position? The staff of in-service education should not be responsible for the evaluation of work performance, but they help to set nursing care standards and identify the elements of nursing practice that will be needed.

Reinforcement in-service classes and practice sessions such as cardiopulmonary resuscitation will be needed. Intensive training courses and practice sessions in the care of the acutely ill, in the implementation of new methodology in the management of nursing care, such as primary care nursing, or in the use of new equipment are elements of in-service projects. Some of these projects may be performed by professional nurses at various levels in the organization. However, all projects should be planned and controlled by the nurse-administrator of the in-service department.

The organizational structure of nursing service will influence the functions and communications of the in-service education department. There is no one way to organize an in-service education program. If nursing service is decentralized, many activities of in-service education and training will be decentralized. However, the nurse-executive or a delegated associate member should be responsible for the overall direction and implementation of in-service education and training programs. The in-service education and training functions, authority, and communications must be clearly identified for the position in each subsystem, and colleagueships between in-service staff members and nursing service managers are crucial for the achievement of quality care.

Directing and controlling in-service programs

The nurse-executive is responsible for selecting an appropriate professional nurse to head in-service programs. The qualifications of this person will depend on the programs required. Since the goal is to meet desired outcomes of quality in nursing, a professional nurse should be responsible for all in-service education and training programs of nursing services. Decisions about nursing employees' educational needs and programming should not be delegated to a nonnurse educator by hospital administration. If this occurs, administrators and nurses are admitting that there is no professional component of nursing.

Nursing is more than a set of techniques and procedural tasks done for patients. The in-service staff must possess knowledge of nursing practices and be totally committed to quality patient care. The characteristics of job descriptions for in-service staff members will depend on the learning and training needs of the personnel and their expected activities to ensure quality nursing services for consumers.

The hospital should provide educational opportunities for professional nurses to acquire new knowledge and skills through enrollment in specific programs in their nursing specialties or in workshops and institutes. Moreover, the staff of the in-service education department should use educational opportunities to update their nursing practices and teaching skills.[35,36a]

A dynamic nursing service organization offers nursing assistants and professional nurses opportunities to improve and develop their capabilities in their chosen field as they help to achieve nursing service objectives— that is, to provide quality care to every patient.

REFERENCES

1. Anderson, M. I., and Denyes, M. J.: A ladder for clinical advancement in nursing practice: implementation (University Center for health sciences, University of Wisconsin Hospitals—Position Descriptions for nursing clinician, 1972), Journal of Nursing Administration 5:16-22, Feb., 1975.
2. Ayers, R., Bishop, R., and Moss, F.: An experiment in nursing service reorganization, American Journal of Nursing 69(4):783-786, 1969.
3. Bakke, K., Page, M., and Ciske, K. L.: Primary nursing, American Journal of Nursing 74:1432-1438, Aug., 1974.
4. Baldridge, J. V., and Burnham, R. A.: Organizational innovations: individual, organizational, and environmental impacts, Administrative Science Quarterly 20:165-176, 1975.
5. Berwind, A.: The nurse in the coronary care unit. In Bullough, B., editor: The how and the expanding nurse role, New York, 1975, Appleton-Century-Crofts, Inc., pp. 82-95.
6. Blair, E. M.: Needed: nursing administration leaders, Nursing Outlook 24:550-554, Sept., 1976.
7. Brown, E. L.: Keynoter challenges nurses to achieve comprehensive care, NLN Collaboration Convention Journal, pp. 1-3, June 11, 1975.
8. Bullough, B.: Influences on role expansion, American Journal of Nursing 76:147-148, Sept., 1976.
9. Cassidy, J. T.: The advanced nursing practitioner: a dilemma for supervisors, Journal of Nursing Administration 5:41-42, July-Aug., 1975.
10. Ciske, K. L.: Primary nursing: an organization that promotes professional practice, Journal of Nursing Administration 4:28-31, Jan.-Feb., 1974.
11. Colavecchio, R., Tescher, B., and Scalizi, C.: A clinical ladder for nursing, Journal of Nursing Administration 4:58, Sept.-Oct., 1974.
12. Conway, M. E.: Management effectiveness and the role-making process, Journal of Nursing Administration 4:25-28, Nov.-Dec., 1974.
13. Daubenmire, M. J., and King, I. M.: Nursing process models: a systems approach, Nursing Outlook 21:512-517, Aug., 1973.
14. Davis, L. E., and Taylor, J., editors: Design of jobs, Baltimore, 1972, Penguin Books.
15. Dickson, P.: The future of the workplace (the coming revolution in jobs), New York, 1975, Weybright and Talley, chapters 1 and 2.
16. Fulmer, R.: The new management, New York, 1974, McGraw-Hill Book Co.
17. Gaynor, A. K., and Berry, R. K.: Observations of a staff nurse: an organizational analysis, Journal of Nursing Administration 3:43-49, May-June, 1973.
18. Haase, P. T.: Pathways to practice, American Journal of Nursing 76:806-809, May, 1976; 76:950-954, June, 1976.

19. Hannah, K. J.: The computer and nursing practice, Nursing Outlook **24**:555-558, Sept., 1976.

20. Hicks, H. G.: The management of organizations: a systems and human resources approach, ed. 2, New York, 1972, McGraw-Hill Book Co., chapters 2 and 17.

21. Hrebiniak, L. G.: Job technology, supervision, work-group structure, Administrative Science Quarterly **19**:395-410, Sept., 1974.

22. Keller, N. S.: The nurse's role: is it expanding or shrinking? Nursing Outlook **21**:236-240, April, 1973.

23. Knopf, L.: Debunking a myth, American Journal of Nursing **74**:1416-1421, Aug., 1974 (based on United States National Institutes of Health: From student to R.N.; a report of the nurse career-pattern study by L. Knopf. DHEW pub. no. NIH 72-130 Washington, D.C., United States Government Printing Office, 1972).

24. Koontz, H., and O'Donnell, C.: Essentials of management, New York, 1974, McGraw-Hill Book Co., pp. 170-208.

25. Koontz, H., and O'Donnell, C.: Principles of management, ed. 6, New York, 1976, McGraw-Hill Book Co.

26. Likert, R.: The human organization, New York, 1967, McGraw-Hill Book Co., chapter 10.

27. Luthans, F.: Introduction to management, New York, 1976, McGraw-Hill Book Co.

28. Luthans, F.: Organizational behavior, New York, 1973, McGraw-Hill Book Co., chapters 6, 7, and 8.

29. McGann, M. R.: The clinical specialist: from hospital to clinic, to community, Journal of Nursing Administration **5**:33-37 March-April, 1975 (and reactions to McGann in same issue).

30. McGriff, E., and Simms, L.: Two New York nurses debate the NYSNA 1985 proposal, American Journal of Nursing **76**:930-935, 1976.

31. Maas, M. L.: Nurse autonomy and accountability in organized nursing services. In Stone, S., Berger, M. S., Elhart, D., Firsich, S. C., and Jordan, S. B.: Management for nurses, St. Louis, 1976, The C. V. Mosby Co.

32. Marram, G.: The comparative costs of operating a team and primary nursing unit, Journal of Nursing Administration **6**:21-24, May, 1976.

33. Marram, G. D., Bevis, E. O., and Schlegel, M. W.: Primary nursing: a model of individualized care, St. Louis, 1974, The C. V. Mosby Co.

34. Miles, R. E.: Theories of management: complications for organizational behavior and development, New York, 1975, McGraw-Hill Book Co., chapters 4 and 5.

35. National League for Nursing, The Department of Hospitals and Related Institutional Nursing Service: Four approaches to staff development, pub. no. 20-1578, New York 1975, The League (papers presented at CHRINS Meeting during 1975 NLN Convention, New Orleans, Louisiana).

36. Nehls, D., Hansen, V., Robertson, P., and Manthey, M.: Planned change: a quest for nursing autonomy, Journal of Nursing Administration **4**:23-27, 1974.

36a. News: ANA's continuing education in full swing; agencies, activities approved, American Journal of Nursing **77**:34, Jan., 1977.

37. Nuckolls, K. B.: Who decides what the nurse can do? Nursing Outlook **22**:626-631, Oct., 1974.

38. Perrow, C.: Hospitals: technology, structure, and goals. In March, J. G., editor: Handbook of organization, Chicago, 1965, Rand McNally & Co., p. 948.

39. Petit, T.: Fundamentals of management coordination, New York, 1975, John Wiley & Sons, Inc., chapters 4, 12, and 13.

40. Poulin, M. A.: Nursing service: change or managerial obsolescence, Journal of Nursing Administration **4**:40-43, Aug., 1974.

41. Reif, W. E., and Tinnell, R. C.: A diagnostic approach to job enrichment, Division of Research, Graduate School of Business Administration, Michigan State University, MSU Business Topics, Autumn, 1973, pp. 29-37.

42. Rotkovitch, R.: The A.D. nurse: a nursing service perspective, Nursing Outlook **24**:234-238, April, 1976.

43. Shelty, Y. K.: Leadership and organization character, Personnel Administration, pp. 14-20, July-Aug., 1970.

44. Short, L. E.: Planned organizational change, Division of Research, Graduate School of Business Administration, Michigan State University, MSU Business Topics, Autumn, 1973, pp. 53-61.

45. Sills, G. M.: Nursing in medicine, and hospital administration, American Journal of Nursing **76**:1432-1434, Sept., 1976.

46. Simon, H. A.: Administrative behavior, ed. 3, New York, 1976, The Free Press, chapters 7, 8, 10, and 11.

47. Somers, J. B.: A computerized nursing care system, Hospitals **45**:93, 1971.

48. Stevens, B. J.: The head nurse as manager, Journal of Nursing Administration **4**:36-40, Jan.-Feb., 1974.

49. Stevens, B. J.: The problems in nursing's middle management, Journal of Nursing Administration **2**:35-38, Sept.-Oct., 1972.

50. Thompson, J.: Organizations in action, New York, 1969, McGraw-Hill Book Co.

51. Thompson, J.: Technology, policy, and societal development, Administrative Science Quarterly **19**:6-21, March, 1974.

52. Volante, E. M.: Mastering the managerial skill of delegation. In Stone, S., Berger, M. S., Elhart, D., Firsich, S. C., and Jordan, S. B.: Management for nurses, St. Louis, 1976, The C. V. Mosby Co.

53. Zielstorff, R. D.: The planning and evaluation of automated systems—a nurse's point of view, Journal of Nursing Administration **5**:22-25, July-Aug., 1975.

10 Organizing—an organization structure

As shown on the organization chart, formal organizational positions are symbolized by boxes, and lines of authority are symbolized by straight, solid, connecting lines (Figs. 6-3 and 10-1). A formal traditional structure may be viewed as a structure of authority relationships. In a formal organization the top authority (the Board of Trustees) divides its authority and delegates it to subordinates, who repeat the process, generating a hierarchy in the expected pyramidal form (Fig. 10-2).

Structuring authority, power, accountability, and responsibility relationships involves three types of authority—line, staff, and functional—that can be delegated. These elements of authority are presented in this chapter. The development of management theories, including the bureaucratic type structure and the systems approach, have been presented in Chapter 6.

PURPOSES OF FORMAL ORGANIZATION STRUCTURES

A formal organization structure is designed to establish efficient, logical, and effective interrelationships between individuals of the enterprise to attain objectives. An effective structure reaps the advantages of specialization, technology, and the division of work when the optimal use of the expertise and skills of individuals is realized and when their activities can be coordinated to facilitate the achievement of goals of the enterprise.

Argyris[4] states that any type of organization is formed by people to attain goals that can best be met collectively. As previously mentioned, in structuring positions, nurses join a health institution because they expect their participation in it will satisfy some of their personal and professional goals (see Chapters 7 and 9). Designing an organizational structure requires goal-directed effort and an awareness of the influence of sociotechnical concepts and technology on individuals' positions and their performance.

DETERMINING THE SPAN OF CONTROL

In every health organization the question is, How many subordinates can an immediate superior supervise? The span of management is often referred to as the number of hierarchical levels under the top executive officer in the system.

A wide span of control has two to four levels and is referred to as a flat or horizontal organization structure, whereas a narrow span of control has many levels and is referred to as a tall structure (Figs. 6-2, 10-1, and 10-2). Thus, span of control is associated with hierarchical levels and departmentalization within a system.

The concept of span of control involves the coordination of individuals' activities by the superior, focusing on superior-subordinate relationships and authority, to attain a systematic integration of all activities in the system.[24,35]

Background of span of control concept

How wide a span of control should be goes back to antiquity. Jethro, Moses' father-in-law, observed the problems Moses was having in leading the Israelites out of Egypt. Jethro suggested to Moses that he appoint rulers of thousands, rulers of hundreds, rulers of items, and concern himself with

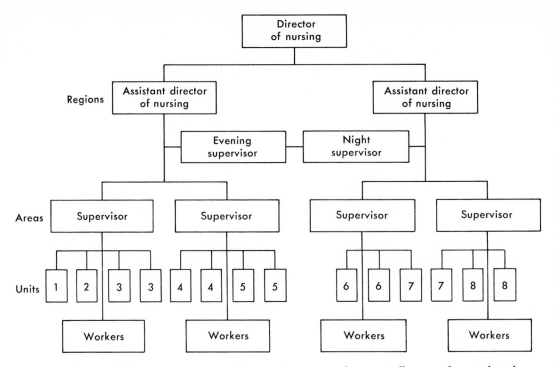

Fig. 10-1. A tall nursing service organizational structure has a small span of control with several necessary hierarchical levels. This structure is usually organized by title and rank. Unit groupings and supervisory positions are organized geographically. The supervisory staff and workers' activities are not based on specialization in nursing.

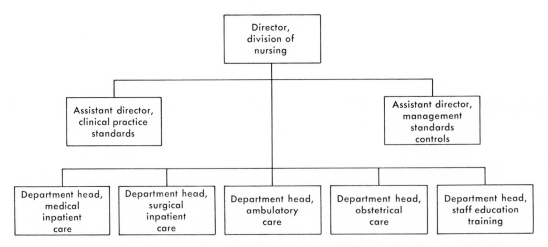

Fig. 10-2. Horizontal and vertical dimensions in the flat organizational structure permit a large span of control. The functional form of organization promotes effective use of nursing resources by drawing on specialized skills and training and ensures coordination within each specialized nursing care area in the care of patients. It provides professional reinforcement of professional nursing practice and provides advancement opportunities for nurse-practitioners within their specialized area of practice. Semiautonomous departments and their units must have clearly defined lines of communication and authority in meeting the goals of the division of nursing service.

important decisions to resolve major problems[14] (see Chapter 6).

Henri Fayol[15] recommended that one department head command only a small number of subordinates, while a foreman command 20 to 30 workers (see Chapters 3 and 6).

V. A. Graicunas,[19] a French management consultant, perpetuated the concept of the number of workers per supervisor by developing a mathematical formula to determine the ratio of subordinates to an immediate superior. Graicunas also stressed that the number of unit or departmental relationships a supervisor had was a more crucial consideration than merely numbers. Frequently this concept does not apply in practice. Supervisors and superiors have many potential relationships but can exercise only a few at one time. In general, if numbers are considered, some propose four to eight subordinates at the upper levels and 18 or 20 at the lower levels.

Gerald Bell's[35] study in 1967 indicates that the span of control is unrelated to the closeness of supervision but is determined principally by the nature of work and technology. His study signifies that the quantity of organized manpower devoted to supervision is affected by the complexity of the subordinates' jobs and the competence and training of the subordinates.

Peter Blau's 1968 studies[8] indicate that a narrow span of control may be indicative of much upward communication rather than close downward supervision. Thus, the closer the contact, the more supervisory time will be consumed per subordinate and the smaller the span will be. Today most organization research does not focus on span of control as a normative prescription but rather as an indicator of the quality of the organization's resources delegated to supervision.

Factors to be considered

Division of activities by departments or by grouping units and the creation of multiple hierarchical levels are not completely desirable for all systems. Many levels increase operating costs, and more manpower resources are delegated to managing and coordinating intradepartmental and interdepartmental activities.

Less supervisory contact is required with the use of well-defined objectives and standards and carefully designed roles with appropriate authority when individuals understand what is expected. A well-trained professional nursing staff requires not only less time from its superior but also fewer contacts with superiors. On the other hand, when plans cannot be made accurately and when subordinates must do much of their own planning, they may require considerable guidance in decision making from their superiors.

Nursing service administrators should set clear standards and policies to guide subordinates in decision making. The staff must understand the operating process and goals of the nursing service system. The top administrator's ability to communicate goals and directives clearly and concisely tends to increase an administrator's span.

Face-to-face contacts are necessary in handling many solutional problems and in appraising an individual's performance and discussing it with him or her. Face-to-face conferences with groups involved are often the best way of resolving problems and directing subordinates. Conferences provide a superior with a direct "feel" as to how subordinates think about the objectives, standards, and policies in relation to their job. This participative approach between subordinates and superiors conserves resources by reducing individual face-to-face contact.

In our technological age of health care delivery the exact number of levels in a nursing service system will depend on the effect of underlying variables and their impact on the time requirements of effective managing. Implicit in the span of control is the necessity for the coordination of manpower resources, authority, responsibility, and accountability. These establish the framework for much of traditional management theory.

A highly trained technical and professional nursing staff at the lower levels of the hierarchy tends to decrease the need for continuous supervision. As previously mentioned, individuals who are well oriented to their roles and understand what is expected of them work effectively within a long span of control.

LINKING THE HIERARCHICAL STRUCTURE

For the bottom-up approach to organizational design to be effective the hierarchical structure must provide ways of integrating each sociotechnical system with the systems above and below it. Rensis Likert,[26] in the early 1960s, developed a model that shows how every participant functions as a linking pin for groups in the hierarchical structure. In this model the organization is conceived of as a system of vertically overlapping groups, connected by individuals who occupy key positions in two groups. By virtue of their roles, these individuals serve as linking pins between groups and hold together the hierarchical structure. The application of this concept in nursing service is shown in Fig. 10-3. An effective supervisor at the first level, a clinical nurse supervisor at the middle level, and a department head or top administrator must be able to function well "upstream" as well as "downstream."

According to Petit's concept,[38] all professional nurses must be skilled in both leadership and membership functions as well as in their roles. Supervisory nurses must be effective both as supervisors and as subordinates. Likert[26] identifies the various aspects of group processes that determine how effectively the hierarchical structes of a production system are integrated through linking pins. This concept of integration has implications for nursing service.

Robert Kahn[22] and his colleagues took the linking pin concept a step further through their model of overlapping role sets. As previously mentioned, each status is a position in a social system, and associated with each status is a role—the behavior expected of the individual occupying the position. A role set is the set of individuals, superiors, subordinates, peers, and others with whom a supervisor or administrator has role-related relationships. Thus, the linking pin function

is performed by individuals who play roles in two or more role sets.

DIFFERENTIATION OF ORGANIZATIONAL ACTIVITIES

The total tasks of the nursing service division are differentiated so that its departments and units can be responsible for the performance of specialized inpatient and outpatient care activities. According to Petit,[38] differentiation segments the organizational system into subsystems (see Chapter 6). For example, the medical, surgical, pediatric, obstetric, and inpatient care units, as well as ambulatory care, possess particular attributes in relation to the requirements of their clients.

In any health organization, differentiation occurs in two directions—the vertical specialization of activities, represented by the vertical organizational hierarchy, and the horizontal differentiation of activities, referred to as departmentalization (Fig. 10-2). Vertical differentiation establishes the management role structure from the bottom level to the top officer, and the basic communication and authority structure. On the other hand, the horizontal differential defines the basic departmentalization. Together they make up the formal organization structure of the system.

Vertical differentiation (hierarchy)

As previously discussed, the vertical division of work to various positions establishes the hierarchy and the number of levels in the organization structure.

Traditionally, in the formal organization, vertical specialization is established by specific definitions of roles for various positions with status differences between levels. Positions in vertical dimensions determine the line authority over the lower positions in the hierarchy. The higher up in the hierarchy, the broader the planning and decision making. Traditionally, top executives are concerned with major strategic decisions, and those at the lower levels are concerned with technical operations. Thus vertical differentiation of work tends to create an organizational pyramid since each superior has more

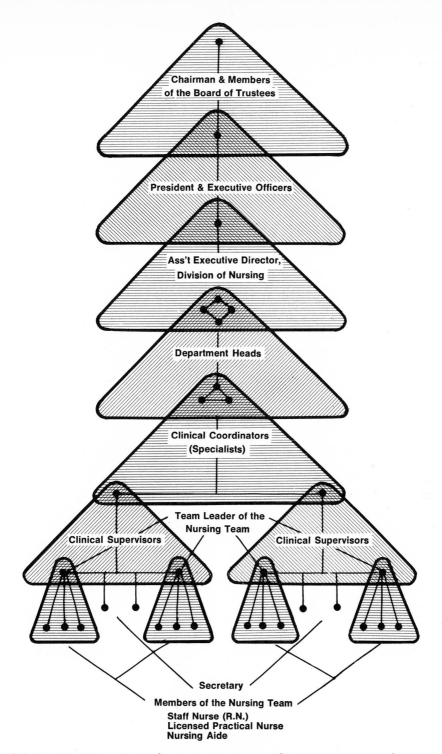

Chairman & Members of the Board of Trustees

President & Executive Officers

Ass't Executive Director, Division of Nursing

Department Heads

Clinical Coordinators (Specialists)

Team Leader of the Nursing Team

Clinical Supervisors

Clinical Supervisors

Secretary

Members of the Nursing Team
Staff Nurse (R.N.)
Licensed Practical Nurse
Nursing Aide

Fig. 10-3. Participative pattern of organization in providing nursing care and services for patients. An organization can function best when its personnel are linked together as members of a highly effective work group with mutual objectives within a management system that links the groups together into a total organization by means of persons who hold overlapping group membership. Interaction between individuals, as well as in the groups, takes place when the groups are well knit. Within this structure the linking process provides for accomplishment of management by objectives. The vertical line communication channels are linked with the lateral structure designed as councils.

than one subordinate, and the structure tends to broaden at its base (Fig. 6-2).

Horizontal differentiation (departmentalization)

Division of activities in any organization by units or departments may be created according to function, homogeneity, similarity of services, or territorial location. In most health care delivery systems, various types of departmentalization exist. In general, most nursing service departmentalization is done to facilitate the grouping of patients in terms of the nature or similarity of the medical and nursing specialization required or the territorial location (Figs. 10-1 and 10-2).

The appropriate division of the management of nursing care services aims to attain a better quality of patient care through benefits derived from specialization. It is through departmentalization that a system expands horizontally. Koontz and O'Donnell[24] emphasize that the division of work according to occupational specializaton is an economic rather than a management principle.

In medium and large hospitals and medical centers the nursing service system is divided into inpatient care and outpatient semiautonomous departments or units. Each department may consist of various units for the care of clients requiring an intensive, moderate, or minimal amount of nursing care and the expertise of professional health teams. Other special services such as emergency, surgeries, and ambulatory services support the principles of specialization technology and division of labor.

Departmentalization aims to provide a better arrangement and control of the facilities, equipment, and materials required to perform the necessary services. It also provides a setting for the intensive training of students and nursing service personnel as well as for research.

Division of activities through departmentalization or modifications should provide effective communication vertically and horizontally between health professionals and others in the total system. It should promote more accurate accountability of resources and of individual performances in accordance with standards of nursing care practices.

If work activities cannot be grouped to attain nursing service objectives, departmentalization should not take place. A logical grouping of nursing service activities must result in the attainment of nursing service objectives; otherwise it does not serve a useful purpose.

Considerations in departmentalization or its modifications. Each department and unit must have a clear definition of the results expected, as well as of the activities to be undertaken to accomplish defined goals and objectives (see Chapter 7).

The nursing service administrator should explicitly define the standards, policies, and scope of decisions to be undertaken by top administration and those to be handled by departments and their subunits. All nursing service members should understand how each subsystem must function to attain the objectives of the department and those of the total system.[5]

Without defined intradepartmental and interdepartmental management responsibilities and authority, the functional semiautonomous departments or units may become small empires that conflict to the point of detracting from organizational goal attainment. The problems of coordination become more complex with the existence of many departments. Autonomy may promote an attitude of independence that can result in a subunit's drifting away from the overall organizational goals. A control system, as previously mentioned, must go hand-in-hand with decentralizing authority.

The nursing service participative approach through its councils and committees determines overall nursing service objectives, standards, and policies and promotes unity of purpose within the division of nursing service. The nurse-executive must plan with departments to prevent duplication. Long- and short-range department or unit plans must be approved by the top executive team of the nursing service system (see Chapter 8).

Departmentalization offers greater autonomy to the department head and staff, along with a clearer recognition of performance standards. In some situations department heads and staff are motivated to a better performance in their specialties.

CENTRALIZATION AND DECENTRALIZATION

There are many interpretations of centralization and decentralization concepts. The dispersion or degree of delegation of responsibilities, power, and authority to lower levels of an organization is the only analytical use of the centralization-decentralization concept.[29,32,38]

Other basic types of centralization-decentralization are the territorial, geographical, or functional division of operations. These types have been discussed under departmentalization.

Optimal degree of decentralization

The organization chart does not reflect how much decision making is retained at the top and how much is delegated to the lower levels. Research literature[28,34] indicates that top executives may support decentralization verbally but in actuality make most or all of the major decisions. Frequently, top executives centralize authority and power at the top either directly or through a formal structure or policies—informal instruction, budgetary control mechanisms, or through the submissive attitude on the part of subordinates.

Institutions make use of both centralization and decentralization. These concepts differ only in degree. Decentralization of a nursing service system does not mean complete autonomy for decision making. If a system operated under complete centralization, subordinates would have no responsibilities, power, or authority. In that situation the system would accomplish nothing. On the other hand, complete decentralization is also impossible, since it would result in a complete lack of coordinated, organized activity.

In general, decentralization attempts to focus on the importance of the human element and to incorporate behavioral ideas into the organization structure. It provides for the participation of professional nurses in decisions that affect the practice of nursing in their specialties and in the management of their services to their clients. Moreover, decentralization tends to increase the motivation of individuals at the middle and lower levels.

Through applying a large degree of decentralization, the nursing service system can gain the benefits of professional participation through greater involvement in decisions in the implementation of programs and projects. The nursing staff in department subunits know the primary nursing care activities required to meet their nursing objectives. They can develop an effective division of work and recommend an effective role structure.

On the other hand, the central administrative staff possesses broad knowledge concerning the standards of practice and management principles and are aware of the environmental variables and overall goals of the entire nursing service system and of the institution. Thus, the nurse-executive working closely with department heads provides those in the middle and lower levels with information and direction toward decisions that enhance overall goals.

More effective decisions are possible because of the speed and firsthand knowledge that decentralization provides. Decentralization also serves as an excellent experience in decision making for those in the lower levels. In a decentralized setting, top administrators have more time to focus on creative innovations and policy making. Decentralization offers a less complex and less costly organizational control system.

Department heads and supervisors are obligated through their job design to communicate their staffs' opinions and recommendations for changes in standards, policies, and structure to accomplish a defined objective. Nurse-executives are responsible for reviewing, analyzing, and communicating final decisions to their subordinates.

Organizationally, decentralization supports several management principles.[24] They are as follows:

1. Operating decisions should be made as

near the point of operations as the competence of personnel permits.

2. All subparts of a system are designed and operated as components of the total system and in harmony with the hospital structure and policies.
3. All parts of the system must blend with freedom to develop and adapt to changing situations.

Decentralization of decision making requires the careful delegation of authority to qualified professional nurses who are experts in their specialties and understand the delegating, coordinating, and controlling processes of management (see Fig. 9-1).

Centralization

Centralization of authority in decision making produces uniformity of policy and action, reduces the risks of errors by subordinates, and uses the skills of central and specialized experts. Thus centralization tightens control of operations.

The introduction of computer informational systems is beginning to alter the balance of advantages between centralization and decentralization. Some researchers[29] argue that computerized information will foster greater centralized planning and control. Others disagree. They believe that there is much more to centralization than just centralized information systems. Others support the idea that available, sophisticated, informational technology will have some impact on the degree to which delegation of authority is necessary,[44] but it is uncertain when and how much influence the computer will have on organization structure.

The power of labor unions and collective bargaining have contributed to greater centralization in medium and large health institutions.

There are great advantages to be gained by the centralization of particular controlling activities involving personnel, accounting, and information services. Centralization contributes to the development of uniformity and more standardized procedures.

Nursing service exists for the patients whom the hospital system serves. For this reason, nursing service functions closely depend on those of the total system. The nursing service structure's scope, flexibility, and freedom to change are closely related to the development of the most appropriate design to perform the practice of nursing and care activities delegated to the departments of nursing services.

Faulty identification

In some situations the decentralization system promotes faulty centralization of decision making among professionals and other groups in a unit or department. Individuals tend to identify with a group when evaluating a problem and selecting a course of action in terms of the consequences for their specific group. The design of a decentralized system must minimize decisional biases from the principle that undesirable effects of identification are those that prevent individuals from making correct decisions. Decisions must be balanced against other values outside a particular unit or department. For this reason top administration must evaluate decisions from the standpoint of efficiency and effectiveness rather than adequacy.

Summary

Decentralization does not absolve the nursing service administrator's responsibility and authority for decision making to attain the goals of the system. The nursing service administrator is responsible for introducing overall plans and policies that coordinate and integrate activities.

Administrators should recognize that the centralization of decisions is powerful in the coordination of plans and controls, but they also should realize that centralization does not have the powerful coordinative qualities of staff members.

The nursing service executive staff should set up a mechanism to establish how much authority is to be concentrated or dispersed. It is necessary to create a balance between decentralization and centralization in order to share authority on decision making between the top and lower levels of a system. The extent of delegating authority in aspects of planning, policy, and control-making decisions depends on how the decisions will affect the objectives of the system as a whole.

STAFF AND LINE CONCEPT OF ORGANIZATION

It is sometimes difficult to define the terms "line" and "staff." In this age of specialization the traditional concept of line and staff creates confusion concerning the nature of authority relations. Consultants say that more difficulties, friction, and loss of time and effectiveness stem from a misunderstanding of this concept. Some have suggested that an organization discard line and staff and base its structure on the tasks of functional responsibilities of workers. Much

of the confusion stems from conflicting definitions regarding line and staff functions.[9,20]

The application of the scalar process assumes that formal authority is accompanied by technical competence and power. Researchers recognize that technical expertise and authority might not be equal and therefore recommend staff specialists to supplement the technical competence of the supervisor or department head who maintains scalar authority.

Authority relationships among various functions, whether vertical or horizontal, are the main arteries and veins that keep the system and its parts alive and healthy. It is impossible for nurses and other employees to work effectively within the structure unless they understand the authority relationships

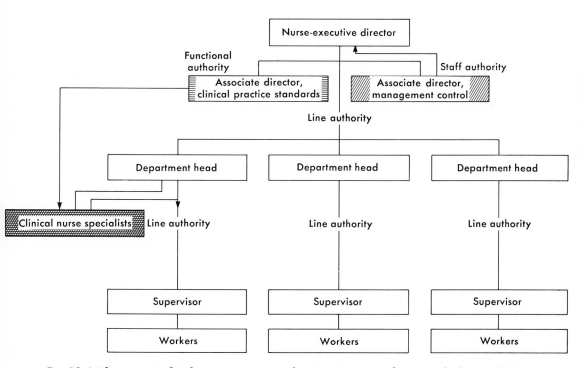

Fig. 10-4. Three types of authority may exist in the nursing service division. The line authority of each position has authority over lower positions in the hierarchy. Line authority is the backbone of the hierarchical structure. The staff authority of the specialist serves the line structure in an advisory capacity without authority to put recommendations into action. Functional authority permits the specialist in a given set of activities, such as nursing practice and standards, to enforce directives within a limited and clearly defined scope of authority. The nursing service division must clearly define the functions and scope of authority for both staff and functional positions. Nurses serving in staff positions should be active participants in the nursing service council.

of the line and staff structure of their hospital.

Line authority

The line structure, consisting of the direct (vertical) relationships, connects the positions and tasks of each level with those above and below it. The line functions and authority derive from the scalar principle of relationships in which a superior exercises direct supervison over a subordinate (Fig. 10-4).

The line functions and duties are usually those that directly affect the accomplishment of jobs to be done on a floor or a department. In other words, the supervisor (superior) of the floor, in relationships with the staff nurses (subordinates), directs, guides, and instructs them for achievement of objectives. The director of nursing is a superior officer over the supervisor (subordinate). At the same time the executive officer of the hospital of his or her associate is the superior over the director of nursing (subordinate) for accomplishment of functions and duties.

An organization could not operate without individual on-line positions. It has been said that line authority is one of the "glues" that keeps the structure together. Line structure is indispensable to all organized efforts. It provides channels of upward and downward communications and links the various parts of activities together through appropriate connections with the ultimate point of authority in the organization. The gradation of the span of authority within the relationships can be viewed as a bottom-up set of interactions between individuals and groups who are delegated specific functions.

One sees this interacting process by viewing the relationships of the nursing team at work on a floor. The nurse is assigned the functions of the leader of a nursing team under the direction of the supervisor of the floor. To accomplish the objectives of the team, to create a smooth working unit, to blend the efforts of all members, and to coordinate the care and services for each patient, the team leader (superior) accepts a leadership role with specific authority relationships. The supervisor and all members

of the staff must understand and work within the authority relationships to coordinate efforts, produce quality of care, and gain personal satisfaction from their efforts (Fig. 10-1).

Staff authority

The formal staff organization has been used since antiquity. As previously mentioned, Moses' father-in-law Jethro took a staff role acting as a consultant to solve problems in organizing the Israelites. Frederick Taylor supported staff organization (see Chapter 6).

The flow of staff authority (with few exceptions) is upward to the top executive, who then exercises line authority in putting recommendations into effect (Fig. 10-5). In studying and helping to resolve problems, staff individuals may consult with line supervisors and department heads and have them, if possible, agree with their proposals before they take them to their peers. A nurse-executive is more likely to accept staff proposals that meet the approval of the subordinates who must implement them.

Line personnel can seek advice from staff members and either accept or reject their recommendations. Staff authority relationships refer to those functions and tasks that help the line to work more efficiently and effectively in the accomplishment of objectives.

In some nursing service divisions, staff members act as aides to the top nurse-executive. They may be viewed as an extension of the executive but do not have responsibilities down the line of command. Staff positions in nursing service may focus on staff education, personnel work, and accounting functions or on other functions such as quality assessment that require expertise. With line-staff positions, line members are relieved of functions that can be accomplished more effectively from a centralized position.

FUNCTIONAL AUTHORITY

Functional authority is a type of formal authority that permits specialists on a given set of activities such as accounting, per-

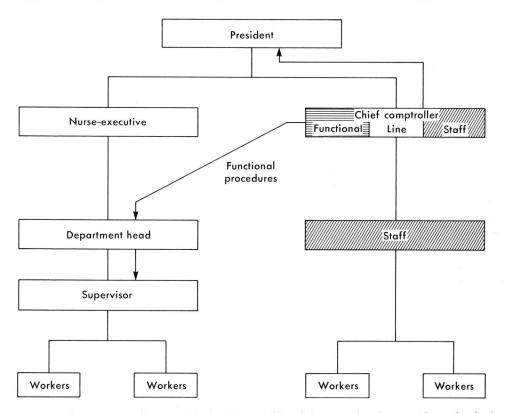

Fig. 10-5. The position of comptroller has line, staff, and functional authority. This individual has line authority within his own department and reports to his line superior. He serves in an advisory (staff) capacity to the top executive officers including the nurse-executive and her immediate assistants. The president of the organization delegates to the comptroller functional authority for setting specific procedures for the line administrative and supervisory members to follow and implement. The personnel director has line, functional, and staff responsibilities.

sonnel, materials management, or engineering to enforce their directives within a limited and clearly defined scope of authority.

Functional organization was developed to reduce problems of coordination of staff advisory authority by permitting orders to flow directly to lower levels (Figs. 10-4 and 10-5). For example, in an institution the comptroller may serve as a line, staff, and functional authority at the same time but for different phases of the organization's activities. The comptroller may give budgetary accounting advice (staff) to the nurse-executive or department head, supervise his own accounting department (line), and set specific accounting procedures for the supervisory staff with his own specialist authority (functional).

Today staff specialists are the experts in their particular specialty, and top executives depend on them to study the problems, present the alternatives that might be adopted, and help make major decisions. Nurse specialists can contribute in setting and implementing standards to improve clinical practice and the delivery of nursing service (Fig. 10-4).

Lower managers' acceptance or rejection of staff recommendations that may or may not be representative of the wishes of the executive officer can create a more complicated set of relationships than the traditional simple line-staff type of structure. Frustration may lead to a power struggle and create a poor environment for interaction. It is no longer possible to delineate clearly between line and staff relationships. Nursing service professionals have many functional responsibilities in the patient care system.

The service departments' and top managers' functional authority relationships are changing and becoming more clearly identified in the hospital system. Functional authority refers to the authority control that resides within a specialized staff and is exercised within other operational units.

Functional authority is the power that a position or a department may have delegated to it involving specified processes, practices, or policies. Functional authority is not restricted to managers of a particular type of department. In some situations functional authority may be exercised by line, service, or staff department heads because they are usually specialists whose knowledge becomes the basis for functional controls.

Functional authority allows wide variations as compared with the traditional, line, pyramidal structure in which the relationships are based on the unity-of-command concept, with authority directed from only one supervisor and each subordinate responsible to only one superior for his total activities. In the modern hospital system, nurses communicate with many superior and staff officers delegated specific functions within the system.

Clarification of functional and staff authority

Confusion and frustrations arise when functional authority relationships are not clearly identified and established within the management process. Without clear identification the hospital that uses a functional staff can severely damage the line (unit-of-command) structure.

In this age of specialization, functional staffs and specialists in clinical and business areas are frequently delegated authority involving line officer activities. Understanding and clarity of functions are necessary to prevent multiple rather than unified action (Figs. 10-4 and 10-5). The growth in the use of executive and functional authority has complicated the organizational relationships of the total line structure. Functionalization

of management, if carried to extremes, destroys the department head's and supervisor's jobs.

It should be mentioned that when the director of nursing and supervisory staff lose their authority to plan, organize, staff, and direct the activities within the division of nursing, they can no longer manage. To some extent this occurs when an administrative executive has functional authority over some part of another administrative officer's job. When the executive manager requires nursing service to follow a procedure without consultation with the division head and assigns additional tasks to the units, he is interfering with some of the nursing service director's prerogatives. This is also the case when the executive officers and medical staff decide the type, when, where, what, and who of a new health service requiring considerable nursing care services, without the participation of nursing and others in the preplanning of the program. This type of authority control interferes to some extent with the authority of the supervisory staff of the department and promotes fear and distrust of the system.

Positive approach to staff and functional authority

With increased sharing of functions between specific individuals and groups, the relationships of the staff specialists and executives with functional areas of control and direction must be clarified with all department heads and other supervisory personnel. Functional authority is accomplished when the staff member and the middle- or top-level managers are delegated specific authority in the structure and present suggestions relating to methods, processes, and policies that should be followed by all subparts of either the staff or line departments. For instance, with the approval of the top executive officer, the personnel director may issue directions or instructions prescribing particular procedures to be followed such as appraisal standards for measurement of performance, handling of grievances, terminations, position controls, wage and salary scales, and personnel wage increases. The comptroller is given authority to decide the kind of accounting records of manpower to be kept by the nursing service departments. The materials-management department, in consultation with health professionals and scientific engineers, may prescribe and initiate standard inventory methods and controls for all supplies and equipment used in patient services. The environmental safety system is delegated functions concerning electrical hazards, inspection of units, and evaluation of accidents and errors in procedures. The nurse specialists with expertise in a specific area are delegated functional responsibilities for quality of patient care.

Information and directions should be transmitted through the supervisory line structure to give a basis for units of command and maintain group participation at each level within the department and its subunits. Staff and functional authority should be clarified, especially when they converge on a department. This is necessary not only from the viewpoint of the individual's understanding of the staff and functional types of authority but also for those who are receiving the authorized instructions and directions for implementation.

Authority of the nurse-specialist or nurse-coordinator

Recently nursing services have employed nurse-practitioners in the position of clinical specialists or clinical nurse-coordinators who possess expertise in clinical patient care and in a nursing specialty. In some hospitals the nurse specialist has no authority to initiate actions to improve the clinical care of patients. This has created frustrations and conflicts among nurses and physicians within the structure.

There are several management principles to be considered before employing a nurse-practitioner in any position. The job description of the position should clearly define the exact nature and limits of authority. It provides the guidelines by which the person will work and identifies the position role with others contributing to the management of patient care (see Chapter 9). In a structure in which line and staff positions are not in-

tegrated the person in this new position may have difficulties because of a lack of understanding of line and staff functions of the position. Cooperation is established through routine interactions and the development of relationships practiced over a period of time. The nurse-specialist must be clinically competent but also possess managerial leadership abilities in the nursing care system.

The demands of a situation influence how a nurse-practitioner will be able to function at a specific level of the hierarchy. Thus the qualities, nature, characteristics, knowlege, and skills required for successful achievement of goals in a particular area or program must be carefully determined before the assignment of the nurse. Nurse-leaders, physicians, and executive administrators for professional services should be briefed on the positions of nurse-practitioners and understand and promote the management of the health team concept (see Chapter 9).

It appears evident that the nurse-practitioners, as a nurse-specialist or clinical coordinator, should have line or functional authority within the boundaries of the functions of the job (Figs. 10-1 and 10-4). This is important because *the art of managing cannot be a separate function from the art of nursing.* Quality nursing requires that the expert nurse will incorporate the management principles of planning, organizing, staffing, directing, and controlling.

The weakness of delegating functional or staff authority to such positions is that it usually subjects subordinates to the frustrations of multiple direct supervisory commands unless all members understand and accept each other's role and scope of authority. In general, subordinates dislike having to choose between their immediate line supervisor and the functional specialists if there are conflicting orders. In practice, when conflict of authority arises, the line authority tends to prevail. The subordinates, supervisor, and team leaders tend to consider the clinical specialist or coordinator as an important source of guidance. Acting as a staff consultant and informal teacher, this nurse may be limited in efforts to improve overall nursing practice and the delivery of nursing services. The nurse with expertise in a nursing specialty has a great responsibility to assist in the measurement of the quality of nursing services and to help make decisions affecting patient care. The prime reason for line authority is to help make the system work for patient care. In the future, perhaps, the nursing service system will free all nurse-practitioners to concentrate on the nursing processes of health care.

The nursing service organization's design for administrative strategies and jobs through which it hopes to be effective is closely related to the nature of the external environment (see Chapter 6; Fig. 8-2). Nursing service leaders must consider the nature of clients, human resources, competition, the sociopolitical environment, and technology (see Chapter 9).

The larger environment in which institutions operate plays an important role in the way organizations design jobs, direct and supervise members, and make decisions. Due to rapid changes within the health system and a somewhat unstable environment, a so-called organic type of organization may be better than a mechanistic type.[25,46]

Today, top professionals in line positions cannot be knowledgeable in all things. They need assistants with specialized knowledge and skills. Communications must be lateral between persons of different rank. The focus of communications is based on giving and receiving information and advice. Nurses with special expertise and skills tend to be committed to specific tasks and value the progress made toward organization objectives. Today, nurse-leaders are challenged to design jobs and a structure that have less hierarchy of control.

ORGANIZATION CHARTS

An organization chart may be viewed as a drawing that depicts what executives desire to become a reality concerning formal relationships of people in the various positions. A chart usually shows who supervises whom and how various jobs are linked together to make a cohesive, coordinated system (Figs. 10-2 and 10-5). The main channels of communications within the various levels of the

hierarchy show the downward flow of authority and responsibility and the upward flow of accountability.

Advantages. The process of drawing up master and subsidiary charts impels executives to think more specifically about the intermediate middle- and lower-line relationships. The nursing service organization chart is considered an important supplementary tool of the total hospital master chart. The chart is useful in orienting new members of the staff and in describing the structural design to members of the staff, high-level professionals, and those outside the hospital. It provides a quick visual illustration of the structure and communications.

Through the formal committee organization the nursing service professional staff can design an organization chart that indicates existing role and organization structures and relationships. As Prouty[39] points out, such a project can be a learning experience for all staff members and the nurse-administrator. Revision of an organization chart (when changes in positions and structure have taken place) can help show all nursing personnel and other departments the new relationships, responsibilities, and authority of various individuals toward the attainment of goals. The use of an organization chart as a design tool is of value in showing positions and relationship one would like to have in the organization.

Limitations. Organization charts may be used to denote the status or rank of members from the board of trustees and president down to the lower level. However, a position on the chart alone does not make for high status. The authority, power, and number of subordinates that a person has also determines influence, rank, and status.

The degree of responsibility or authority cannot be determined by the size and position of the boxes on the chart.[9] For example, directors of nursing may be shown to be on the same level as all other department heads, even though they have more delegated complex functions and authority than some other department heads.

It is difficult to show the degree of decentralization in relation to delegation of decision-making authority. For example, clinical nurse-specialists may be shown on a line from the middle level down to the lower level in the care of clients. However, the chart does not indicate their power and authority in decision making. It is difficult to determine line and staff positions and authority as one views the many light and dark lines shooting in various directions from one box to others.

The chart is a valuable tool, but a static one. It does not attempt to illustrate the highly dynamic process of human interaction. Any chart provides a restricted view of an organization and is a static model, not the organization itself.

INTRODUCTION OF MODERN STRUCTURAL MODELS

Hospital management is beginning to modify its traditional organization structures. The elements of the system approach are being introduced (see Chapter 6). Project and program organization structures, the most common departure from classical organization structures, are used to solve specific problems and accomplish particular objectives. The project concept is a philosophy of management as well as a form of organization structure. Cleland and King[9] stress that the project viewpoint is quite different from the functional organization. In the project the chain of command exists to a degree, but the major focus is on the horizontal and diagonal work flow.

Project and program planning have been mentioned in discussing the planning process in Chapters 6 and 8. Another modern structure model is the matrix structure, which comprises a project structure along with the functional structure of the organization.[1,9,28]

Project structures

There are several basic types of project structures. In the individual project the top executive delegates one individual responsibility for a specific project and activities. For example, a nurse-specialist or department head with unique expertise in a particular project becomes the project manager. This person has no assistance but seeks information and ideas from selected members within and outside the departments. The objectives of the project must be approved by the top executive, and all professional nurses must be oriented to the objectives, the phases of the plan, the duration of the project, and the results.[16]

A staff organization project is one that has a manager and a staff to perform project activities, but the primary functional tasks of the projects are performed by line members of the organization.

A third type is the so-called intermix project. Here the project manager has a staff and selected department heads or supervisors who report directly to the director as they carry out project activities. For example, a nursing service organization may wish to develop a quality assurance program, peer review, or a performance evaluation program. During a specific period of time the project members would be relieved of their jobs, usually for several hours each week. During the project the individuals assigned to its activities generally remain accountable to their functional superior for pay, performance, and promotions.

Matrix structure

The matrix structure consists of a project plus the functional organization structure. In the matrix management process, department heads and others in the line have authority in their units. The project members (specialists) are assigned projects along the horizontal structure.

Researchers admit that problems arise in the matrix organization structure. It tends to discourage informal groups and the nurturing of superior-subordinate relationships, and it reduces participant motivation for all members. Leadership is important for its success.

According to Cleland and King,[9] the advantages of the matrix organization outweigh the disadvantages. Some advantages mentioned by Cleland and King are as follows:

It provides flexible manpower utilization because a reservoir of specialists are maintained within the functional structure, either on a part- or full-time basis.

Specialized knowledge and skills are available to all programs on an equal basis. Personnel with appropriate knowledge and skills can be transferred from one project to another.

When matrix members are no longer needed, they may return to their functional positions or be assigned to a particular area of nursing. Matrix organization can change the functions of middle and top positions concerning planning, directing, and evaluating standards of nursing practice and management. Matrix organization is an element of the systems approach placed on the traditional (vertical) structure.

Matrix organization: management by exception and management by objectives. The concept of management by exception was first introduced by F. W. Taylor, "the father of scientific management," and aimed to use all available human resources within an organization to attain defined objectives.

With the scientific management approach, arbitrary power and arbitrary decision making cease. Every problem becomes the province of scientific investigation for decision making, and the personal exercise of authority is almost eliminated. A common superior is selected to resolve problems if a satisfactory level of attainment is not being met. Today management by exception comprises measurements, projections, observations, selection, comparison of data, and definite phases of action toward the attainment of objectives.

Management by objectives, previously discussed in Chapter 6, and management by exception encourage individuals' involvement in the selection of goals and their attainment.

In the work place of a health care system the matrix organization may be faced with nonacceptance on the part of highly trained professionals who may feel frustrated when faced with frequent organization changes. Moreover professionals prefer to be allied organizationally with their own professional group. Recently, faced with rapid technological advances, institutions began to introduce project and program organization and matrix

organization using representatives of various interest groups through horizontal and lateral channels.

Committee structure

The common and inescapable organizational form is the committee structure. A committee is a group of individuals who meet by plan to tackle a specific subject. It is not an informal work group that occurs spontaneously without a definite design.[18]

Some executives and staff members view committees as an unfortunate but inescapable part of our organized system and believe that an organization will never free itself from the committee structure. To a great degree, committee and team decision making are a direct consequence of increased specialization and technology.[10,17,34,37]

Nurse-executives should carefully determine when a group decision applies. In some cases an individual decision is deferred because of personal reluctance to risk decision making on a particular sensitive subject.

Definition. Committee refers to all kinds of formal groups and task forces elected or appointed within an enterprise.[43] A formal committee structure is composed of selected individuals. Each committee has official status and administrative approval, defined objectives, functions, clearly stated directives, and procedures for maintaining and selecting members and presenting recommendations or implementing decisions.

Advantages. A committee can be an excellent means of transmitting information and ideas up or down the hierarchy. It provides an opportunity for motivated and interested members to participate as a group in creative activities and to agree on a plan for the attainment of objectives.

A committee can be used to collect and combine the authority and power of several individual members to make or implement a desired decision. Note that the arbitrary use of authority discourages initiative. After consultation with staff members the nurse-executive should determine the direction and the objectives of the organization, but she should also encourage as much autonomy as possible in the methods used to attain them. How-

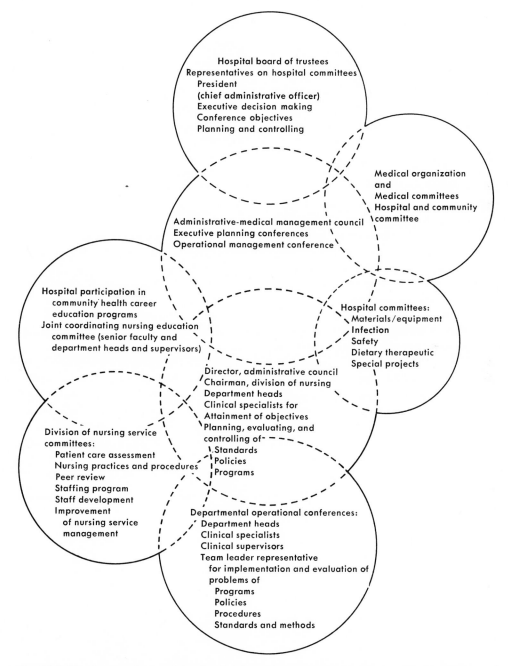

Fig. 10-6. Nursing service participation in a lateral communications system for coordination of activities to attain objectives becomes more effective when the overlapping groups of each subsystem contribute their ideas through an established system. Councils and group conferences of the division of nursing work together to accomplish nursing objectives and participate with other hospital groups in the patient care system to provide for an effective performance in the care of patients.

ever, limiting authoritarianism by the establishment of decision making must be carefully done to secure the best decisions.

A committee can perform an effective coordinating function by means of bringing persons together for agreement on a course of action that will involve individuals at various levels of the nursing service organization (see Chapter 11).

Through a committee structure, the nurse-executive and department heads can get work done, secure feedback, and evaluate staff members' behavior by listening to their presentations (Fig. 10-6).

The committee structure creates communication channels to and from committees through which other members may submit their ideas and suggestions. This builds group acceptance for decisions and their implementation.

Disadvantages. Some executives and researchers believe that the committee decision-making process is not as feasible in practice as in theory. Others believe that the decision-making process should involve individuals at the lowest possible level who have the technical capacity and expertise to make decisions. This type of organizational approach would almost eliminate the need for committees within the formal structure.

As emphasized in Chapter 9, the job design of nursing positions at the lower and middle levels should provide authority and power for decision making to attain patient care goals, to coordinate activities, and to improve nurse-patient relationships.

Decisions made by a committee are often made by the most dominant member present. This type of group decision making can be destructive, since the dominant member may not be the best qualified person to make the decision but only the strongest personality in the group. On the other hand, a member who does not participate in decisions shifts responsibility as a group member.

The cost of committees in terms of members' efforts, time, preparation, and materials can become expensive. Committee output (outcomes) should be compared with manhours and material inputs.

Indecisions may occur in the absence of defined objectives or in the presence of conflicting viewpoints. When a committee chairperson does not use appropriate leadership skills, the group tends to be unproductive and its enthusiasm and input decrease. Productive committee action may be thwarted by a minority's refusing to accept the majority viewpoint.

Administrators have difficulty enforcing effective accountability against a committee. Some members may shunt personal responsibility by stating, "It was not my decision; the decision was made by the committee." In many organizations, committees are perpetuated long after their specific purpose has ceased to serve the existing goals of the organization.

Making a committee work. The nurse-executive has the job of pulling everyone together to attain goals through the committee structure.

When the organizational structure is modified to accommodate new growth and development, and decision making is made at the lower levels, top management relinquishes some of its authority and power. The planned conferences between supervisors and their superior will take care of delegated operational plans, such as the staffing plan and the preparation of budgets.

The nurse-executive must determine what objectives and functions can be handled more effectively by a committee than through the line processes.

The nurse-executive should consider the following factors:

1. A committee should not be formed unless the nurse-executive is absolutely certain that it can accomplish definite decisions that will be better than his or her own. Persons in leadership roles should never transfer their decision-making responsibilities onto a committee.

2. Committee members should be selected carefully. Individuals should not be selected to enhance their personal status. They should not be note-pad doodlers. Committee members must indicate interest in the attainment of nursing service objectives, be alert to changes needed in the nursing care process, and have expertise and experience related to the functions of the com-

mittee, group, or task force. The nurse-executive should consider the groups that will be involved in the implementation of a decision. For example, nurse-practitioners should have great input on a quality assessment committee.

3. The confidentiality of the functions of a particular committee should be considered. For example, a temporary committee to investigate and develop initial planning for major organizational changes requires a select group that can focus on the objectives and keep discussions within themselves and with the nurse-executive.

4. The degree of authority and decision-making power to each committee must be precisely spelled out. A committee is expected to produce definite actions and cannot depend on persuasion alone. Shall a committee be given power to recommend or to make a decision by majority rule or consensus? What committees will have authority to assign its members to specific activities? Each committee must be given a clearly stated directive regarding its functions, authority, and power in decision making.

5. The committee members should be told how much assistance they can secure from top administration or other departments in the way of background data, information, and opinions. The nurse-executive must provide the information needed to help make decisions and attain objectives.

6. A three- to eight-person committee with one chairperson is usually more effective than a larger committee. A large committee has difficulty in working as a single unit. A large group tends to develop factions, making agreement difficult.

7. The specific time of meetings must be defined for each committee. The mechanism of reporting recommendations and report of meetings to the nurse-executive also must be defined.

8. The designated committees, their goals and functions, the names of each committee, and their dates and time of meetings must be circulated to each nursing unit at the beginning of each fiscal year.

9. The responsibilities of the chairperson such as the selection of appropriate meeting place and the provision of materials, documents, agenda, and minutes must be defined to members.

10. If indicated, the nurse-executive should provide for conferences on leadership skills for chairpersons since their role is crucial in producing actions.

11. The nurse-executive should let the committee do the work assigned to them.

In summary, the nurse-executive should keep in mind that committees *can* be extremely useful when used carefully.

Types of committees and groups in nursing service. The kind of standing committees, task forces, and institutional committees with nursing service input depends on the objectives of nursing service and the total system, as well as on the primary focus of short-term plans.

Nurse-executives and their staff who view nursing as a process try to develop a committee structure that blends actions to improve the quantity and quality of nursing services for their clients. The focus is on clinical nursing care and the nursing systems in the delivery of services.

Horizontal expansion and delegation of authority and power to nurses at the lower and middle levels can increase members' interest and motivations toward the improvement of patient care.

Standing committees. Stevens[41] compares two different standing committee structures, based on specific concepts to attain goals. Many nursing service organizations have standing committees to improve the quality of nursing care and evaluate performance, and a systems approach to improve the delivery of nursing services.

There is no one best form for a standing committee structure. The important goal of nurse-executives is to develop standing committees that will assist them and all staff members toward the achievement of nursing service objectives at a particular time.

Group conferences. The size and structure of the division of nursing and the kind of restructuring taking place within the system influences formal group conferences and their design. As previously mentioned, such group formations must meet specific objectives and show productive results. Effectiveness of group conferences, although difficult to assess, can be measured in the improved individual members as well in a group's reduced problems of communication and the outcome of projects and programs.

Administrative council. Based on the participative approach in planning, coordinating, and controlling inputs of the total nursing division, the nurse-executive may create an administrative council. This type of council provides a means of communication between the nurse-executive and his or her immediate associates in administrative matters that affect the entire nursing division in the attainment of goals and objectives. For example, this group may assist the nurse-executive in structuring a standing committee such as the patient care evaluation committee or nursing service management improvement committee. They may recommend a project committee be established to investigate the initiation of primary nursing care or a staff development program in clinical nursing.

The council may include the nurse-executive as chairperson, the inpatient care department heads, staff development director, and representatives of the nurse-specialists group. At some scheduled meetings the nurse department heads of the surgeries, the clinics, and ambulatory care may participate in those meetings. The chairperson of a nursing project or task force may present a progress report and discuss committee recommendations. This type of council provides a means of communication between the nurse-executive and his or her immediate associates as well as a sharing of information. It also provides mutual support in the initiation of changes that will affect the entire nursing division.

Supervisory group conferences. Supervisory group conferences are usually designed to resolve immediate management problems in the nursing care of patients. With decentralization and with first-line supervisors (head nurses) participating in decision making as a function of their position, this type of head nurse conference may not be necessary. For example, when the first- and second-line clinical supervisors participate in the decision making of the staffing plan of their respective units with their superior (department head), or when they are members of standing committees, the need for such group conferences is reduced. Such groups should exist only if they serve a useful purpose.

Interdepartmental committees. Nurse-ex-

ecutives should work closely with top administration in determining the nursing input on interdepartmental committees. They should know the goals, functions, authority, and power of such committees and must guard against wasting nursing service resources.

In general, interdepartmental or interdivisional committees aim to coordinate activities and operations to attain the objectives of the total system and to resolve conflicting goals between nursing and other departments such as dietary, pharmacy, materials management, or personnel. In many situations the supervisory staff and team leaders possess more accurate information needed to evaluate recommendations than do persons at the top level of the nursing division. Standing interdepartmental committees should not exist unless they serve a valuable purpose.

For example, the material management department head may be chairperson of a committee delegated to keep equipment, materials, and supplies up to date and to evaluate the utility, costs, and effectiveness of new products. Supervisory members and nurse-practitioners can be productive members of such a committee. Nursing service should have input on the safety committee, hospital peer review, or the personnel committee.

Task force groups. With the introduction of innovations and approaches to meet the clinical needs of patients and those of the staff, the nursing division may design temporary committees to investigate and recommend solutions for a specific problem or to restructure an aspect in the management of nursing services. A temporary committee may be patient-centered, personnel-centered, or interdepartmental.

The membership of a task force committee depends on the kind of problem to be studied. Members should be selected regardless of position for their knowledge and experience associated with the problem or project. The task force must utilize the organization's best expertise as well as resource individuals outside the nursing organization. Projects using the PERT approach (see Chapter 6) and the matrix system use a task force committee approach.

Another interdivisional committee may be used when a nursing education program and its major clinical facility are part of the same parent enterprise or when faculty members of a community college use the facilities for clinical student experience. This committee may be composed of faculty members and those department heads and the nurse-executive involved in the use of the facilities during the coming semester who meet three times a year. During the semester, faculty members work closely with the nursing department to resolve ongoing arrangements.

Summary. In sum, committees are an investment of individuals' efforts, and human resources must not be wasted. Committees must exist only to meet specific objectives and result in productive outcomes. To succeed, members of each committee must be selected carefully on the basis of their potential contributions to the attainment of committee objectives.

STRUCTURING AUTHORITY, POWER, AND ACCOUNTABILITY

The structuring organization and plans emerge from the philosophy and objectives of the nursing service system (see Chapters 7 and 8). If the philosophy and objectives focus on the nursing care process of patients, the positions will not be task oriented to maintain a system. The supervisory and administrative staffs' interaction with their work groups will focus on clinical performance in patient care rather than on personnel and things.

The aim of administrators will be to have nurses use authority, power, and accountability to improve the quality of patient care and to create a social work environment to attain definite objectives.

An effective organization must coordinate and integrate its activities. This is accomplished when members adjust their behavior to meet organizational needs. The major mode of compliance is for one person to direct another's behavior. This mode creates a relationship between the person who directs and the one who follows the

instructions. The principal modes of compliance are frequently termed authority, influence, power, leadership, and control.[33] These terms may be used interchangeably, but each has a specialized meaning.

Systematically arranged position descriptions, organization charts, standard operating policies, and rules are essential documents within each system. However, when members in various positions begin to act, react, and interact, much of the actions tend to take place in the white areas between the boxes of a chart.

Professional autonomy

As previously mentioned, professional autonomy for nursing care is the right of self-determination and governance without outside control. Thus, autonomy for nursing care requires the decentralization of decision making to the nurse-client level (see Chapter 9). In recent years there has been evidence that the nurse-executive is gaining more autonomy in the hospital system. Unfortunately, the average staff nurse, team leader, and first-line supervisor are given little authority for professional decision making in the care of their clients. Secondly, in our bureaucratic organizations, many leaders are unwilling to recognize that it is the organizational system and not the nurse that impedes the development of an autonomous and accountable collegial nurse-practitioner.[31]

In a bureaucratic, traditional environment the scope of authority and accountability of professional nurses as employees is defined too rigidly and narrowly down the chain of command. Nurses are delegated some management authority but have not been made responsible for their own patients over an extended period of time. Focus has been on the maintenance of the system and so-called management tasks. Decision making, as previously mentioned in job design, is concentrated at the level of the superiors, not at the first level with the nurses and patients.[36]

Nurses should understand how organizations operate by distributing authority that sets the stage for the exercise of power. They should recognize the importance of personality factors and use their strengths and limitations in decision making to improve the quality of the nursing service system.

Authority in the management of patient care

Authority is defined as the right to decide or to act. Thus, authority is the right to command. Barnard's[6] concept of authority stems from the authority relationship with the subordinate. Workers tend to establish individual areas of acceptance open to them, as well as areas of resistance. There are many reasons why one individual decides to accept directions from another. When authority exists, the subordinate accepts as legitimate that another person can tell him what to do.

Sources of authority

Within the hierarchy of an organization, authority flows from the top downward. The president comes into possession of his authority from the board of directors of the institution. The supervisory members are delegated their authority from their superiors.

Authority may also flow from subordinates to supervisors and upward to the president. This type of authority is termed bottom-up authority. It does not flow through the formal structure of the organization. For example, some staff nurses may not give bottom-up authority to their supervisor yet support the objectives of the nursing service system. The nurse-executive may not receive complete bottom-up authority from all members of the organization for the primary nursing care plan but, may receive enough bottom-up authority from the staff and others and enough top-down authority to initiate the plan. Thus, to exercise authority effectively, the nurse-executive must receive enough general support from subordinates and from superiors.

Individuals will grant authority to superiors in an organization because of rank, personal qualities, position, and tradition. In the organizational line of command it may not be the person that we accept, but the role or position.

Delegation of authority

In organizations, delegation of authority refers to the process by which a superior gives an immediate subordinate the authority to do a job. For example, a nurse-executive has a clear understanding with department heads that they have the power to make decisions and to act within explicit limits.

However, this authority relationship does not relieve the nurse-executive of his or her responsibilities, but merely permits him or her to share these responsibilities with competent subordinates. The department head assumes responsibility and is accountable to the nurse-executive for decisions and actions.

Likewise, supervisors should have a clear understanding with superiors and subordinates of what power is delegated to different persons to make decisions and to act within a defined scope of authority. Team-leaders and staff nurse-practitioners also should know the limits of their decision-making power in the care of patients. Each nurse must have sufficient authority to attain personal nursing care goals and establish effective nurse-patient relationships.

The structure should provide organizational interdependent responsibilities for collective action involving patient-care problems, peer consultation, and the maintenance of the nursing system. Functionally, professional nursing autonomy and accountability cannot be viewed as separate entities.

Attitudes toward authority

At all levels of an organization, nurses by definition depend to some degree on the favor of superiors. To delegate responsibility and authority effectively requires that an individual understand the dependency patterns of others. Some nurses may seek excessive dependence; others may seek independence to the extent that they forget they are working in an interdependent system for the attainment of quality care for patients.

Superiors, regardless of their roles, must learn to support subordinates and to view their behavior as a reflection of the different behavioral attitudes people display toward authority figures and not as a nuisance. Kiev[23] states that dependent behavior should neither be encouraged nor discouraged but handled appropriately for each situation.

Delegation of authority brings unavoidable risk, but assuming risk is an unavoidable part of a professional nurse's role. If professional nurses are to gain influence in the patient care system they must be competent in the art and skills of delegating responsibility and authority to others.[22]

THE POWER SYSTEM

Positions in the nursing service organization should identify the rights and scope of authority the person may use to accomplish the objectives of that job. Authority is a source of power. Administrators or supervisors may have the authority to do something but lack the ability (power) to do it. On the other hand, nurses may have the power or influence to get something done but lack the authority to accomplish it. Such conditions tend to create instability and conflict in an organization.[40] Professional nurses in the clinical care of patients and those managing the nursing system need authority as well as power.

Elements of power

According to Zaleznik,[45] an individual's power basically consists of three ingredients: (1) the scope of formal authority given to the individual's position; (2) the authority given for needed expertise and the reputation for competence in attainment of desired objectives; and (3) the combination of respect and popularity from others. Through this capitalization of power the individual internalizes his sources of power. Such individuals know they have power and influence, assess it from a practical point of view, and are willing to risk their personal esteem to influence others to gain a particular objective. The risk in using power is that an individual is expected to perform effectively and get results. When he fails to perform and get results, his power base begins to decrease in direct proportion to earlier opinions others had about him.

Power and influence are forces that exist between persons and operate in social interaction. Power is stronger than influence because with power an individual endeavors to bring about potential actions of others by commanding or exerting influence. Moreover, power also depends on how people perceive one another and the situation they are sharing, as well as the ability to command.

Does each nurse accept legitimate power on becoming a member of the nursing service organization? Do others in the organization accept and expect each nurse to have power to attain nursing objectives?

A nurse who has the necessary expertise and knowledge can emerge as a powerful leader. However, this nurse may not have relevant authority to balance the power. In another situation, a head nurse may have power due to nursing knowledge and skills and leadership in improving patient care, regardless of the differences in financial compensation and authority. Does the nurse administrator give this nurse the necessary scope of authority, encouragement, and support to attain personal nursing goals?

In hospitals, expert power is frequently in the hands of physicians, accountants, and other individuals who have been associated with the hospital for years. Employees in the departments of nursing and medicine, as well as informational systems managers, have professional and functional power. Such power should be used to develop constructive, positive ends and colleagueships for the effective coordination of activities.

Coercive power is another kind of power based on fear. The perennial carrot-and-stick approach may get only short-term results and alienate those punished, although in some situations there is a need for coercive power and the ability to distribute rewards.[18] Psychological punishment should not be overlooked. For example, if people want very much to join a group, they will permit themselves to be influenced by the superior (leader) so that they are not punished by being denied admission to the group.

Reward power is recognized. Since a superior may give rewards, subordinates will allow that person to influence their behavior.

Rewards, the opposite of coercive power, may be monetary or verbal.

Coalition and group power

In large organizations there is an informal organization that may be powerful. It is a coalition of individuals with a common bond that can exert a forceful influence for good or ill.[22]

Likert[26] has shown that cohesive groups with high peer loyalty show less variation in productivity than do those with less cohesion. If group goals are in line with those of the system, the nursing care will be superior; if not, the work of the group tends to be below acceptable standards. A cohesive work group, when properly motivated, tends to perform effectively in the absence of their supervisor.

Personality power may be given to people who are physically attractive or have other personality features. Some individuals willingly yield to their influence. Etzioni[13] states that referent power is personal rather than position power. It connotes power with, rather than over, and involves emotional identification and affiliation with a superior.

Power may be viewed as both positive and negative. Negative power is the domination of others, submission of one person to another, and the use of many manipulations to gain an end. Negative power is destructive and dangerous to an organization.

On the other hand, individuals can develop and make use of positive power. Individuals with a positive power motive inspire others to move with them, thus sharing the power. Positive power is not based on coercion but on the identification of goals. For example, the effective supervisor (head nurse) does not dominate the work-group; the group recognizes the need for leadership and power and willingly follows directions. This is similar to the type of philosophy that McGregor and Maslow promoted (see Chapter 7). It is a challenge to achieve this kind of leadership in an organization.[11]

Tactics to improve power

Management researchers have offered suggestions to improve power to control and direct the actions of others.[42] Individuals should form alliances with others above them at their level, and below them in the organization who seem to have those characteristics and abilities that the organization wants. Such alliances help first and middle supervisors gain the respect of their subordinates, who then know that these supervisors have access outside a specific work area.

An effective leader is cautious in deciding when to seek advice. In seeking advice people should not show others any weakness in themselves or their positions.

Supervisors and administrators should continuously be aware of what the organization is looking for and try to grow with these needs. They should maintain contacts outside the organization that contribute to their sense of flexibility and maneuverability within the organization.

Individuals should be able to identify those people who have important and frequently confidential information. They should seek information that other people need so that they can supply information and add to their own power. Thus, supervisors or nurse-executives seek out informal channels rather than holding explicitly to formal channels.

There is definitely an art in the ability to compromise and forget insignificant points while being willing to stand up for those points that are important. A successful administrator recognizes the stakes involved and the potential alienation and power that people have so as to move with the flow action that is most important. Frequently, individuals may win one decision but in the process create enemies and thus lose the battle.

A successful leader should be able to sell a plan. Enthusiasm, a technique dealing with nonverbal communication, is an important way to assist the leader in committing others to the plan (see Chapter 11).

Confidence is something that others see in a leader. There are techniques, skills, and tactics that leaders can develop so that others will view them as confident. In reporting to peers and subordinates, individuals should speak and write optimistically to produce a feeling of confidence. This will enhance their power positions.

In summary, professional nurses in any position need both authority and power in the practice and management of nursing. To develop effective colleagueships with others with authority and power, nurses should understand clearly the power and politics that are used by various groups and individuals within the system. They should be skilled in using techniques to sell their plans to others. Nurses should recognize the value of pooled authority and positive power for the attainment of nursing goals.

PROFESSIONAL NURSES' ACCOUNTABILITY AS EMPLOYEES

Position design and organization structure define the objective and functions for each position concerning to and for whom the person in the position is responsible. To a great degree responsibility is retained within the worker. Individuals accept responsibility within themselves when they agree to perform the tasks of the job. For example, when nurses do not agree with the conditions of an assignment and are unwilling to accept responsibility, they should reject the assignment. In doing so they accept the risks of refusal in accordance with their interpretations of the responsibilities and accountability for nursing practices.

Nature of accountability in institutions

Nurses employed in hospitals and other agencies have the legitimacy of the institution to support their practice. They have job descriptions and nursing policies and procedures that help define the limits of their practice. Frequently, nurses refrain from their professional code of ethics and responsibilities by limiting their practice to carrying out physicians' written orders.

Nurses are accountable to the employer and to the physician. They are accountable to clients through their physician and their superiors by means of the chain of command in the organization. To support the accountability of nurse-practitioners in specialty units, administrators, physicians, and nurses have developed limits of nursing responsibilities in specific situations in the care of patients and a protocol to be followed so that patient care will be performed appropriately.

In discharging accountability in patient care, the professional nurse is expected to provide written documentation in reporting an inappropriate action performed by others in the care of a patient. Such action by a nurse involves a high personal risk, particularly if it involves a physician. Thus, most nurses are reluctant to document such actions.

The nurse is held liable to the extent that the actions taken are consistent with the functions stated in the job description. However, a nurse's obligation is not sufficient to ensure coordinated performance within an organization. Thus, through the chain of command, accountability flows upward through an organization.

Trends toward an accountability process

For many years, professional nurses have used the ANA Code for Nurses to describe the areas in which nurses are accountable. In recent years a statement of philosophy, a description of practice, and standards of nursing practice have been defined by each specialty nursing group (see Chapter 5). In each institution there is a need to improve the documentation of nurse practice.[1,3]

Passos[36] distinguishes between accountability and evaluation. Accountability refers to an external process for determining the productivity of an individual, group, or enterprise. Evaluation refers to an internal process developed and conducted by and for the benefit of professional peers.

There are many questions to be asked and answered before all professional nurses are required to account for their own acts. Moreover, liability in nursing must be accompanied by the willingness of nurses to have their performance monitored, reviewed, and evaluated by their peers.[21]

MacDonald,[30] discussing quality assurance in an institutional nursing service, stresses several priority needs to create a climate conducive to quality delivery and measurement. It is true in a client-patient-centered nursing delivery system that the need to focus nursing service operations toward nursing practice, the need to consider the impact of manpower, methods, materials, and machines on the quality and quantity of nursing output, and the need to recognize that nurses must develop standards of practice all are necessities to develop a mechanism for the evaluation of such elements.

The nursing profession is developing a methodology for monitoring the quality of nursing care. According to Jelinek,[21] a measurement approach should focus on structural process and outcome approaches.

To establish quality assessment, programs must involve the total nursing staff. It is the nurse-practitioners at the operational level who should identify specific criteria for the accountability of their actions in the care of their clients with the support and guidance of their peers.

THE WORKABLE ORGANIZATION

There is no universal theory of organization design. However, individuals in the role structure must use the organization structure to implement operational processes to attain goals, rather than be used by it.

In reality an organization structure seldom has all the characteristics essential for an effective, dynamic process of human interaction.

The formal communication system takes place within the defined hierarchical authority structure of the system. It also provides a variety of channels such as conferences, scheduling, meetings, and records. Communications as a management process through the formal and informal structure is discussed in Chapter 11. In most organizations both the formal and informal overlap, and the personnel are members of both organizations.

An effective nursing service organization can be compared to a renowned philharmonic orchestra. The traditional roles and structure of nursing service can hamper the expertise, creativity, and innovative output of the nurses who make up the orchestra.

All professional nurses (musicians) perform. The outcome of the care of their clients depends on the knowledge, skills, and experience they possess to meet patients' needs. Members of the nursing orchestra have different roles from their colleagues. Yet all members in the areas in which they work must be free to make their own judgments. However, they must be somewhat restricted if total nursing care (sound) is to be appreciated and applauded by clients, consumers, and others.

The nurse-executive (the conductor) and the organization plan (the score) provide the overview support and direction necessary to bring the members together to attain their defined goals.

The future type of modern organization as we now envision it is far from certain.[7,27] However, with increased technology and pressures from environmental forces, structural and organizational processes will continue to change. No doubt the modern bureaucratic system will remain, but with more emphasis on functional systems and innovations.

REFERENCES

1. Abdellah, F. G., Beland, I. L., Martin, A., and Matheney, R. V.: New directions in patient-centered nursing: guidelines for systems of service, education, and research, New York, 1973, The Macmillan Publishing Co.
2. Anders, R. L.: Matrix organization: an alternative for clinical specialists, Journal of Nursing Administration **5:**11-14, June, 1975.
3. Anderson, E. H., Bergersen, B. S., Duffey, M., Lohr, M., and Rose, M. H.: Current concepts in clinical nursing, vol. IV, St. Louis, 1973, The C. V. Mosby Co.
4. Argyris, C.: Management and organizational development, New York, 1971, McGraw-Hill Book Co.
5. Arndt, C., and Huckabay, L. M.: Nursing administration: theory for practice with a systems approach, St. Louis, 1975, The C. V. Mosby Co., chapters 2 and 4.
6. Barnard, C.: The functions of the executive, Cambridge, 1938, Harvard University Press, pp. 73, 168-169.
7. Bennis, W. G., Benne, K. D., and Chin, R.: The planning of change, ed. 2, New York, 1969, Holt, Rinehart and Winston, Inc., pp. 139-142.
8. Blau, P., and Schoneherr, R.: The structure of organization, New York, 1970, Basic Books, Inc.
9. Cleland, D. I., and King, W. R.: Systems analysis and project management, ed. 2, New York, 1975, McGraw-Hill Book Co.

10. Cooper, S. S.: Committees that work, Journal of Nursing Administration 3(1):3-10, 1973.

11. Cribbin, J.: Effective leadership, New York, 1972, The American Management Association, chapter 6.

12. Drucker, P.: Management: tasks, responsibilities and practices, New York, 1974, Harper & Row, Publishers, Inc.

13. Etzioni, A.: Modern organizations, New Jersey, 1965, Prentice-Hall, Inc., pp. 75-93.

14. Exodus 18:17-26.

15. Fayol, H.: General and industrial management, London, 1949, Sir Isaac Pitman & Sons, Ltd., p. 55.

16. Fox, D. H.: A contemporary organizational design for maternal and infant care projects, Journal of Nursing Administration 5:26-33, May, 1975.

17. Ganong, W. L., and Ganong, J. M.: Reducing organizational conflict through working committees, Journal of Nursing Administration 2(1):12, 1972.

18. Gellerman, S.: Management by motivation, ed. 2, New York, 1968, The American Management Association.

19. Graicunas, V. A.: Relationship in organization: papers on the science of administration, New York, 1937, Institute of Public Administration, pp. 181-187.

20. Herbert, T.: Organization behavior—readings and cases, New York, 1976, The Macmillan Publishing Co., pp. 235-245. See ref. 42.

21. Jelinek, R. C., Haussman, R. K. D., Hegyvary, S. T., et al.: A methodology for monitoring quality of nursing care, pub. no. (HRA) 74-25, Washington, D.C., Jan., 1974, United States Government Printing Office.

22. Kahn, R. L., Wolfe, D. M., Quinn, R. P., and Snoek, J. D.: Organizational stress: studies in role conflict and ambiguity, New York, 1964, John Wiley & Sons, Inc.

23. Kiev, A.: A strategy for handling executive stress, Chicago, 1974, Nelson-Hall, Inc.

24. Koontz, H., and O'Donnell, C.: Principles of management, ed. 6., New York, 1976, McGraw-Hill Book Co.

25. Lawrence, P. R., and Lorsch, J. W.: Organization and environment, Boston, 1969, Division of Research, Harvard Business School.

26. Likert, R.: The human organization: its management and value, New York, 1967, McGraw-Hill Book Co., chapter 10.

27. Lippitt, G. L.: Hospital organization in the postindustrial society. In Nursing digest, Wakefield, Mass., 1975, Contemporary Publishing, Inc., pp. 49-60.

28. Luthans, F.: Introduction to management, New York, 1976, McGraw-Hill Book Co.

29. Luthans, F.: Organizational behavior, New York, 1973, McGraw-Hill Book Co.

30. Macdonald, M. E.: Quality assurance in an institutional nursing service. In Quality assurance—a joint venture, pub. no. 15-1595, New York, 1975, The National League for Nursing.

31. Malone, M. F.: The dilemma of a professional in a bureaucracy, Nursing Forum 3(4):58, 1964.

32. Marciniszyn, C.: Decentralization of nursing service, Journal of Nursing Administration 1(4):17, 1971.

33. Mass, M. L.: Nurse autonomy and accountability in organized nursing service, Nursing Forum 12(3), 1973. Vol. XII, No. 3, 1973. (Reprinted in Stone, S., Berger, M. S., Elhart, D., Firsich, S.C., and Jordan, S. B.: Management for nurses, St. Louis, 1976, The C. V. Mosby Co., pp. 34-47.)

34. Massie, J. L., and Douglas, L.: Managing: a contemporary introduction, Englewood Cliffs, N.J., 1973, Prentice-Hall, Inc., chapters 6 and 17.

35. Ouchi, W., and Dowling, J. B.: Defining span of control Administrative Science Quarterly 19:357-365, Sept., 1974.

36. Passos, J. Y.: Accountability: myth or mandate. In Nursing Digest, Wakefield, Mass., 1975, Contemporary Publishing, Inc., pp. 78, 83.

37. Perrow, C.: Complex organization, Glenview, Ill., 1972, Scott, Foresman & Company, pp. 4, 165-167.

38. Petit, T.: Fundamentals of management coordination, New York, 1975, John Wiley & Sons, Inc.

39. Prouty, M.: Making an organizational chart, Journal of Nursing Administration 4:32-35, Jan.-Feb., 1974, Prentice-Hall, Inc.

40. Robbins, S. P.: Managing organizational conflict: a nontraditional approach, Englewood Cliffs, N.J., 1974, Prentice-Hall, Inc.

41. Stevens, B. J.: The nurse as executive, Wakefield, Mass., 1975, Contemporary Publishing, Inc., chapters 3 and 7.

42. Tannenbaum, R., and Schmidt.: How to choose a leadership pattern, Harvard Business Review 51(3):162, 1973. Also published in ref. 20.

43. Webber, J. B., and Dula, M. A.: Effective planning committees for hospitals, Harvard Business Review 52(3):133, 1974.

44. Wortman, M. S., and Luthans, F.: Emerging concepts in management, New York, 1969, The Macmillan Publishing Co.

45. Zalenznik, A.: Power and accountability. In Developing executive leaders, Cambridge, 1972, Harvard University Press. (Reprinted in Stone, S., Berger, M. S., Elhart, D., Firsich,S. C., and Jordan, S. B.: Management for Nurses, St. Louis, 1976, The C. V. Mosby Co., pp. 13-33.)

46. Zaltman, G., Florio, D. H., and Sikorski, L. A.: Innovations and organization, New York, 1973, John Wiley & Sons, Inc., p. 171.

11 Communication in nursing services organization

This chapter deals with the influence a communications system can have on the quality of nursing services rendered to patients in a health care institution. Attention is given to the concepts, mechanisms, and barriers of the communication process.

In health care organizations, executives and other professionals discuss the need for effective communication, but often concepts are not understood. As a result the mechanisms of communication are not used effectively. As we observe the functioning of the nursing services organization, every task of nurses at any level involves communication. Nursing involves the sharing of information as well as understanding and interpreting the information transmitted and received.

COMMUNICATION NEED INCREASED

A generation ago the successful nurse-administrator directed a relatively simple nursing organization. Nurses appeared to have the capacity to be all things to all people. The director discussed problems with his or her supervisors on a daily basis and closely guided their actions. Head nurses knew all their patients because they remained on the same unit during their several weeks of hospitalization. Nurses knew physicians' general routine orders. Nurses and physician did not depend on many different individuals to perform specific patient service tasks. In general, the formal authority structure and other tangible factors such as status and power controlled the mechanisms of communication. In many situations nurses accepted the authoritarian

approach based on their attitudes, beliefs, and values.

In today's complex, structured health care organizations, many nurses recognize the value of an effective two-way communication system in improving patient care services. They also recognize that the structure and job design of the organization can support or restrict the communication process (see Chapters 9 and 10). Nurse-administrators and department heads can no longer make effective decisions without the assistance of others who have information about a problem or subject.[46]

Today, professional nurses are involved in human and labor relations, the development of quality and quantity nursing service standards, the assessment of nursing care, and a whole list of other technical aspects of health care operations. Thus, as members of the health or hospital management team, nurses can play a vital role in improving patient care services. However, nurses' effectiveness depends to a great degree on their awareness of communication concepts, their positive approach to communication, and their skill in using its mechanisms.[25,32,38]

THE HEALTH CARE ORGANIZATION AS AN INFORMATIONAL SYSTEM

In our so-called sophisticated and organized society, communication has become a crucial component in managing the internal activities of a health care organization. It is also vital in the exchange of information between an institution and others in the external environment (see Chapters 4 and 5).

Communication can play an important role in the managerial functions of planning, decision making, organizing, directing, and controlling. Nurses and other related health professionals are recognizing that the communication process is a prerequisite in defining and assessing patient's problems, in carrying out a plan of care, and in documenting actions.

In health care institutions the need for effective communication has been intensified by dynamic technology, advances in science, sociocultural events, the employment of many different professional and technical work groups, and the demands and pressures to render patient care services to all consumers at a reasonable price (see Chapters 3, 4, and 6).

Today, nurses are involved in three major communication approaches: (1) the organizational approach, (2) the interpersonal approach, and (3) the technological and scientific informational approach.[22,27,34]

Through the formal and informal structures of a health care enterprise, communication flows may be multidirectional—vertical, lateral, and diagonal. Communication takes place between two or more individuals, between a superior and groups, and between a group and other groups. Structurally, the system may be perceived as a configuration of communication patterns. In some enterprises, nurses view the communication system as multivariable.[20]

In a dynamic nursing service organization that creates a social climate of trust and empathy and is problem-solving oriented, the decision-making process consists of many interrelated messages between superiors and subordinates. These exchanges contribute to final decisions on particular subjects. Through the problem-solving approach, new information regarding other subjects may be transmitted to other individuals for their input.[4]

The interpersonal theory is applied in communication. One may find great differentiations of power, status, and rank between individuals and groups within the system, resulting from increased specialization in a health care organization. Various professional and technical groups have different self-interests, goals, attitudes, abilities, and expertise. The communication process is also influenced by the physical and social nature of the institution itself.[20] Major tangible and intangible factors that create barriers and group conflicts to effective communication will be discussed later in this chapter.

Administrators and department heads are challenged to use techniques that keep status and power differences between groups to a minimum and to keep channels open and unrestricted between individuals and groups.[30] Power and authority are discussed in Chapter 10, and personal goals are mentioned in Chapters 7 and 9.

The communication process can facilitate the interdependency of one unit on another, resulting in mutual understanding, coordination, and cooperation for the attainment of objectives. Effective communication flows between nursing service units and departments can produce a coherent, dynamic organization for improving nursing and other patient care services. On the other hand, ambiguous and inadequate information or too much knowledge of each other's activities may stimulate intradepartmental and interdepartmental conflict.[41]

The advances made in the treatment of diseases, the introduction of national health care regulations and standards of patient care services, and the use of more complex appliances and equipment have increased the demand for information exchanges between groups within and outside the institution. Administrators complain of informational overload that is costly, time consuming, and confusing. Nurses complain about the endless amount of paper work.

Computer technology is taking on an important role in communication.[23,29,51] Computer technology has been applied in the assessment of patients' conditions and needs, in the implementation of medical records, maintenance medication, and unit-management systems, and in management control systems and continuing training and education programs.[2,12,14]

Some institutions have a fully automated system that provides data instantly on request at terminals located in units, as well as at physicians' offices and agencies outside the institution. These terminals are connected to a computer center by broad band telephone lines that are capable of transmitting many messages simultaneously.

Message exchanges between physicians, between physicians and nurses, and between nurses and other units via the computer provide for effective planning and organizing of patient care services, for conservation of resources, and for more accurate documentation.

It should be mentioned that a successful automated computer program requires joint planning by professionals and others who will use the system and equipment with the computer specialists and programmers.

The planners of computer systems should determine the objectives, priorities, procedures, schedules, job functions, and the content of orientation and training programs for the staff. Training programs should focus on what the system is expected to do, how the equipment is to be used, and the importance of communicating problems as they arise. It should be emphasized and understood that individuals, as senders or receivers, must interpret and assimilate raw information. Knowledge requirements, perception, and listening are essential components in transmitting and receiving information.

It is evident that the nurses of the future will be challenged to use their knowledge, perceptions, and skills to improve the communication process in nursing services. Communication is basic in providing quality patient care.

DEFINITION AND MEANING OF COMMUNICATION

The word *communication* is derived from the Latin word *communus*, which is translated as *common*. The basic forms of communication are by signs (sight), by sounds (hearing), and by written words (reading).[7,21]

Language, a systematic communication by symbols, is a universal characteristic of the human species. The origin of language is

unknown, but scientists generally agree it has been in use for about 7,900 years.

The meaning of semantics

The field of semantics consists of three basic aspects: (1) the relation of words to the objects indicated by them, (2) the relation of words to the interpreters of them, and (3) the formal relation of signs to one another in symbolic logic. The study of general semantics focuses on the ways in which meanings of words influence human behavior. It examines the mental act that the hearer forms when a word is spoken. S. I. Hayakawa[21] has contributed much to our understanding of communication.

Different people use different words. Our past training, personal interests, goals, and background color the words we use, and our personal perceptions based on beliefs, attitudes, and values influence our communication. We select certain words and gestures to communicate with because they project a mental picture in our minds. The receiver of our message translates it as he understands it. Communication does not take place until the receiver possesses a meaningful understanding of the sender's words or gestures.[44]

For example, in a health care organization an executive views the word *policy* as a broad statement or guide. Subordinates may interpret it as a specific rule that could prevent them from satisfying a personal goal. Researchers and professionals use specific words and symbols in their work. When they communicate with other groups they must use words that are meaningful for that particular group. A nurse-executive, department head, or clinical specialist may know a great deal about a subject, but if ideas are not transmitted in meaningful language that receivers can understand, communication will not take place.[4]

Ambiguous information does not motivate a receiver to take the action desired by the sender. Some nurses who have been in a particular specialty or unit for several years may use jargon when they communicate with new employees or others outside their territory. Unless receivers feel confident and secure they will not ask questions to clarify the meaning of words used. Thus, a communication barrier is created.

Words are carriers of and barriers to meaning. Berlo[7] emphasizes that meanings are in people, not in words, since words have no meaning in themselves. There meanings are denoted by the sender (source) and the receiver. Communication may be viewed as a dialogue in which the source endeavors to manipulate the receiver. This is counterbalanced by the receiver's influence on the source.

Defining communication

Communication may be defined as a meaningful exchange and understanding of ideas, statistical data, opinions, or emotions from a source to a receiver to produce intelligent desirable actions that will accomplish organizational objectives.

In nursing service organizations, individuals, groups, things, authority levels and line, staff, and functional positions can be linked together so that personal goals are recognized and organizational objectives are accomplished.[1,3]

Some readers may regard the preceding statement as unrealistic because most nursing services organizations are structured along classic organization concepts. Perhaps the acceptance and application of the communication process by all nurses as basic to improving the management of nursing care and as effective communication will become a reality.

The major goals of communication are to create effective changes, as desired by superiors, in subordinates' behavior, their knowledge and skills on the job, or in their attitudes and personal goals for the attainment of an organization's objectives. Subordinates also may be the source of messages to their superiors to create effective changes in their management decisions.

ELEMENTS IN THE COMMUNICATION PROCESS

For centuries scholars and scientists have attempted to explain the communication process. Aristotle viewed communication systems as including the speaker, the speech, and the audience. Since the 1900s, management experts have contributed to the development of the concepts and mechanisms of communication in enterprises.

In the 1960s, Berlo[7] presented a communication model consisting of the following elements—source, message, channel, and receiver. Other experts[42] accepted this model but added the element of feedback. (Fig. 11-1).

Understanding the concepts and the relationship of the elements as a progression of events is necessary for effective communication to take place.[4]

Source

This is the first step of the communication process. The term *source* refers to one or more individuals or groups who initiate the process. For example, the source may be the board of directors acting for the institution or a clinical coordinator when he or she counsels or praises a subordinate's performance (Fig. 11-1). The source can be nonhuman, such as a computer or electronic monitor.

The source's responsibility is to initiate the first message. To do this the source makes several decisions that include (1) the selection of the raw information such as an idea, facts, or statistics, (2) the selection of the individual or thing that will receive the message, (3) the selection of the language, form, and style of the message, and (4) the selection of the mechanism for transmitting the message.

In most organizations the source initiates a message when he or she feels that the state of authority, influence, or objectives of the organization have been disturbed. When everything is running smoothly there are fewer messages traveling through the system. Specific types of messages are sent to certain receivers when functions appear to be unbalanced. For example, a source will initiate messages to certain receivers when a strike is pending, when operating costs are rising rapidly, when turnover or absenteeism has increased, or when a patient's condition indicates changes in the plan of care.

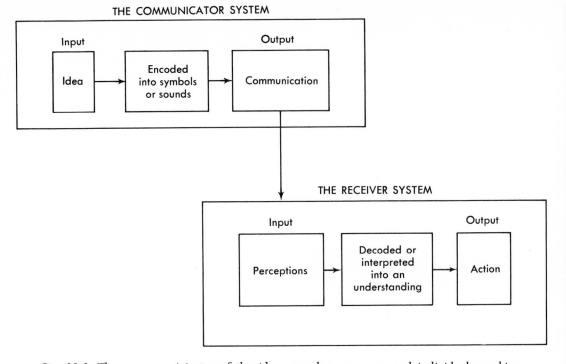

Fig. 11-1. The source, originator of the idea, may be one or several individuals working together or a nurse-executive acting in an administrative role. The process of communication is seen as the interaction between the source (communicator) and the receiver. However, the effects (action) are the changes in receiver behavior that occur as a result of the transmission of a message. Feedback is a response by the receiver to the source's message. (From Bailey, J. T., and Claus, E. K.: Decision making in nursing—tools for change, St. Louis, 1975, The C. V. Mosby Co.)

The source decides what mechanism will transmit the message to the receiver. If communication is to be oral, the source decides the best time and place to transmit the message, considering the number of receivers, the demands of their jobs, their personal characteristics, and the purpose of the message.

The source should be aware, if possible, of any existing physical or psychological barriers that could create difficulties in communicating with the receiver. On the other hand, the source may select and transmit the message in written form through formal channels.

Message

As previously discussed, raw information such as an idea, facts, or statistical data must be converted into meaningful language for the receiver to understand. The term *encoding* refers to the translation of raw information into a meaningful message. For example, the translation of figures, signs, or symbols in appropriate form, the selection of words in normal conversation, or the conversion of signals of an electronic apparatus is a part of the encoding process.

In the preparation of a verbal or written message the source should mentally answer several questions. For example, what objectives are to be attained? Is the message to inform, persuade, instruct, praise, or reprimand? To whom do I want to communicate my message, and what are the characteristics and attributes of my receivers?

A source prepares a message according to his or her perceptions of self, to his or her concepts of position and status in the organization, to the image of the receiver, and

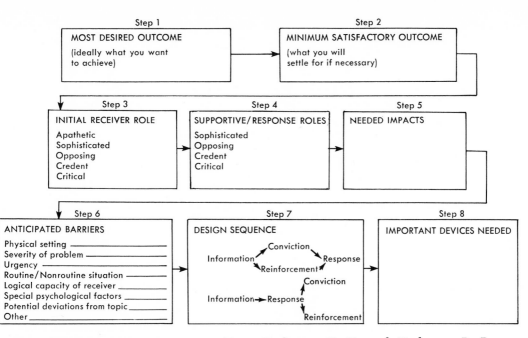

Fig. 11-2. Person-to-person size-up. (From Vardaman, G. T., and Vardaman, P. B.: Communication in modern organizations, New York, 1973, John Wiley & Sons, Inc.)

to the expected feedback of the message from the receiver. The source also recognizes such interpersonal feelings of the receiver as the need for security, empathy, and trust. Unfortunately, the source who is highly channel oriented will fail to consider the receiver and focus primarily on the means of transmission. Hence, the communication process will be less effective. The message should aim to keep information flow at a reasonable level and prevent distortion from entering into the communication process.[8,11]

Verbal and nonverbal messages. These mechanisms provide for direct contact of the source and receiver. Oral communication provides the best opportunity for the source to appraise the degree of understanding of the meanings exchanged and to ask questions to further clarify the transmitted message. The responsive behavior of receivers—what they say or do not say or do—provides evidence for the source to judge whether or not the message has been understood.

Nonverbal forms of communication such as a smile, a nod, or a clenched fist may speak as loudly as words. However, the source should interpret nonverbal communications in terms of the realities of the place and time.

Researchers emphasize that direct verbal communication is a most effective mechanism, even though the meaning of the spoken word is usually less accurate than the meaning of the written word. Nurses in middle and lower levels and their coworkers use oral and nonverbal mechanisms to communicate their messages to others. Department heads and executives transmit many messages at conferences and committee meetings (Figs. 11-1 and 11-2).

Written messages. Written messages include reports, policies, rules, statistical data, newsletters, and memos. Most reports, policies, and procedures aim to support the organization's need for conformity, stability, and predictability. Written material can be checked for accuracy before it is transmitted. However, it is difficult to keep policies, standards, and procedures up to date and to clarify their meaning at the time they are transmitted to the receiver. Executives and supervisory staff members have the problem of making certain that the receiver has read the message (see Chapter 8 for policies and rules).

Need for accurate information

Nurses at various levels of hierarchy must have accurate information such as statistical, managerial, and medical data to make correct decisions and to give meaningful reports to their superiors for decision making. For example, a department head cannot develop a new staffing plan without past data and current inputs and outputs pertaining to patient occupancy rates, classification of patients in relation to their needs, and manpower inputs.

Nurses should recognize their responsibility to get the information they require to function effectively in their jobs and to give what is needed to their subordinates for their jobs. Administrators depend on the quality, amount, and rate of relevant information that reaches them. Subordinates depend on the efficiency with which their superior can assess information for decision making.

Group conflicts often result from an insufficient though accurate exchange of information, as well as from distorted facts. Conveying information accurately and clearly can reduce a receiver's uncertainty about some event or experience. Poorly written policies or numerous memos are costly and create confusion.[33]

Channel

A channel is the means by which the source selects the way the message will travel to the receiver. The channel aims to bring together the source and receiver and is the way the message is physically transmitted—via oral, written, or specific signs. Media channels are means of transmitting messages such as films, radio, newsletters, and policies that enable a source to contact many receivers.[49] Interpersonal channels are those that involve a face-to-face exchange between a source and a receiver.

Problems in formal channels. In an organization, formal channels established by the organization are used to transmit most messages related to the professional functions of staff members. The formal authority network within an organization influences the effectiveness of communiction.

As information passes downward through the hierarchical levels, individuals interpret the message differently. This presents problems for superiors who, by definition, work through others and depend on their subordinates to interpret information and direct others. In addition, a nurse-executive depends on nurses at various levels to channel upward critical information so that the decisions can be made to improve their functions and work environment. In channeling upward information, whatever clinical coordinators on the units consider relevant will determine what is transmitted upward to their department head, who then interprets the information and influences what the executive receives. The information that has moved upward through the channel has been greatly filtered. The perceptions of department heads and their supervisory staff can restrict an accurate flow of information and introduce biases into information that is communicated. This often causes distrust, hostility, and conflicts.

According to Lorsch and Lawrence[33] and Robbins,[41] conflict between groups may occur when communication channels deviate from the formal hierarchical structure and when source-receivers differ in knowledge, beliefs, and social status. Conflict is also created when members use the "grapevine" instead of formal authority lines or bypass authority levels when transmitting information.

Receiver

The message is passed from the source side to the receiver side of the process (Fig. 10-6). The receiver must *decode* the message—that is, to interpret and understand it. Decoding requires specific knowledge, perception, and listening on the part of the receiver. The message must assist the receiver in performing a particular task of the job. For example, the clinical coordinator must be able to understand the meaning of quality assessment standards and methodology to appraise nursing services and improve performance.

Feedback

Feedback is a response to the source's message. A dynamic positive feedback results in effective two-way communication. It informs the source that the desired outcome of the message has been achieved.

When information is new to the receiver, it may create a different kind of response from that of a customary feedback. For example, a personnel director's report to administrative and supervisory staff on the high turnover rate of nurses may initiate much feedback. Those responses may produce innovative actions to reduce the resignation of nurses. The more nurses are feedback oriented, the more effective the communication process will be for both the source and the receivers.

Responses in oral communication

Feedback can give rapid responses indicating to the source that a problem exists. For example, a team leader may say to the clinical coordinator, "What you are telling me now contradicts what is written in the policy manual"; or a new staff nurse may say to an instructor, "Your instructions about how to make out the peritoneal dialysis fluid balance sheet are not clear to me." Such feedback initiates two-way communication.[15]

Premature evaluation may take place by a source or a receiver during feedback. To prevent a receiver from forming opinions based on insufficient information, the source should state the key facts of the message and then present the details of each factor. The initial identification of the major fact tends to increase the possibility that the receivers' responses will be based on a clearer understanding of the message. Repetition of the key points may not remove agitation and tension completely, but it reduces their influence on communication effectiveness.

As previously mentioned, feedback implies that the source has gained some information about the receivers prior to initiating communication with them. This information is used to design effective feedback. If the source has false assumptions about the receivers, any efforts to reach a desired feedback response tend to be less effective.

The feedback element provides an opportunity for the source to alter the original message to obtain some intended changes in the receivers' behavior or attitutdes. Because negative feedback creates friction and in some situations hostility between the source and receiver, the source should endeavor, if necessary, to reach a satisfactory compromise with the receiver.

Effective listening

Effective listening is important in understanding verbal responses. When we interview a potential applicant for a position, counsel a subordinate, or present a plan to a superior, effective feedback only takes place when the source can recall what the receiver said and when the receiver participates actively in evaluating and responding to the messages transmitted by the source.

As one moves up the hierarchy, the skills of listening and evaluating feedback become vital elements of the job. Valuable attributes of an effective leader include the willingness to listen carefully and thoroughly and the ability to abstract key ideas and interferences expressed by receivers.

Self-interest and attribute differences influence feedback

Communication experts[16,30,35] indicate that false assumptions occur more often when the source and receivers have different educations, status, or beliefs. Homophily is the degree to which the source and the receiver have similar attributes. Heterophily means the degree to which source-receivers are different in certain attributes. Feedback between heterophilous source-receivers is often difficult and can lead to distorted information. However, feedback between heterophilous source-receivers has the potential of transmitting new information, instigating the stimulation of receivers toward pending changes.[42]

In health care organizations, effective feedback between physicians, nurses, and executives can be impeded by differences in academic training, goals, and orientation to patient care services. Simon[45] and others[3] indicate that professionals in an organization tend to perceive that important programs and problems to be undertaken are those that will improve their jobs and units. Self-interest acts as a filter through which messages are received. In other words, we listen to what we want to hear and block out what we do not.

Our perception of a problem can color or exaggerate the meaning of the message. Hence, perceptional differencess between the source and receiver can create a psychological barrier to effective communication. Because both sources and receivers have a self-concept of themselves, an image of other individuals, a perception of their own role, and a self-vested perception, they endeavor to manipulate information to gain their own desired outcomes.

Intragroup and intergroup feedback

Individuals and groups, acting as sources or receivers, tend to abstract unpleasant past experiences with an individual in a particular career classification and apply it to everyone in that same classification, thus creating a barrier to effective feedback.[10] For example, in planning staffing needs for an intensive care unit, the clinical coordinator with support from physicians may state, "All practical nurses are not competent enough to work in our units because they are indifferent to the needs of our patients." The staff nurses on a general unit may say, "All nursing aides are lazy and indifferent." Such statements indicate that perceptions are cumulative based on previous experiences.

Some communication experts point out that a lack of knowledge about others' jobs can impede interdepartmental exchanges for the improvement of services to patients, as well as make unreasonable intraunit and interunit demands. For example, poor interpersonal relations and conflicts between special care units and general care units, or between material management units and nursing, are attributable to ignorance on everyone's part regarding the functions and activities of other units. On the other hand, when staffs understand each other's responsibilities and contribution and units are linked through a problem-solving participa-

tive approach, smooth coordination and relations can exist.[1,13,30]

In studying the sources of conflict between departments in organizations, researchers found that complete knowledge about another department permits self-interest to undermine coordination and cooperation.[30] Complete knowledge or perfect communication does not improve coordination, but increases conflict; whereas lack of knowledge diminishes differences and makes coordination easier. Researchers indicate that conflict may be initiated when separate units have inadequate or distorted information about each other or when units possess complete knowledge.

It should be mentioned that the task demands of individuals' jobs and roles as well as the physical location of their work areas have a great influence on the amount of communication in a group and between groups.

Physical barriers, such as poor means of communication and time constraints, can be removed when known to exist. However, psychological barriers dealing with perceptual differences of source and receivers are more difficult to cope with in developing communication relationships within organizations and agencies in the external environment.

Noise

Noise refers to the interference that takes place between the transmission and the reception of a message, thus influencing the desired effects of the communication. As previously mentioned, semantic problems with language, filtering, and conscious distortion of the message as well as electrical static can be called noise.

INFLUENCE OF ORGANIZATION DESIGN ON COMMUNICATION

The structure and job design of an organization can positively influence the communication process. On the other hand, it may create a negative, constrictive influence on effective communicative relationships between the units of the organization.[49]

Our present modern health care organiza-

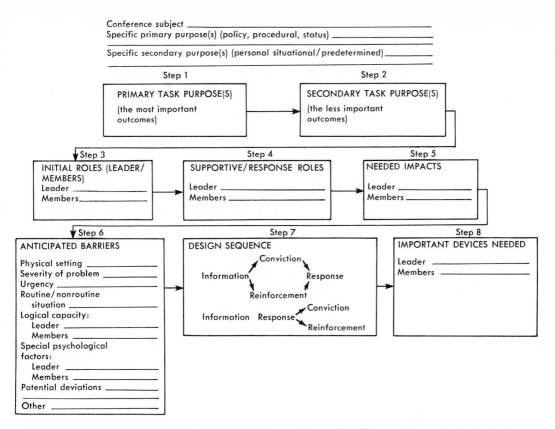

Conference subject _____
Specific primary purpose(s) (policy, procedural, status) _____
Specific secondary purpose(s) (personal situational/predetermined)_____

Fig. 11-3. Conference size-up. (From Vardaman, G. T., and Vardaman, P. B.: Communication in modern organizations, New York, 1973, John Wiley & Sons, Inc.)

tional designs are based on concepts of various management schools (see Chapter 6). Nursing administrators should be aware of the major schools' contributions to improve the communication process (Fig. 11-3).

Scientific management school

The leaders of the scientific management school focused on one-way formal communication to initiate behavioral changes in their workers to improve their performance and thus increase productivity. Taylor[47] believed that individuals respond primarily to economic incentives. He did not recognize the value of the informal group organization on productivity.

Superiors depended on written directives and instructions to obtain obedience from subordinates. The supervisors in the lower and middle levels received scant information

related to their responsibilities and the operations of the enterprise.

In 1911, with the expansion of business enterprises, Fayol[17] recognized the need for horizontal communication to supplement the vertical channel and developed a gangplank concept of communication.

The human relations school

In the late 1930s, Barnard[5] recognized that communication was vital to effective management. He stressed that subordinates must interpret and understand the meaning of a superior's message before authority could be communicated.

By means of the Hawthorne studies, Mayo and others recognized that higher productivity could be attained by attending to the personal needs and goals of the workers (see Chapter 6). These studies indicated that the

		AUTOCRATIC	CUSTODIAL	SUPPORTIVE	COLLEGIAL
FRAMEWORK VARIABLES	Depends on Managerial orientation Employee orientation Employee psychological result	Power Authority Obedience Personal dependency	Economic resources Material rewards Security Organizational dependency	Leadership Support Performance Participation	Mutual contribution Teamwork (integration) Responsibility Self-discipline
	Employee needs met	Subsistence	Maintenance	Higher-order	Self-realization
	Performance result	Minimum	Passive cooperation	Awakened drives	Some enthusiasm
	Morale measure	Compliance	Satisfaction	Motivation	Commitment to task and team

Fig. 11-4. Four models of organizational behavior. (From Human behavior at work: human relations and organizational behavior by Davis, K. Copyright 1972, McGraw-Hill Book Company. Used with permission of McGraw-Hill Book Company.)

informal group organization could influence the attainment of objectives (see Chapter 6).

Through the contributions of Likert,[30] Argyris,[1] and others[37] the concept of two-way communication was introduced as a social process of the organization. Personal motivations and goals of individuals have been discussed in Chapter 6.

The systems school

As discussed in Chapter 6, the systems approach has a degree of formal structure; however, the communication process is a vital component of the organization. It is used to hold units together. Open systems maintain much of their stability and predictability through feedback. Individuals in the administrative hierarchy are the source that evaluates the messages and transmits the appropriate new information to receivers so they can alter their plans and modify the behavior of their subordinates.

Coordination and control are initiated by means of the communication process. Some experts perceive the organizational design primarily as a communication system. Aspects of the systems approach are visible in our modern health care institutions. However, the communication system of this school may cause an overload of information, distort or omit, or create difficulties in interunit coordination of activities.

INFLUENCE OF ORGANIZATION FORMAL STRUCTURE ON COMMUNICATION

Most modern hospital organizations are designed along classic concepts of management (see Chapters 6 and 10). In several institutions, supportive and collegial organizational behavior approaches are being introduced in the traditional structure (Fig. 11-4). The types of organizational behavior operating in an institution are closely interlocked with the communication system.[13,18]

One should be aware of major factors that create structural differences between a bureaucratic enterprise and that of a health care organization, influencing the nursing service structure design and its communicative relationships. The major factors are (1) the purpose, philosophy, and goals, (2) the dual authority and power structure of the controlling body and that of the medical system, and (3) the formal and informal relationships of various health care specialties and the general services of the total organization.

The focus on structure pertains to the nursing service organization as a system in a health care organization. In general, the structure follows the concepts of the total system. A structure may be perceived as an arrangement of components (units) and subsystems (departments) in the organization, with a pattern of relationships as the social system of the organization. This formal, stable structure is composed of many different groups of individuals who are required to work together through hierarchical levels and a division of responsibilities and delegated authority to accomplish goals and objectives. Nursing service goals and objectives of a formal organization and those of its members have been discussed in Chapter 7.

Meaning and purpose of the formal structure

The aim of structure and job design is to provide a great degree of conformity, regularity, and predictability for individuals' behavior in intraunit and interunit activities. Structure can be understood in terms of its size, its degree of formalization, centralization, decentralization, and its delegation of authority. The formal lines of communication—the position description, policies, procedures, rules, and standards that travel vertically and horizontally to subordinates—promote conformity and predictability in individual behavior. However, the structure and job design restricts and controls the ideas, feelings, and actions of all individuals in the organization.[38,39]

Roger and Roger[42] and others in communication research emphasize that the elements of structure belong to the organization and not to the individuals in it. Any type of structure sets the way that individuals will communicate with each other. The classic structure places constraints on nurses and their co-workers in the achievement of objectives by requiring them to work with certain individuals and not with others, to take orders from some individuals and not from others, and in general to act in a way that meets the desired expectations of those with high status and power in the system. It is the organizational behavior model that makes individual and group behavioral patterns so important in the organization.

Multidirectional complex of hospital operations

There is a visible separation between *expertise* required and line authority in the formal structure. This imbalance makes communication more difficult and tends to create conflicts between individuals in line and staff positions. As previously discussed in Chapters 9 and 10, there is a need to clarify roles to effect an appropriate communication process.

The organization structure with a wide span of management control, few levels between the second to top executive, and a clear understanding of roles by all members tends to enhance communication. With few channels for information to travel, there is less distortion and confusion. In a defensive organization structure, focusing on superiority, strategy, command, and control, individuals in the lower and middle hierarchical levels tend to get the impression that all important decisions are controlled by their superiors regardless of their input. This assumption allows inaccurate information to flow upward and information flowing downward to be ignored. On the other hand, in a structure that applies the supportive and collegial behavioral approach, the members are problem oriented, empathize with and trust each other, and regard communication as an essential component for managing people and things to attain goals.

Exception in communication

Exception in communication is the application of management by exception. It can be a dynamic interlocking mechanism between top administrators and subordinates in the units. When applying this principle, supervisory members focus on situations that are out of the ordinary or contrary to policy or standards of practice.[28,43]

For example, the quality of patient care standards or a staffing program is developed and approved by the nursing service organization. The effectiveness of these programs is evaluated periodically by random samples and comparisons between actual results and defined objectives and standards. However, when clinical coordinators or department heads investigate a specific problem because of complaints, they follow the principle of exception in performing their control activities.

The application of the principle of exception reduces detailed communication flows between superior and subordinates. It reduces the amount of time spent in reviewing how results are minimized and provides a climate of trust and openness and a participative approach to decision making.

Horizontal channels of communication

There is a need to formally build a horizontal communication system into the nursing service structure. Studies indicate that a large percentage of a supervisor's communications are via the horizontal source. For example, in the patient care units there is much informal contact with nurses and other professionals who have related patient care responsibilities. Such communications are of primary importance in providing good care to patients. The informal organization will be discussed later.

Committees, conferences, and interdepartmental meetings have been used to promote horizontal communication. Most administrators use these meetings to keep people informed and to coordinate intraunit and interunit activities. Professional groups use the horizontal acommunication system to share information related to their endeavors and to set objectives and standards pertaining to their professional responsibilities within the system. The advantages and disadvantages of committees are discussed in Chapter 10.

Upward channels of communication

In the classic hierarchical structure, except for feedback controls, the upward system is primarily nondirective in nature.[3] In recent years management techniques have promoted upward managerial communication. The grievance procedure, counseling, attitude questionnaires, assist interviews, formal and informal unit-management committees, and suggestion boxes have increased communication upward.

The supportive and collegial organizational approach stimulates upward communication in improving patient care services. Through committee meetings with a nursing staff, administrators have an opportunity to understand the difficulties and frustrations of nurses.

Application of the organizational behavior approach

To improve the quality of patient care and communications between professionals in a health care organization, professionals should build a supportive and collegial environment on the existing traditional structure (as shown in Fig. 11-1).

Likert,[30] Katz and Kahn,[27] and others through their behavioral science research have shown the positive effects of supportive and collegial organizational models. In a hospital environment of specialization, there is a great need to coordinate overlapping functions between nurses and physicians and between nurses and administrators to provide quality patient care.

A successful collegial approach depends on the executives of the system to build a feeling of mutual contribution among individuals at the top and middle levels of the hierarchy of each department. Hence, workers at the lower level will feel that as they perform their activities they make an effective and necessary contribution. In a collegial climate, subordinates view their superiors as contributors to the same goals and therefore accept them in their roles in the organization.

The objective of the collegial structure is *to integrate power rather than command it.* In a collegial environment members tend to produce quality work because they want to and not because they are told to do so.

For the collegial approach to be effective, all staff members in the total system should be introduced to this concept and their respective positions during orientation. The goals of each subsystem, administrative team, health team, and nursing team must be toward *teamwork* to integrate and coordinate intraunit and interunit activities. Thus, communication becomes the crucial element in providing effective, efficient patient care services.

It should be mentioned that the adoption of supportive and collegial organizational relationships and communication does just that, making some so-called autocratic and custodial practices unnecessary. Policies, procedures, and standards are needed to provide a degree of conformity and predictability. However, they play a secondary role as part of the structure.

ROLE AND STATUS PROCESSES IN COMMUNICATION

Nurses should understand the role, status, and power processes that prevail in their work environment. Role, status, and the communicative processes reflect differentiation within groups, although all are closely intertwined with one another.

Scientists in different fields of communication view the term *role* differently.[10,16,43] Role may be defined as the part a person plays in the organization or the way a person in a certain position behaves in different situations. Scott and Mitchell[44] point out that there is some agreement on definition, but the effects of a role on the individual are interpreted differently according to deterministic, particularistic, and interactional points of view (Fig. 11-5).

Schneider[43] and others warn that role collision, role incompatibility and role confusion can disturb a group's role structure, reducing both effective communication and the overall output of all involved.

Role collision occurs when two individuals hold overlapping roles. This may happen if the clinical coordinator and his or her immediate superior have not clarified their respective roles with each other. Role incompatibility or role conflict occurs when an individual is forced to meet expectations for two different roles in different groups. The seriousness of the conflict depends on the nature and degree to which the roles are incompatible, as well as on the hard line with which role expectations are enforced.

Role incompatibility also depends on an individual's ability to adjust to the demands of one role or the other. For example, a nurse may be faced with responsibilities at work and at home. A nurse-administrator

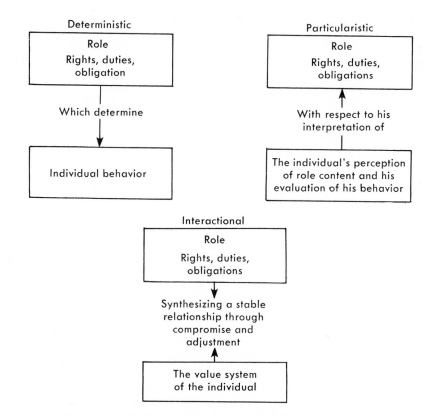

Fig. 11-5. The dimensions of the role concept. (Reproduced with permission from Organization theory: a structural and behavioral analysis. ed. 3, by W. G. Scott and T. R. Mitchell, Homewood, Ill., Richard D. Irwin, Inc., 1976 ©.)

may be faced with a role conflict between carrying out the ethical code of nursing and his or her responsibility as director and the expectations of superiors or the medical staff. Role conflict should be reduced by restricting the demands made in each role and by trying to reach a compromise whenever possible.

Role confusion takes place when an individual discovers inconsistent expectations in other group members concerning the behavior appropriate to a role, especially if there has been no formal agreement that defines the role.[35]

Thus, problems that disturb role structure, especially when an individual holds an important role, can be disastrous to all involved. The social characteristics of the total organization, different individuals' motivation, and the power process all are influential in reducing role conflict. Executives are responsible for designing rational relationships among organizational functions. When roles are clarified, individuals' ability to perceive them more accurately and use them effectively are improved.

Status

Status concerns an individual's relative standing in a group. There are several factors that determine the status of members in an organization. The most important factor in determining an individual's status is his or her level in the hierarchy (scalar status) or his or her job or area of activity in the organization (functional status).

Status symbols are used in health care organizations to indicate relative standing. As hospital organizations have become more complex, the reliance on status symbols has increased. For example, the location and size of an office and its furniture are all status symbols among executives. However, when job titles clearly indicate the individual's position, status symbols are relatively low in importance.

According to Likert,[30] status can have adverse effects on a subsystem's ability to resolve disagreements effectively. Executives or a strong group with considerable status and power express themselves much more freely than do individuals in lower levels. Hierarchical status acts as a strong deterrent on the willingness of group members to speak up and express their ideas. Some individuals in leadership positions do not consider that their status can affect discussions and interactions in the problem-solving process. Other leaders strive to maintain and exploit status. When this happens, members of each group decide that it is best for them to listen only to the leader. They usually agree with the leader's solution without discussing other possibilities.

When a group feels its leader is seeking more status and power, those in the group also compete for status. It is difficult to reduce conflict in groups where the leader seeks to use the power of status.

As previously discussed, the application of the supportive or collegial approach in all phases of problem solving depersonalizes status differences. As Likert[30] emphasizes, all contributions of the group should be viewed as "ours," and the team process separates the member's sense of personal worth from the member's contribution. In a collegial environment the leader uses each member's strong motivational forces created by the desire for a sense of personal worth to promote creative problem solving, to gain an understanding of each member's ideas and group's decisions, and to get commitment to implement decisions (see Fig. 11-3).

Influence of power

The bases of social power proposed by French and Raven,[19] Cartwright,[9] and others[20,25] give us useful insights into an individual who exercises power on another to influence behavior.

The five bases of social power exercised by an individual are (1) *reward* power, based on the receiver's perception that the source is able to mediate rewards for him; hence, the subordinate perceives that compliance to the desires of the superior will lead to positive rewards; (2) *coercive* power, based on the receiver's perception of fear that the source is able to mediate punishments if the receiver fails to comply with the source's desires; (3) *legitimate* power, based on the receiver's perception that the source has a legitimate right to prescribe behavior for the receiver because of the source's position in the organization; (4) *referent* (attraction) power, based on the receiver's identification with the source through admiration of the source's personality; and (5) *expert* power, based on the receiver's perception that the source possesses special knowledge and skills that in turn gain the receiver's respect and compliance.

Group power

According to Likert,[30] Cartwright,[9] and others,[36] group power conceptually includes the possibility of group interaction. In a person-to-person power interaction the source does not use substantial power, which is created by group decision making. Studies indicate that a decision by an entire group to change its behavior is much more effective in producing actual change than are exhortation mechanisms by the source.

Likert's analysis of group power indicates that when person-to-person power interactions turn more to group interaction, a whole new level of influence takes place. The group, as the motive source, creates strong motivations that cause individuals to seek membership in groups whose values, beliefs, and goals are compatible with their own. They want to be respected and valued by members of the group.

As previously mentioned in discussing collegial organizational behavior, strong motivational forces within individuals cause them to change their behavioral pattern toward achievement of the group's goals. This motivational power is based on group problem solving and goal setting. Hence, it creates valuable attitudes resulting in positive group power. In recent years, nurses have begun to recognize the value of positive group power in the achievement of nursing goals in the health care system.

Physician-nurse communication

For decades much research has been directed to physician-nurse relationships and communication as crucial to quality patient care.[6] The evolution of the physician's dominant and authoritative role and nurses' submissive role as they work in an autocratic and custodial environment has been discussed in Chapter 2. In our sophisticated, complex health care organizations there are many new obstacles to effective communication between these two professionals.

Kalisch and Kalisch,[24,25] in analyzing the sources of physician-nurse conflicts, examine the obstacles that stem from within nurses and physicians themselves, from formal and informal organizational design and the characteristics of the institution, and from the perceptions, beliefs, values, and attitudes of our society.

To resolve conflicts positively, both physicians and nurses must turn their inner aggression and anger outwardly and collectively to provide quality patient care. All nurses in an organization must work together competently and confidently to create a structure and job design built on supportive and collegial relationships within the entire nursing service organization.

In a supportive and collegial environment, prepared nurses together can demand and assume accountability for their practices and actions. Such organizational behavior will motivate nurses to secure solutions to their management problems from administration. Highly motivated, prepared, and competent nurses will direct their efforts to improve the quality of patient care services by working with health groups in the community and with their professional associations. In a collegial environment nurses will more likely raise analytical questions about the organization in which they work and thus discover valuable information about the strategies necessary for effectiveness in communicating among themselves and with physicians.

INFORMAL ORGANIZATION INFLUENCE ON COMMUNICATION

The informal organization plays an important role in organizational behavior. The major difference between the formal and informal organization is that the formal organization has prescribed goals and relationships defined by top executives, while the informal organization does not. Today, the two coexist and are closely intertwined. Every formal structure has an informal organization, and every informal structure eventually evolves into some degree of formal organization.[10]

The communication networks of informal groups occur spontaneously and are constantly changing. Thus, the informal structure does not have the predictability of human behavior the formal structure does. It is the formal structure that stabilizes communications, but the informal structure that arouses members to action.

Power of the informal organization and its network

The informal organization involves a group leader, members of the primary group, fringe status participants, and those in out status positions. Thus, the informal organization involves the actual power of participants at the center and others who are in the group but have not been accepted by the decision-making core.

According to researchers[41] there are several informal commmunication networks. The single-chain network begins when the individual at one end communicates with the last individual through intervening group members. The so-called gossip network occurs when one individual communicates personally with every individual in the group. The probability network happens when one individual communicates in a random fashion with others. In cluster-chain networks one person communicates only with others that he or she can trust. Davis[13] and others state that the cluster chain appears to be the most prevalent network in the informal organization.

Value of the informal organization

The informal structure can contribute to the formal organization if leaders in the formal structure use if effectively. Nurses in the lower and middle levels of the hierarchy can use the informal network to make their job easier and to attain unit goals. Because the informal network can disseminate information quickly, nurses can get an idea across rapidly to supplement the formal

downward and horizontal communication. In the units the information organization can give satisfaction and stability to groups.

Because of the inevitability and power of the informal organization, leaders should endeavor to exploit its functions, blending them with those of the formal structure for the attainment of objectives. By paying attention to informal networks, leaders can gain certain information to help them make plans and decisions. The term *grapevine* is commonly identified with the informal communication process.

It is true that the informal system is frequently misused and has negative features such as the spreading of false rumors and destructive information. It is difficult for leaders in the formal structure to initiate a specific type of informal network, but they can indirectly influence the outcomes of informal communications. Nurses should understand group dynamics and the informal organization and take advantage of them whenever possible to attain the system's goals. If the formal organization could meet all the needs of each individual there would be no need for the informal organization.

REFERENCES

1. Argyris, C.: Integrating the individuals and the organization, New York, 1964, John Wiley & Sons, Inc.
2. Arndt, C., and Huckabay, L. M.: Nursing administration—theory for practice with a systems approach, St. Louis, 1975, The C. V. Mosby Co., chapters 2, 8, and 9.
3. Athanassiades, J. C.: The distortions of upward communication in hierarchical organization, Journal of the Academy of Management **16**(2), 1973.
4. Bailey, J. T., and Claus, E. K.: Decision making in nursing—tools for change, St. Louis, 1975, The C. V. Mosby Co.
5. Barnard, C.: The functions of the executive, Cambridge, 1938, Harvard University Press.
6. Bates, B.: Physician and nurse practitioner: conflict and reward, Annals of Internal Medicine **82**(5):703, 1975.
7. Berlo, D. L.: The process of communication, New York, 1960, Holt, Rinehart & Winston, Inc.
8. Brandner, P., and Bayer, M.: Nurse/patient peer practice, American Journal of Nursing **77**:86-90, Jan., 1977.
9. Cartwright, D. P., and Zander, A. F., editors: Group dynamics: research and theory, ed. 3, New York, 1968, Harper & Row, Publishers, Inc., chapter 5.

10. Collins, B. E., and Raven, B. H.: Group structure: attraction, coalitions, communication and power. In Lindsey, G., and Aronson, E., editors: The handbook of social psychology, ed. 2, vol. 4, Reading, Mass., 1969, Addison-Wesley Publications, Inc., pp. 102-204.

11. Conway, M. E.: Management effectiveness and role making process, Journal of Nursing Administration 4(6):25-28, 1974.

12. Cook, M., and McDowell, W.: Changing to an automated information system, American Journal of Nursing 75:46-51, Jan., 1975.

13. Davis, K.: Human behavior at work: human relations and organizational behavior, ed. 4, New York, 1974, McGraw-Hill Book Co.

14. Donabedian, D.: Computer-taught epidemiology, Nursing Outlook 24:749-751, Dec., 1976.

15. Doona, M. E.: A nursing unit as a political system, Journal of Nursing Administration 7(1):29-32, 1977.

16. Elsberry, N. L.: Power relations in hospital nursing, Journal of Nursing Administration 2(5):75-77, 1972.

17. Fayol, H.: General and industrial administration, London, 1949, Sir Isaac Pitman & Sons, Ltd.

18. Frank, R. K., and Frank, I.: The necessity for new colleague relationships between professionals, Nursing Digest 4(3):83-85, 1976. (Condensed and reprinted from Illinois Medical Journal, June, 1975).

19. French, J. R. P., and Raven, B.: The basis of social power. In Cartwright, D., and Zander, A., editors: Group dynamics: research and theory, ed. 3, New York, 1968, Harper & Row, Publishers, Inc.

20. Georgopoulos, B., and Tannenbaum, A. S.: The American general hospital as a complex social system, Health Services Research 2(1):76-112, 1967.

21. Hayakawa, S. I.: Language in thought and action, ed. 2, New York, 1964, Harcourt, Brace & World, Inc.

22. Hicks, H., and Powell, J.: Management, organization, and human resources—selected reading, ed. 2, New York, 1976, McGraw-Hill Book Co., chapters 25-27.

23. Jessamon, D., and Jackson, W.: Functional business communications, ed. 2, Englewood Cliffs, N.J., 1974, Prentice-Hall, Inc.

24. Kalisch, B. J.: Of half-gods and mortals: Aesculapian authority, Nursing Outlook 23(1):22-28, 1975.

25. Kalisch, B. J., and Kalisch, P. A.: A discourse on the politics of nursing, Journal of Nursing Administration 6(3):29-33, (March-April, 1976.

26. Kalisch, B. J., and Kalisch, P. A.: An analysis of the sources of physician-nurse conflict, Journal of Nursing Administration 7(1):51-57, 1977.

27. Katz, D., and Kahn, R. L.: The social psychology of organizations, New York, 1966, John Wiley & Sons, Inc., chapter 9.

28. Kazmier, L.: Principles of management—a programmed instructional approach, ed. 3, New York, 1974, McGraw-Hill Book Co., chapters 9, 10, and 11.

29. Lawler, E., Jr.: Information and control in organizations, Pacific Palisades, Calif., 1976, Goodyear Publishing Co.

30. Likert, R., and Likert, J. R.: New ways of managing conflict, New York, 1976, McGraw-Hill Book Co., chapters 6, 9, and 15.

31. Litterer, J.: The analysis of organization, ed. 2, New York, 1973, John Wiley & Sons, Inc.

32. Longest, B. B., Jr.: Management practices for the health professional, Reston, Va., 1976, Reston Publishing Co., Inc., chapters 6, 7, and 8.

33. Lorsch, J. W., and Lawrence, P. R., editors: Managing group and intergroup relations, Homewood, Ill., 1972, Richard D. Irwin, Inc.

34. Luthans, F.: Organizational behavior, New York, 1973, McGraw-Hill Book Co.

35. Lyman, W., et al.: Behavior in organizations, New York, 1975, McGraw-Hill Book Co., p. 95.

36. Mears, P.: Structuring communication in working groups, Journal of Communication 24:71-79, 1974.

37. Mears, P.: Structuring communication in working groups. In Hicks, H., and Powell, J. D.: Management, organization and human resources, ed. 2, New York, 1976, McGraw-Hill Book Co., pp. 247-255.

38. Miles, R.: Theories of management: complications for organizational behavior, New York, 1975, McGraw-Hill Book Co.

39. Miles, R.: Theories of management: implications for organizational development, New York, 1975, McGraw-Hill Book Co.

40. Plachy, R. J.: Head nurses: less griping, more action, Journal of Nursing Administration 6(1):39-41, 1976.

41. Robbins, S. P.: Managing organizational conflict—a nontraditional approach, Englewood Cliffs, N.J., 1974, Prentice-Hall, Inc., chapters 2, 3, 4, and 6.

42. Roger, E. M., and Roger, R. A.: Communication in organizations, New York, 1976, The Free Press.

43. Schneider, A. E., Donaghy, W. C., and Newman, P. J.: Organizational communication, New York, 1975, McGraw-Hill Book Co.

44. Scott, W. G., and Mitchell, T. R.: Organization theory—a structured and behavioral analysis, ed. 3, Homewood, Ill., 1976, Richard D. Irwin, Inc., chapter 9.

45. Simon, H.: Administrative behavior, New York, 1947, The Macmillan Publishing Co.

46. Smith, C. B.: Communication—an essential of reality. In Hicks, H. G., and Powell, J. D.: Management organization and human resources, ed. 2, New York, 1976, McGraw-Hill Book Co. (Reprinted from Personnel Journal, August, 1974, pp. 601-605, 625.)

47. Taylor, F. W.: Scientific management, New York, 1919, Harper & Brothers.

48. Toffler, A.: Future shock, New York, 1970, Bantam Books, Inc.

49. Vardaman, G. T., and Vardaman, P. B.: Com-

munication in modern organizations, New York, 1973, John Wiley & Sons, Inc., pp. 50-130, 484-486.

50. Wiener, N.: The human use of human beings, ed. 2, New York, 1967, Avon Books, Inc.

51. Zielstorff, R. D.: Orienting personnel to automated system, Journal of Nursing Administration 41(6):14-16, 1976.

12 | Communication media and models for managing nursing care

As we have seen in Chapter 11, individuals in a dynamic collegial organization structure rely heavily on the problem-solving process. An effective communication process demands that professionals be highly motivated, possess specific knowledge and judgment to reach creative solutions, and implement decisions to attain a high quality of services for patients.

The words "scientific" and "systematic" are vital in differentiating between effective problem solving and random attempts to improve management and nursing care. Written informative reports, managerial proposals, written nursing care plans for patients, or structural models of organized nursing all require a positive process of logical reasoning.

GENERAL CONCEPTS FOR REPORTING INFORMATION

There are two basic elements in a written message: (1) *time perspectives* focusing on past, present, and future conditions or events and (2) *thinking perspectives* focusing on descriptive information, conclusions, and implications for evaluation and decision making.[25,33]

As we prepare a written report, document, policy, or procedure, or interview a patient on admission, we may ask, "What happened?" and try to highlight past events over a given period of time.

We also look at the patient's present condition and situation. As reporters we ask, "What is happening now to our plan?" or say, "Mrs. Jones, how do you feel now?" While observing and examining Mrs. Jones,

we listen to and interpret her remarks.

We then begin to consider the future in relation to the situation. We consider Mrs. Jones' problems and her condition and their potential effects on her physical activities, relationships, and attitudes.

Our thinking perspectives involve our own knowledge and judgment of the problem based on accepted generalizations and our own observations. *Observations* focus on those events, relationships, persons, and things that we perceive. *Generalizations* are those judgments made by others. Both must be accurate as possible. The methods and procedures used are those that will provide conclusions and implications for evaluative purposes by sources and receivers. A written message given by an administrator or clinical nurse to others (superiors, peers, or subordinates) will be the input that influences feedback, the quality of decisions made, and the actions taken by others.

DEFINITION AND MEANING OF WRITTEN MANAGERIAL REPORTS

A *report* consists of information that has been carefully gathered and logically presented to cover a specific event, condition, or thing. It is a basic tool for planning and decision making within an organization, although some formal reports involve external parties.

A written message may serve as a record. It may be sent up or down the vertical lines of the hierarchy or horizontally to units and departments of the organization. It may serve as a permanent record such as the patient's chart, or an agreement between parties that is kept for a necessary period of time or in accordance with specific regulations.

A written report gives all individuals involved with the problem or event an opportunity to analyze, weigh, and judge the information as they interpret it and perceive its effects. Written information provides the source with the opportunity to review logically what he or she tried to communicate in words, and aims to initiate action and feedback.

A report should assist others to reach a decision and motivate individuals to a definite course of action for desired outcomes. Written messages are a means to an end, not an end in themselves.[30]

Basic principles for effective written messages

Any type of report must meet certain criteria. It must meet a legitimate need for the communication of particular information. Formal and informal reports must be closely linked to recognized, approved, function-related reasons.

The written message must have a clearcut objective. Perhaps our many complaints about preparing and reading reports stem from the fact that we cannot clearly articulate what various types of reports are supposed to do.

Written reports must be directed to the receiver's ability to decode the information to initiate positive feedback and desired behavior. As previously mentioned, sources (writers or team leaders) must know the kind of information they want to transmit and what forms they want to use. They must also know the characteristics and abilities of the receivers involved.

Necessary formats

Many different types of formats are designed for specific kinds of messages. Formats for routine reports should be used. A well-conceived form will record the necessary information economically, efficiently, and quickly. When standardized formats are built into report styles for specific events, the source can complete reports with ease and usually in the time requested. The receiver can then process and understand them more readily (the format of nursing care plans will be discussed later in this chapter).

Formats for nonroutine reports are necessary, but should be flexible. The format for nonroutine reports should be as simple as possible. Headings, numbers, and topographical aids should permit receivers to follow easily the source's ideas and information. In complex, lengthy reports the format should provide for numeric information, as well as digest material that emphasizes the highlights of the report.[33]

Formats for specific types of reports should follow a logical sequence. The common format may include (1) stating the problem, the recommendations, and the method of implementation; (2) giving background of the event, the reasons, and the solutions; (3) giving past information, present information, or status of the situation, and predicting what will happen in the future; and (4) stating the problem, the limitations, procedures, or methods for the study, the findings or results, and the conclusions and recommendations.

Thus, written reports should be prepared with step-by-step scientific reasoning that may be inductive or deductive in form. *Inductive* reasoning implies the development of knowledge and the formulation of criteria, whereas *deductive* reasoning requires the drawing of inferences from general principles or the application of knowledge an individual possesses.[2,9,28]

Professional nurses as team leaders, primary nurses, nurse-administrators, or clinical specialists should direct their energy and knowledge to the problem-solving process for the achievement of nursing service objectives.

Informal and formal reports

Administrators must make sure that reports are properly coordinated and designed to meet desired outcomes. Thus, they should monitor and update reporting mechanisms in light of managerial changes and new objectives. In our sophisticated nursing service environment in a health care organization, efforts should be made to conserve human and material resources to communicate necessary information among individuals and groups.

BASIC TECHNIQUES FOR REPORTING NUMERICAL INFORMATION

In a health organization numbers are used for several purposes. They serve as names for codes such as position classifications, employees' time-card numbers, and numbers governing inventory control systems. The accounting department with the aid of the computer relies on the function of numbers to achieve its objectives.

Statistical information may be historical, comparative, or predictive. Professional nurses should know how to use statistical information and how to interpret numerical data and detect inaccurate presentations.

Numerical information helps to clarify complex data, identify trends, demonstrate relationships, and emphasize quantative differences. The risks in the use of numerical information involve oversimplification of the information or overemphasis on quantative factors instead of important inherent qualitative factors and relationships. Hence, numerical information may create a biased report.[31]

The major modes for reporting numerical information include graphics, tables, text, charts, pictographs, maps, and overlays.

Graphics

Graphics visually illustrate a large amount of data in various relationships. However, a poorly designed chart may negate the desired outcome. Basic types of statistical graphs include area, bar, column, curve, and line diagrams. The versatile single scale graph is suitable for comparing amounts, subdivisions, and relationships. The column type permits the presentation of two scales and provides easy comparision of related terms having different measurement units. Time and special skills are needed to prepare scale relationships of different units. Curve or line diagrams are the most flexible of all graphic modes.

In the use of line charts, the size of the scale vertically or horizontally can influence the final appearance, as shown in Fig. 12-1. Both line charts presented contain the same statistical information, but the modes used give different value impressions of the information.

Tables

Tables may be used to clarify information by means of columns and rows that facilitate

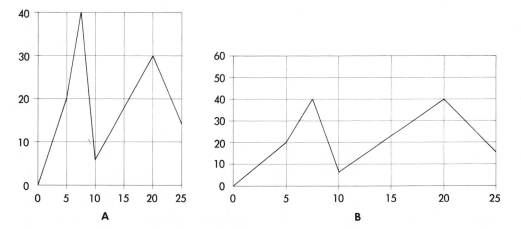

Fig. 12-1. A and **B** A zero point is always used. Both of these line charts present the same statistical information. Condensing the values on the X axis on one and elongating the Y axis gives an impression of much greater fluctuation in the data presented, as in **B** where the Y axis is compressed and the X axis is extended.

comparisons. If tables are used to compare amounts, the two percentages must be based on the same magnitudes of numbers. Hence, percentages must be statistically comparable. It is difficult to portray trends with tables.

Text

Text frequently is used to express a mass of mathematical information because it economizes time, space, and cost. However, it may be difficult for readers to interpret, especially when unfamiliar mathematical symbols are used.

Transparent overlays

Transparent overlays are very effective when presenting information to a group. A base line or bar chart is used to give the scale, grid, title, and so forth. The data are superimposed through the use of different colored transparent overlays. With overlays the viewers can select those overlays that particularly interest them. The specific comparison of data can be made and then removed. By means of overlays the reporter can show ongoing effects of different numeric information.

A visual message by means of graphics and tables must be clear and concise. Titles should be brief, and essential explanations should appear beneath each illustration. Symbols should be appropriate and readable. When the source uses data from other printed sources, credits should be given. Any mode used should present information honestly.

INFORMAL AND FORMAL REPORTS

In a health care organization informal reports range from simple to complex. Informal messages may include accounting, computer data, manpower, and material input and output data. Most informal data reports are presented on preset forms covering daily, weekly, monthly, quarterly, and annual periods. These reports are essentially informative, requiring very little writing of symbols on the form.

As previously mentioned, preset formats save time for both reporters and receivers and result in getting more accurate information to achieve a specific objective. For example, formats may be designed to request a transfer or leave of absence, to report an accident of a patient, a visitor, or an employee, to report an interview of an applicant for a position, or to present an evaluation interview with an employee. Formats are used to collect data in a quality assurance program.

Reports on surveys or studies of a particular situation may be considered informal reports unless sophisticated research techniques are applied.

Formal research has become an important tool of the scientist in various disciplines. Today research finds its way into a health organization by means of education and scientific programs conducted by university staffs, governmental agencies, and professional associations. Formal nursing research involved in nursing practice and models to provide nursing services to consumers is just beginning to penetrate the nursing services in health care institutions.

Formal research follows a definite format and style and uses rules designed to safeguard the findings.

AUTHORIZED ORIENTED MEDIA

In general such documents include impersonal legislative or regulatory constraints on individuals or an organization. For example, a health care organization receives legislative and regulatory documents from national, state, and local governmental agencies in the form of guidelines and codes. Institutions also receive guidelines from approved professional associations involving standards of operations to achieve a good quality of patient care (see Chapters 4 and 5).

Formal contracts usually stem from outcomes of informal, complex proposals. Commitments to conditions or actions include the acceptances of specified circumstances or conditions. For example, a professional staff or a nursing service organization will become committed to provide a dynamic teaching environment for students in nursing, based on a formal contract between the college or university and the hospital. Or, the hospital will make a commitment to staff members to reimburse them for credits earned in an approved education program.

Commitments

The contract specifies job requirements for the position and may include conditions that would result in termination of the contract.

Commitments to codes of conduct pertain to ethical and professional standards to which organizational members subscribe. For example, a hospital states that professionals required in a unit or clinic in the direct care of patients and the nursing service organization accept the ANA code for nurses.

MANUALS FOR NURSING SERVICES

Manuals, discussed in Chapter 8, are basically guides to action. Specific types of information are bound together in an appropriate manner to communicate specific information for particular purposes. Different kinds of written information in manuals may be classified as (1) managerial information, (2) specialized information, (3) general information, and (4) public relations information.

Managerial information

Managerial information includes policy manuals, administrative handbooks, and managerial guides. These manuals include position descriptions, personnel benefits and opportunities, goals and objectives, structure design, and codes of conduct. The manual for professional nurses and technical nurses should emphasize the independent role of nurses and the dependent role based on a collegial approach.

Specialized information

A specialized information manual suitable for various departments and their units should include the highly technical procedures and instructional guides in the direct care of patients.

This manual should also clarify the roles of specialists such as clinical nurse specialists, members of the in-service department, and consultants of staff departments in the entire system. The specialized manual should emphasize the statements of professional nursing practices and standards. It should clarify the structure mode of nursing service operating in the units, including the nursing care plan.

The major role of other departments for providing technical and nontechnical tasks should be clarified.

General information

General information manuals include for example the employee handbook for all members of the institution. It gives an introductory statement of the goals, philosophy, and objectives of the institution, and the general organization structure, goals and functions of the various departments, and benefits and opportunities for its members.

Public relations information

The public relations handbook provides information to patients, their families, and visitors. It clarifies the objectives of the institution and provides guidelines concerning services offered, safety measures, and communication mechanisms. It explains the patient questionnaire to be completed at time of discharge. This manual aims to reinforce the organization's goals and trustworthiness.

Automated written communications

As mentioned in Chapter 11, automated written communication media is becoming an important source in the medical, nursing, and managerial operations of a health care organization. Automation mechanisms for processing final written output include the automatic typewriter, data processing, printing, and reprography. In the near future, nurses will be more closely involved in automated communications.[6,7,10,32,38]

NURSING CARE PROCESS—WRITTEN NURSING CARE PLAN

In recent years, many staff nurses, nurse-administrators, and nurse educators have given reasons why the traditional written nursing care plan is not effective in planning and communicating care for patients.[5,11,20] Studies indicate that the traditional formats and methodology do not promote a collegial problem-oriented approach between nurses or between nurses and other professional members of the health team.[13,18,23,24]

Experience and literature indicate that much confusion exists concerning the concepts and objectives of nursing care plans. Most nurses agree that the traditional care plan is inadequate for quality control, nursing diagnosis, nurse accountability, and research. Confusion exists as to the meaning of terms such as nursing diagnosis, assessment, and intervention. Block[4] asks if we are concerned with poorly defined terms in nursing or with our lack of agreement over meaning and consistency in their usage.

Observations and review of nursing care plans in hospitals indicate that many nurses fail to write care plans. Frequently the original written plans are not kept up to date.[16] The information on the nursing record does not portray a continuous and comprehensive assessment and plan of action to help the patient in all aspects of his or her health-illness continuum. Regardless of the team or primary nursing model of organization, most nurses complain about the format and the lack of time to write care plans. In general, nurses spend less and less time charting other than required information such as medication and treatment.

In the technological environment of a health care organization many proposals are being presented to change the methodology and management of nursing care. In today's society, nursing services must be able to identify and verify that the role of professional nursing and its activities are of value to health consumers. Nursing must be able to validate that it can in fact effect change in client adaptation. Thus, there is a need to focus on the nursing care process and new organizational patterns to facilitate professional nursing practice in serving patients' needs.

Changing concepts in nursing

The concepts of the role and activities of nursing have undergone many changes since Florence Nightingale's concept of nursing. Historically, the care and comfort activities of meeting the basic needs of individuals have always been a part of nursing. The "laying-on of hands" with a purpose continues to be a part of nursing.

Prior to the 1940s, great emphasis was placed on the nurse's skill of observation. Nursing diploma programs focused on patient care *tasks* to assist the physician in the care of patients. The nurse reported observations, not judgments, and the physician in turn determined the patient's plan of care.

As the scope of medicine expanded and the patient load increased, nurses were delegated more and more medical and hospital tasks (see Chapter 2). Nurse educators and directors of nursing began to focus on the independent role of nursing and the activities involved. In recent years, theorists have presented many models of nursing concerning the view of man, the goal of nursing, and the nursing process. Roger,[25] Roy,[27] Auger,[2] Gragg,[9] and others have contributed much to the development of nursing approaches that can predictably result in quality nursing care.

Today, theorists support the use of a problem-solving–based nursing process that results in a client-centered goal of nursing and accountability of the profession of nursing as a scientific discipline. Nursing is service oriented for health consumers.

Goal of nursing care

To provide an effective nursing care model for rendering nursing care one must accept nursing's primary goal. Nursing exists to help each patient adapt to changing situations of health and illness. This means that nursing assists the patient to adapt to changes occurring in himself, as a member of a family, and as a member of society. Nurses must be able to identify as accurately as possible the individual's level of adjustment to his problems and determine how he or she can best cope with these problems. Thus, the nurse's role is to help each patient adapt to changes in health, illness, and environment.

To be an effective agent for the patient the nurse must gather data, define problems as they occur, and select an appropriate approach to meet his or her needs. Because patients cope with their problems in different ways, the nurse must continually assess and plan with each patient in consultation with other professionals who also serve the patient.[13]

Problem-solving approach to nursing diagnosis

Nursing practice is becoming increasingly sophisticated as knowledge is developed and applied in meeting patients' needs. Gragg,[9] Roy,[27] and others describe the application of scientific principles and problem solving in nursing (Fig. 12-2). In general, nurses use a simplified version of the inductive approach

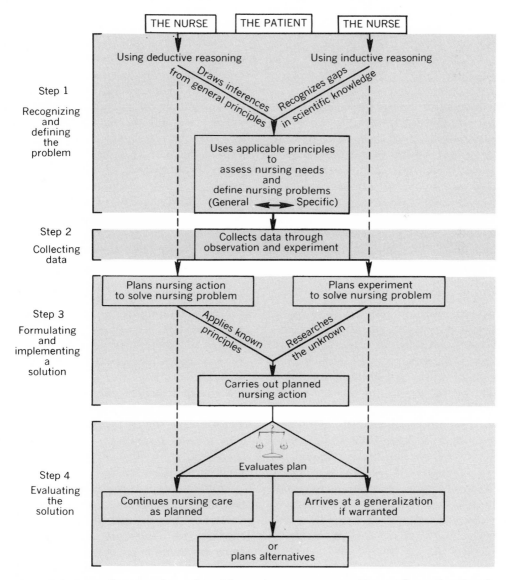

Fig. 12-2. Scientific principles and problem solving in nursing. (From Elhart, D., Firsich, S. C., Gragg, S. H., and Rees, O. M.: Scientific principles in nursing, ed. 8, St. Louis, 1978, The C. V. Mosby Co.)

based on their knowledge, experience, and observations of each patient.

Frequently, nurses define terms differently, and words have different meanings to different nurses. Mundinger and Jauron[20] have described how a group of primary nurses were able to formulate a meaningful definition of nursing diagnoses and base their nursing actions on them. At the conclusion of their efforts their nursing diagnosis read as follows:

Nursing diagnosis is the statement of a patient's response which is actually or potentially unhealthful and which nursing intervention can help to change in the direction of health. It should also identify essential factors related to the unhealthful response.[20]

The nursing diagnosis can be the key to planned change in the nursing process. The identification of factors that create undesirable responses and prevent the patient's adjustment to desired changes suggest what the goals will be for that patient.

Hence, diagnosis is a process of identifying patient responses, guiding patient actions, and recording related factors where nursing can intervene with some predictability to change a patient's response.

Changes in recorded information

Notes written on the progress sheet by the nurse who is problem oriented will differ from those written by the nurse who is task oriented.[9] For example, the task-oriented nurse might write, "10:00 AM: Mrs. Smith ambulated in room." On the other hand, the problem-oriented nurse might write, "10:00 AM: Mrs. Smith ambulated in room with assistance of Miss Jones, R.N., for second time after surgery. She walked around her room for 10 minutes, denies having excessive pain or any dizziness, but states feeling some weakness."

The task-oriented nurse's action to relieve pain could be written as, "9:00 PM: medicated for pain on left side." The problem-oriented nurse would write, "9:00 PM: Mrs. Smith has throbbing pain in left side at site of wound with dull pain extending from ribs to iliac crest. Medication given; after 30 min-

utes indicated relief but still had dull pain on application of light finger pressure near wound area."

In some patient situations the nurse may correctly identify a patient's undesirable response, but it cannot be changed. For example, the surgical orthopedic patient who must be kept in traction, the eye patient with eye patches on both eyes, the patient with chronic back pain, or the laryngectomy patient who has communication disability related to loss of speech all present situations that may require nurses to rethink and redefine nursing diagnoses so that their planning and action will help patients adjust to their specific problems.

Nursing diagnoses usually change more frequently than medical ones. For example, for an acutely ill patient in the coronary intensive care unit, the nurse's diagnoses will focus on chest pain, nausea, and weakness related to myocardial infarction and on life-saving activities. However, when this patient is being rehabilitated he will react more to his living environment. The nurse's diagnosis may then be irritability related to enforced physical inactivity or anxiety related to loss of job or future relationships with his wife and family.

Conceptual problems of the nurse

The perceptions of nurses, based on training, education, experience, and beliefs, influence how they view their responsibilities for making and recording a plan of care for each patient. The problem-oriented nurse recognizes that there can be more than one right plan and realizes that many different methods may bring the same desired outcomes. Thus, the nurse is more confident in commiting knowledge and judgment on care to the written care plan.

Problem-oriented nurses endeavor to find the best plan for their patients and not necessarily the one that will gain a superior's approval. Also, nurses feel at ease with peers and supervisors in a collegial approach since all members work together to achieve the agreed objectives.

Problem-oriented nurses recognize (based on knowledge and experience) that it is impossible to completely control all patients' outcomes. Even though planning and the organization of nursing care aim to decrease risks and overt actions that will be detrimental to patient outcomes, nurses recognize that a degree of uncertainty exists in all activities.

Because the practice of nursing is based on the physical, biological, behavioral, and social sciences, a nurse cannot predict with absolute certainty all outcomes of patient care. Problem-oriented nurses accept the concept of nursing intervention, knowing that a good plan may fail. Staff nurses and their superiors recognize that failure is not the only standard used to evaluate nursing judgment recorded on the written plan of care.

The goal of nursing by means of a nursing diagnosis and plan of action is accomplished through the nurse's observations, judgments, and creation of a relationship of empathy and trust with the patient. A problem-oriented approach to the practice of nursing and an organizational collegial approach can facilitate the documentation of skilled nursing care.[35]

A concise, pertinent, and continuous nursing care plan for each patient must be coordinated with the patient's medical plan of treatment. The identification of nursing problems with appropriate documented nursing actions should be an integral part of a patient's health record. The patient's health record completed by health professionals is a document of the care provided to a patient for payment of services. Professional nurses are responsible for documenting the nursing care given. Such records validate nursing contributions to consumers of health services.

Changing rationale toward nursing care plans

With the rapid scientific and technological advances in health care organizations, nurses in clinical practice and nurse-educators and administrators are now emphasizing nursing diagnoses, methods of documentation, and communication mechanisms (see Chapter 4).

Influences promoting change. In the ex-

ternal environmental boundaries of health care systems, state and national legislative actions emphasize the importance of nursing diagnoses and the potential value of a diagnostic classification system for nursing. Since 1970, many states have completely revised or greatly amended their nurse practice acts.

The 1972 New York State Nurse Practice Act[21] describes nursing as more than assistance to the medical profession. The new definition states that the professional nurse "diagnoses and treats human responses to actual and potential health problems." Many states' nursing practice acts outline and legally establish the independence and accountability of the practice of professional nursing (see Chapter 4).

The generic Standards of Practice published by the American Nurses Association in 1973 clearly emphasize the nursing process.[1] The ANA Standards of Nursing Practice include the collection of data, nursing diagnoses, goal setting, plan of nursing care, nursing action, reassessment, and revision of plan. The ANA Standards of Nursing Practice for the different nursing specialties support nursing diagnoses and assurance of quality care (see Chapter 5).

The 1976 Manual of the Joint Commission on Accreditation of Hospitals states standards concerning written care plans.[12] Standard III reads:

Written nursing care plans and administration policies and procedures should be developed to provide the nursing staff with acceptable means of meeting its responsibilities and achieving projected goals. . . . Nursing care policies and procedures should be consistent with professional recognized standards of nursing practice and shall be in accordance with the Nursing Practice Act of the State.

Standard IV of the JCAH Manual states:

There shall be evidence established that the nursing service provides safe, efficient, and therapeutically effective nursing care through the planning of each patient's care and the effective implementation of the plans.[12]

The two major reasons that professional nurses should use a problem-oriented nursing process are that (1) the goal of nursing is primarily for the *individual* and that (2) the profession of nursing is service oriented and thus accountable for its independent services to each patient.

In recent years, specialized professional nurses have worked together to develop a typology of diagnoses that describes the scope of nursing and communicates the nature of nursing services in the care of patients. With the support of administration, nurses in hospitals should accept the challenge of experimentation to improve the diagnostic process. Several approaches to improve nursing diagnoses and communications between health care professionals will be summarized.

DIAGNOSTIC CLASSIFICATION SYSTEM FOR NURSING

The First National Conference in the Classification of Nursing Diagnoses, sponsored by St. Louis University, was held in October, 1973. This conference was followed by a research study and a second national conference in March, 1975. Gebbie and Lavin[8] report on the proceedings of the first workshop and describe the basic process used to develop a taxonomy of nursing diagnoses. At this workshop, 100 nursing diagnoses in 30 broad areas of patient care were identified. These descriptions gave the critical attributes and shared characteristics of phenomena. Other groups are developing taxonomies.

Bircher[3] presents a category system showing the subcategories and their relationships and the steps of the process that would be accomplished by means of intervention and evaluation. He believes that a workable taxonomy would provide potential points of reference, purpose, and direction and would facilitate communication and collaboration in nursing practice, nursing education, and nursing research.

Roy[28] states that "a standardized typology of nursing diagnoses would not only serve the interests of practicing nurses, educators, and researchers, but would also clarify—for nurses and others—the nature of the phenomena with which nursing is concerned."

Roy emphasizes that category sets must be relevant to the purpose of the classification system. They must be comprehensive and complete, including problems experienced in various environmental settings such as inpatient, clinic, and home care and in all age groups. Each set must be clearly defined.

The category sets of nursing diagnoses must be useful and provide for the insertion of new items into the system. They must be comparable with related systems and able to be computerized.[38]

Thus, a diagnostic classification system for nursing would consist of a list of summary statements about patient problems based on an organizing principle.

THE PROBLEM-ORIENTED RECORD (POR)

The problem-oriented model (POR), also known as SOAP, stems from the problem-oriented medical record (POMR) that was introduced by Dr. Weed in 1968.[37] Weed based his POMR system on the concept that a core of behavior should be taught, rather than a core of knowledge that required a memory-dependent system. Weed's POMR system is based on developing the physician's capacity to extract data from source material and to analyze the data in a systematic, thorough, efficient way to achieve objectives. The POMR system has four major elements: (1) subjective data, (2) objective data, (3) assessment, and (4) the plan for each problem and progress notes and related data.

Few hospitals have adopted the POMR system completely. Unfortunately, the traditional patient care record is source oriented, organized according to the source of data supplied by physicians, nurses, and laboratories. Individuals using the source-oriented record must mentally retain and sort data about any one patient problem. Many educators and nurse-administrators state that POR has important potential for documentation by all health disciplines including nursing.

A logical format of the POR process of assessing and planning to meet each patient's problems has evolved under the SOAP model.[29] This four-part model consists of (1) subjective data, which involves the patient problem and how he views it and feels about it; (2) objective data, which includes the physical and biological and laboratory findings as well as other relevant findings associated with the problem; (3) assessment, which comprises a continuous on-going evaluation of the patient and his problems, noting changes as they occur and using established criteria for assessment; and (4) the plan developed for diagnosis, therapy, and patient teaching.

Application of POR system to nursing care plans

According to Mitchell,[19] McCloskey,[17] and others the SOAP format can help resolve the problems and frustrations facing professional nurses in planning and communicating nursing care of patients via traditional written care plans.

The major components of the POR record system are as follows:

• The database, as previously mentioned, includes information known about the patient at time of entry into the health care system. It also includes the physician's history, physical examination, nursing history-interview, and assessment. It may include laboratory data and other information from other sources.
• The table of contents for the record. This is the *problem list* derived from the database as well as problems formulated by the health team members, the primary nurse, or the clinical nurse specialists. Each problem is defined, labelled, and numbered. As professionals work with the patient, subsequent data, care given, and progress are recorded in relation to each numbered and titled problem. There will be differences on what the nurse or physician constitute as the patient's problem.[39]

Yarnall and Libke[40] state that a problem may be perceived as anything that bothers the patient, threatens his health, or requires some form of management. Physicians focus on problems concerning medical diagnoses and therapies in the treatment of disease; whereas nurses focus on the physiological, safety, and belonging self-esteem or self-actualizing needs that relate to actual or potential health problems of the patient.

Mitchell[19] suggests that the plans should be written on the initial progress note in relation to each identified problem. Such plans correspond to the initial medical and nursing orders regarding patient management.

In some institutions the care plans are written in the progress notes and nursing orders on the order sheet. By means of SOAP format the nurse can communicate a diagnosis, a plan of care, and a rationale to other professionals on the health team. The nurse's orders are written on a combined physician/nurse's order sheet. The secretary takes off the nurse's and physician's orders. An activity sheet is used to ensure that all orders are carried out. In some institutions the traditional Kardex becomes the nursing activity list. Other institutions use a daily printout from a computer. The patient's activity sheet should be kept at bedside. It makes the patient feel that he or she is part of the plan of care.

Narrative notes are used to record progress, identify and clarify new problems, or resolve old problems. On the flow sheet or graphic form the secretary records repetitive or serial data such as daily weight, serum enzyme values, or episodes of incontinence. When data on flow sheets or graphic forms indicate resolution of a problem or occurrence of a new problem such as abnormal rise in temperature or blood pressure, the nurse records a note on the progress sheet.

New problems requiring nursing input are numbered, titled, and added to the problem list if they have not been previously identified by other health team members.

As noted, the recording of a patient's problem is descriptive and precise, stating observations and judgment in support of action taken. The narrative notes on the progress record can be organized under the problem number using the format of SOAP: Subjective data, Objective data, Analysis, Plan.

The problem-oriented record is a patient's care plan, not a nurse's or a physician's care plan. It provides a tool by which all health team members can see their patient as an individual needing their services and fosters colleagueships between physicians and nurses.

It is suggested that one professional nurse be accountable for the nursing care of a patient: the initial plan, ongoing assessment, nursing diagnosis, and the recording of problems and actions taken on the progress and order forms of the patient's record. This does not mean that this nurse will not consult with others, but that this nurse alone is responsible and accountable for seeing that the patient's plan of care is carried out. However, this does not exclude others from communicating with the patient and his family. The nurse has the informal conference for communicating with co-workers, assisted by a clinical coordinator and a clinical nurse-specialist to determine a plan of action for a patient's complex problem. Organized management models will be discussed in Chapter 13.

AUTOMATED INFORMATION IN NURSING CARE

In recent years hospital administrators and physicians have shown through projects that automation can facilitate operations and improve patient care. In some institutions, automated recordings of nursing observations have been developed. Studies have been conducted using automated nursing notes with such headings as sleeping, elimination, eating habits, and appearance.

Another research approach has been a questionnaire using a cathode ray terminal, like a television screen on which alphabetical and numerical characters appear. The terminal is activated by a conventional keyboard on which a list of choices is displayed. The nurse, interviewing a patient on admission, selects the number on the keyboard identifying the patient's answer to the questions. The nurse also records observations. For example, if the nurse records that the skin area is inflamed, the terminal will display a further list of choices indicated by the nurse. This process continues until the computer has sufficient information about the problem. When the nurse signals completion of the

entry, the computer processes the information and provides a narrative printout for the patient's record. The computer updates each patient's nursing care and indicates orders at the end of each tour.

A set of nursing diagnoses and nursing care for meeting patients' needs can be stored in the computer memory bank and adapted for individual patients. Automation, a process-centered system, has numerous advantages, but professional nurses must be aware of its limitations in meeting the goal of nursing. Computers are merely machines with capabilities and outputs that depend on the programmers' input—primarily on the nurses who are accountable for the services given to the patient.[10,39]

It is evident that in the near future professional nurses will develop new methodological bases on a collegial problem-oriented approach for diagnoses and documentation of a plan of action for each patient. The patient's record will then be used for the quality control and accountability of the professionals who serve them.

REFERENCES

1. American Nurses Association: Standards of nursing practice, 1973, Kansas City, Mo., The Association.
2. Auger, J. R.: Behavioral systems and nursing, Englewood Cliffs, N.J., 1976, Prentice-Hall, Inc., chapter 7.
3. Bircher, A. V.: On the development and classification of diagnoses, Nursing Forum 15(1)10-29, 1975.
4. Block, D.: Some crucial terms in nursing: what do they really mean? Nursing Outlook, 22:689-694, Nov., 1974.
5. Ciuca, R. L.: Over the years with nursing care plan, Nursing Outlook, 20:706-711, Nov., 1972.
6. Cook, M., and McDowell, W.: Changing to an automated information system, American Journal of Nursing 75:46-51, Jan. 1975.
7. Cornell, S. A., and Garrick, A. G.: Computerized schedules and care plans, Nursing Outlook 21:781-784, Dec., 1973.
8. Gebbie, K. M., and Lavin, M. A.: Classification of nursing diagnoses, St. Louis, 1975, The C. V. Mosby Co.
9. Gragg, S. H., and Rees, O. M.: Scientific principles in nursing, ed. 7, St. Louis, 1974, The C. V. Mosby Co.
10. Hannah, K. J.: The computer and nursing practice, Nursing Outlook 240:555-558, Sept., 1976.
11. Harris, B.: Who needs written care plans anyway?

American Journal of Nursing **70:**2136-2138, Oct., 1970.

12. Joint Commission on Accreditation of Hospitals: Nursing services in accreditation manual for hospitals, Chicago, 1976, The Commission, pp. 121-125.

13. Kramer, M.: Nursing care plans: power to the patient, Journal of Nursing Administration **2**(8): 29-34, 1972.

14. Likert, R., and Likert, J. G.: New ways of managing conflict, New York, 1976, McGraw-Hill Book Co.

15. Little, D., and Carnevale, D.: The nursing care planning system, Nursing Outlook **19:**164-167, March, 1971.

16. McCloskey, J. C.: The nursing care plan: past, present, and uncertain future (a review of the literature), Nursing Forum **14**(4):364-386, 1975.

17. McCloskey, J. C.: The problem-oriented record vs. the nursing care plan: a proposal, Nursing Outlook **23:**492-495, Aug., 1975.

18. Mayers, M. G.: A systematic approach to nursing care plan, New York, 1972, Appleton-Century-Crofts, Inc.

19. Mitchell, P. H.: A systematic nursing progress record—the problem-oriented approach, Nursing Forum **13**(2):187-210, 1973.

20. Mundinger, M., and Jauron, G. D.: Developing a nursing diagnosis, Nursing Outlook **2:**94-98, Feb., 1975.

21. New York State, Nurse Practice Act, Education Law, Title VIII, the professions, article 139—nursing, Albany, 1972.

22. Niland, M. B., and Bentz, P.: A problem-oriented approach to planning nursing care, Nursing Clinics of North America **9:**235-245, June, 1974.

23. Palmer, M. E.: The nursing care plan: a tool for staff development, Journal of Nursing Administration **4**(3):42-43, 1974.

24. Polisin, H. E.: Nursing care plans are a snare and a delusion, American Journal of Nursing **71:**63, Jan., 1971.

25. Roger, E., and Roger, A.: Communication in organizations, New York, 1976, The Free Press.

26. Rosenberg, M., et al.: Comparison of automated nursing notes as recorded by psychiatrists and nursing personnel, Nursing Research **18:**350-357, July-Aug., 1969.

27. Roy, C.: Introduction to nursing and adaptation model, Englewood Cliffs, N.J., 1976, Prentice-Hall, Inc.

28. Roy, C.: A diagnostic classification system for nursing, Nursing Outlook **2:**90-94, Feb., 1975.

29. Schell, P., and Campbell, A. T.: POMR—not just another way to chart, Nursing Outlook **20:**510, Aug., 1972.

30. Scott, W. G., and Mitchell, T. R.: Organization theory—a structured and behavioral analysis, ed. 3, Homewood, Ill., 1976, Richard D. Irwin, Inc.

31. Schneider, A., Donaghy, W., and Newman, P.: Organizational communication, New York, 1975, McGraw-Hill Book Co., chapters 5 and 7.

32. Stein, R. F.: An exploratory study in the development and use of automated nursing reports, Nursing Research **18:**14-21, Jan.-Feb., 1969.

33. Vardaman, G. T., and Vardaman, P. B.: Communication in modern organizations, New York, 1973, John Wiley & Sons, Inc., chapters 5, 6, and 13.

34. Vincent, P.: Some crucial terms in nursing—a second opinion, Nursing Outlook **23:**46-48, Jan., 1975.

35. Vitale, B. A., Schultz, N. V., and Nugent, P. M.: A problem-solving approach to nursing care plans: a program, St. Louis, 1974, The C. V. Mosby Co.

36. Wagner, B.: Care plans—right, reasonable and reachable, American Journal of Nursing **69:**986-990, May, 1969.

37. Weed, L.: Medical records, medical education and patient care: problem-oriented record as a basic tool, Chicago, 1971, Yearbook Medical Publishers.

38. Wesseling, E.: Automating the nursing history and care plan, Journal of Nursing Administration, May-June, 1972. In Journal of Nursing Administration staff, editors: Planning and evaluating nursing care, Wakefield, Mass., 1974, Contemporary Publishing, Inc.

39. Yarnall, S. R., and Atwood, J.: Problem-oriented practice for nurses and physicians, Nursing Clinics of North America **9:**215-228, June, 1974.

40. Yarnall, S. R., and Libke, A.: A problem-oriented system for patient care and medical records, University of Washington School of Medicine Syllabus, ed. 3, 1972, University of Washington.

13 Nursing staff assignment designs

One important function of professional nurses at the first level of nursing services is organizing the activities of the staff into a workable pattern to meet patient needs. The daily pattern of organizing follows the structured design adopted by the organization to meet defined objectives. The structured design can enhance or constrain the staff in providing quality nursing services (see Chapters 9 and 10).

The nursing staff assignment design should establish effective relationships between the activities to be performed, the workers to perform them, and the necessary physical and social factors. In the modern hospital setting, nurses are encountering increasingly difficult problems as medical technology becomes more complex and functionalization more extensive. Professional nurses are obligated to implement an effective staff assignment design to achieve low-cost excellent patient care.

In nursing services the basic designs for the assignment of staff members in the care of patients are case, functional, team, and primary care nursing. Depending on the type of nursing service organization, its philosophy, objectives, and a variety of operational conditions one finds variations and combinations of these designs.

CASE NURSING

The total care of each patient is assigned to one member of the nursing staff. In the 1920s the head nurse assigned nurses and students to specific patients. In some institutions a private duty nurse gave total care to a patient as directed by the patient's physician. The head nurse or an assistant directed, supervised, and evaluated the care given to meet each patient's need.

FUNCTIONAL NURSING

The functional method of assignment stems from the classic scientific management approach, which stresses efficiency and economy to attain goals (see Chapters 6 and 10). The method for division of labor is a highly mechanistic, rigidly controlled system. Procedural descriptions for standards of care are precisely defined. The use of written care guidelines is still an important communication tool to assure an appropriate level of care.

The functional method is task oriented.[2] The charge nurse assigns specific tasks to each worker who is responsible only for his or her assignment. In the early 1950s, patients were cared for by a few registered nurses, some practical nurses, and many nursing aides. Registered nurses performed many managerial and nonnursing duties. The hierarchical structure of nursing services became stereotyped. Although some authority and responsibility was shared, for the most part staff nurses worked as directed. There was much waste in the use of nurse manpower.

By means of the functional design the medication nurse, the treatment nurse, and the bedside nurse were created. Patients were fitted into a design that provided little flexibility to meet their personal needs.

The functional design operates on a standard set of procedures, focusing on the method with little consideration for the psychological aspects of managing either patients or personnel. However, it should be mentioned that even today, some workers gain personal satisfaction in a task-oriented environment. They feel more secure and at ease in performing repetitive tasks with skill and efficiency.

In crisis situations, professional nurses can gain satisfaction from task-oriented activities. In general, however, their level of personal satisfaction is decreased over a period of time.

TEAM NURSING

Following World War II, consumers of health care demanded more and better care. In the 1950s, nurse-educators and nurse-administrators introduced the team nursing concept in an attempt to meet increased demands for nursing services, to better utilize the knowledge and skills of professional nurses, and to increase both patient and nurse satisfactions.[7] Unfortunately, team nursing has been practiced in many ways and not always in accordance with the principles on which the concept was based.[8] The objective of team nursing is to provide comprehensive and continuous nursing and to promote individualized nursing care by means of the nursing care plan and team conferences. Team nursing requires all team members to participate in executing and evaluating care plans. Thus, it emphasizes the need for cooperation, coordination, and teamwork.

The identification of each patient's problem and the care plan are the foci for determining the tasks to be performed by each member of the team. The team leader, a registered nurse, assigns the duties to the members of the team at the beginning of each shift, plans and coordinates the care for each patient, and serves continuously as a resource person for team members. In certain situations the team leader performs some nursing care.

In general units the size of the patient group for each nursing team, usually 10 to 15 patients, depends on the patients' problems and nursing care needs and the stability of the staffing plan. Thus, the assignment method is associated with patients and is problem rather than task oriented.

The concept of nursing functions on a continuum is basic to the assignment pattern. For example, simple tasks required to meet the physical responses of a patient classified as convalescent may be performed by a nursing aide. However, the total needs of the patient are the responsibility of the team leader. It is assumed that the team leader who works with a small number of patients and assistants can match effectively available manpower resources with patient care needs.

Without meaningful patient care plans and team conferences, team nursing becomes only another method of getting the work done. The rigid traditional management process displaces the objective of team nursing to provide comprehensive and continuous nursing care to each patient. The total care of the patient becomes fragmented. For example, the team leader role may be assigned to as many as 8 to 12 different nurses during a patient's 5-day hospitalization in a unit.

To better serve patients and use professional nurses and team members in providing clinical care, some nursing services have made organizational changes.[2,3] The restructuring includes the revision of job descriptions for the head nurse, team leader, and team member positions, as well as of the overall staffing patterns. Nurse coordinators are responsible for supervising and coordinating in their areas, planning and managing nursing care for patients, and handling non-nursing activities such as clerical duties delegated to nursing. Their responsibilities focus on the clinical care of patients by means of care plans for each patient. Their management responsibilities focus on the interpretation of nursing practices and communications between team members and related health services. Another of their responsibilities focuses on evaluating the nursing care given by the staff members and working with peers and superiors for the ongoing improvement of nursing practices and the coordination of plans to improve the total system. Team leader and team member positions are defined with the same performance responsibilities.

In our sophisticated health care setting, it is evident that nurse accountability and nurse autonomy cannot take place if the nursing care design is fragmented and nursing tasks are performed by many different members with varying abilities.

PRIMARY CARE NURSING

In the early 1970s primary care nursing was instituted in hospital settings by nurses dissatisfied with fragmented care, lack of direct patient contact, and their agreement with patients' complaints about their care. Several studies in the 1960s indicated that the time devoted to direct patient care had not automatically produced better patient care. Ciske,[5] Manthey,[10] Maas,[13] and others have contributed much to the understanding and implementation of primary care nursing and the identification of the dimensions of professional practice, as shown in Fig. 12-2.

Primary care nursing is founded on the philosophy that patients, not tasks, are the central focus of professional nurses. Also, the accountability of nurses for their patients is crucial to providing quality nursing care. Primary care nursing may be defined as a comprehensive, continuous, and coordinated nursing process for meeting the total needs of each patient. This must be accomplished through the efforts of a qualified primary care nurse who has autonomy, accountability, and authority to act as the chief agent for clients.[4]

The primary care nurse accepts responsibility for the total care of four to six patients during their hospitalization on the unit. The number of patients the nurse cares for depends on the type of care needed, the nurse's capabilities and expertise, and the rate of patient turnover. The primary nurse always interviews the patient on admission, formulates a nursing diagnosis, and issues nursing orders.

This nurse is responsible for coordinating patient activities directly with physicians, patients' families, other department workers, and health community agencies on preparation for patients' discharge or necessary special services. The primary care nurse may be called at irregular hours to initiate crucial changes in patients' nursing needs.

The staff nurse is an associate nurse while caring for a patient whose primary care nurse is off duty. Practical nurses and nursing aides are nursing assistants in the care of the patients. When the primary care nurse is off duty, the nursing staff is responsible for following the primary care nurse's documented plan of care for each patient.

The primary care nursing design restricts the use of abilities to other patients on the unit. However, it permits the assignment of other staff members to patients who require their services. The quality of care depends on the effectiveness of the ongoing nursing care plan and the clarity of orders. Thus, the patient's needs and satisfaction depend greatly on the knowledge, judgment, leadership skills, and motivational level of the primary care nurse.

The selection of primary care nurses, their preparation, and in-service training are important factors for effective primary nursing care. It should be mentioned that the primary care nurse should be a registered professional nurse. How can the practical nurse, regardless of motivation and experience, be held accountable to the practices of professional nursing?

Studies indicate that there are fewer errors in care reported by the primary care nursing group than by the team nursing group.[12]

Data gathered from questionnaires completed by patients indicate that patients cared for by primary care nursing groups were more satisfied with their care than those cared for by nursing team groups.[11]

From a structural viewpoint the efficiency of primary care nursing can provide the impetus to restructure the hierarchical chain of command, eliminate traditional middle level supervisory positions, and delegate responsibility, accountability, and authority to a staff nurse in the position of a primary care nurse (see Chapter 9).

Primary care nursing requires a qualified clinical coordinator in the unit or area who is able to act as the facilitator, consultant, and motivator to the staff. Studies indicate that restructuring nursing services for the implementation of primary care nursing by professional nurses can be accomplished without increased patient costs.[11] Note that nursing should follow the personnel pattern of other disciplines. When qualified clinical nurse-specialists or primary care nurses with appropriate experience accept a clinical nurse-coordinator position in a unit, they should receive adequate financial rewards.[15] Talented professional nurses should be kept in the clinical area with patients.

In the restructuring of assignment design from the functional team to primary care nursing, the traditional position of the staff nurse, the head nurse, and the administrator must change. As emphasized by Maas[13] and others, the objective is to move authority for all decisions affecting nursing practice from the organizational chain of command to the professional nurse peer group (Fig. 13-1). The staffing pattern and assignment design should focus on authority and accountability from the tours of duty and geographical units to the care of individuals over an extended period of time.

By delegating authority and accountability of nursing care to practicing professional nurses, developing peer evaluation of performance, and operating in an organizational collegial structure, nursing services may be able to meet their objectives.[2,16,17]

In this social environment nurse-administrators become the innovators, motivators, and supporters of staff members and act as

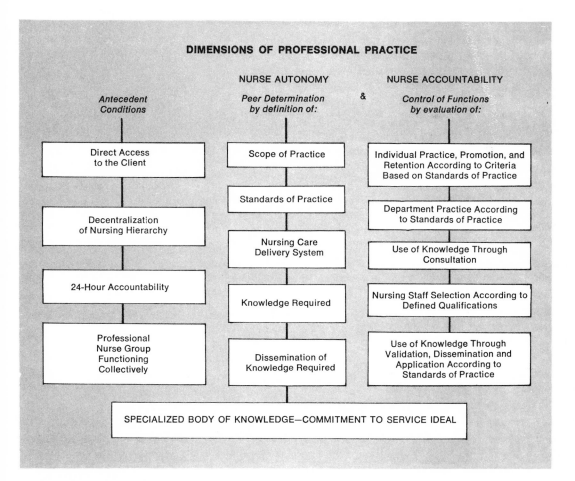

Fig. 13-1. Dimensions of professional practice. (Copyright December 1975, The American Journal of Nursing Company. Reproduced with permission from the American Journal of Nursing Vol. 75 No. 12.)

the *source* to improve the quality of patient care services as they work with other health professionals in and out of the institution.

THE UNIT MANAGEMENT SYSTEM

Due to the complexity of patient care services and the need to use manpower and material resources effectively and economically, many hospitals have taken away most of the nonnursing tasks from nursing personnel. In addition, the use of automated systems has helped to provide and control services.

In the units the employment of receptionists and unit service coordinators frees the clinical coordinator to become more clinically involved. It also frees staff members to implement the nursing care plan for their patients. The number of receptionists (secretaries) and unit coordinators depends on the kind and number of nonnursing duties completed on each unit during a 24-hour period. Activity studies can help determine the position and the duties involved.

For an efficient and economical unit management system, planning input should come from the unit manager and the clinical coordinators of units and receptionists. The receptionists, unit coordinator, and nursing staff should appreciate and understand each other's roles and needs. Each must be willing to work toward mutual goals—serving the needs of patients. Nurses must perceive the unit personnel as providing essential inputs to meet their nursing activities. Unit coordinators and receptionists must perceive their jobs as helping nurses cope with patients' problems.

An effective unit management system requires setting standards for supplies and equipment, formulating written requests, recording information, and describing each position and stating its duties.

Often the difficulties that a receptionist faces are due to nursing staff's failures. For example, a member might use an unnecessary amount of linen or supplies, forget to write down which patient used the item, not return the used equipment to its designated area when it is no longer needed, or not record the patient's temperature on the designated sheet. On the other hand, the unit coordinator and receptionist should communicate verbal or written information that influences their plan of patient care.

To provide better communication and decrease conflicts between unit management and nursing, some administrators make the unit coordinator and receptionist directly responsible to the clinical coordinator of the area or unit. This depends on the size of units, the architectural plan of the institution, and the work-flow of unit management activities.

However, a unit management system does not relieve nursing of its responsibility to use material resources properly and economically and to contribute suggestions to make it an efficient, effective, and supportive system for patient care.

REFERENCES

1. Anderson, M.: Primary nursing in day-by-day practice, American Journal of Nursing **76:**802-805, 1976.
2. Ault, L. D., and Mackay, C.: A systematic approach to individualizing nursing care, Journal of Nursing Administration **7:**39-48, Jan., 1977.
3. Bowar-Ferres, S.: Loeb center and its philosophy of nursing, American Journal of Nursing **75:**810-815, May, 1975.
4. Ciske, K.: Primary nursing: an organization that promotes professional practice, Journal of Nursing Administration **4:**28-31, Feb., 1974.
5. Ciske, K.: Primary nursing: evaluation, American Journal of Nursing **74:**1436-1438, Aug. 1974.
6. Doeffler, R. J.: Patients' perception of care under team and primary nursing, Journal of Nursing Administration **5:**20-26, March-April, 1975.
7. Douglas, L. M.: Review of team nursing: Mosby's comprehensive review series, St. Louis, 1973, The C. V. Mosby Co.
8. Kron, T.: Team nursing -- how valid is it today? Journal of Nursing Administration **1:**19-22, July-Aug., 1977.
9. Lane, H. C.: Promoting an independent practice, American Journal of Nursing **75:**1319-1321, Aug. 1975.
10. Manthey, M.: Primary nursing is alive and well in the hospital, American Journal of Nursing **73:**83-87, Jan., 1973.
11. Marram, G. D., et al.: Cost-effectiveness of primary and team nursing, Wakefield, Mass., 1976, Contemporary Publishing, Inc.
12. Marram, G. D., Bevis, E. O., and Schlegel, M. W.: Primary nursing: a model for individualized care, St. Louis, 1974, The C. V. Mosby Co.
13. Maas, M., Specht, J., and Jacox, A.: Nurse auton-

omy: reality not rhetoric, American Journal of Nursing 75(12):2201-2208, 1975.

14. Page, M.: Primary nursing: perceptions of a head nurse, American Journal of Nursing 74(8):1435-1436, 1974.

15. Rotkovitch, R., editor: Quality of patient care and role of clinical nursing specialists, New York, 1976, John Wiley & Sons, Inc., chapter 18.

16. Santorium, C. D., and Sell, V. M.: A patient centered nursing service. In Journal of Nursing Administration staff, editors: Organization of nursing care, Wakefield, Mass., 1975, Contemporary Publishing, Inc. (Reprinted from Journal of Nursing Administration July-Aug.,1973.)

17. Tucker, S. M., Breeding, M. A., Canobbio, M. M., Jacquet, G. D., Paquette, E. H., Wells, M. E., and Willmann, M. E.: Patient care standards, St. Louis, 1975, The C. V. Mosby Co.

14 | Staffing program for quality nursing care

Health consumers, demanding more quantity and quality care, reduced costs, and more functionalization and specialization, are forcing professional nurses in hospitals to implement a staffing program that will result in quality care and the efficient use of personnel at a reasonable cost.

An effective staffing program for nursing care establishes meaningful interrelationships between quality staffing patterns, workloads, and the organizational structure.[5,6,12] This requires that nurses resolve major staffing problems through the problem-solving process.[24a]

MAJOR COMPONENTS OF A STAFFING PROGRAM

The development of a staffing program and the assignment of personnel requires professional nurse groups to consider six major components that influence the quality and quantity of care. They are as follows:

1. The philosophy and goals of the hospital, the services offered to health consumers, and their desires and expectations of care.
2. The goals, objectives, and organizational structure of nursing services to meet the nursing care needs of patients.
3. The standards of nursing care practices to provide quality care, and management criteria for effective and efficient utilization of personnel.
4. The application of methodology to determine the kind and amount of nursing care required to help each patient along his illness-health continuum.
5. The development of personnel sched-

ules to meet the measured care needs of patients, the personal goals of the staff members, and career development of the staff members.
6. The evaluation of nursing service input and its impact upon quality of care.[20]

Staffing and assigning personnel for patient care and the organizational staffing program are basic components of a budgetary and an evaluation program.

Goals, objectives, and standards

In developing a patient-centered staffing program, professional nurse groups first should review the nursing service statement of goals and objectives (see Chapter 7). All staff members must understand them and regard them as meaningful.

Professional nurse groups should answer the following questions: (1) Does the organizational structural design support the implementation of individualized nursing care? (2) Does the design provide for effective communication between the nurse-doers of nursing care and their superiors? (3) Does the organizational behavioral approach motivate and support staff nurses and permit them to participate in decisions influencing their role in nursing care?[24]

Professional nurse groups should agree on their definition of a standard for clinical nursing practice.[30] Do they support the qualifications and standards of nursing practice as set forth by the American Nurses Association (Chapter 5)? One objective of the nurse group may be to hold professional nurses accountable for their acts of practice. Another objective may be to use professional nurses' input in carrying out patient-oriented functions and other activities to improve the quality of patient care.[19,20]

An objective of nursing service staffing programs may be to provide care consistent with the AHA Standards for Safe Patient Care as set forth by the Joint Commission on Accreditation of Hospitals.[1] A nursing service staffing program must include an adequate number of *qualified* professional and nonprofessional personnel to meet the standards set forth by the AHA and the ANA.[3,8]

Job descriptions for nurse career patterns

Job descriptions should indicate the level of practice expected from the professional and technical nurse. Will the staffing program aim to use appropriately the knowledge and skills of nurses for clinical nursing care? Does the program permit appropriate rewards for good clinical nursing care performance by members? Will the program promote the employment of professional nurses for patient-centered direct care activities?[2,6] (See Chapters 9 and 10.)

In recent years professional nurse groups have accepted an objective to reclassify professional nursing positions toward meeting the clinical needs of patients.[10,17] The peer review process has been used. Other groups have accepted an objective to render care by means of primary nursing care design without increasing human resource expenditures (see Chapter 13).

The outcome in meeting objectives changes the traditional task-oriented activities of nurses to problem-oriented functions in meeting care needs of patients. It also should decrease hierarchical levels of the structure and the delineation of traditional supervisory positions.

Managerial criteria

One objective of a staffing program is to provide employee satisfaction.[34,35] As discussed in Chapters 6 and 7, the hierarchy of personal needs of individuals as defined by Maslow[24] and Herzberg[21] indicates that the lower needs of job security, adequate working conditions, and reasonable work schedules must be met before an individual attains higher achievement goals.

A staffing program and the assignment schedules of personnel should clearly define management policies and procedures. For example, professional nurse groups should state the number of professional nursing hours to be allocated to direct nursing care during each shift in various units, or a policy should state that no employee on a unit will be assigned to another patient unit or area for which he or she has not been trained or is not qualified. Thus, workloads, personnel vacations, number of consecutive workdays, and related matters must be clearly defined and understood by the staff.

An acceptable staffing program reflects the objectives of the in-service training and continuing education programs, professional direction, supervision of direct care, and management of nursing services. A criteria may state that all nursing service personnel working full- or part-time shall be enrolled in an appropriate orientation and training program in accordance with their position prior to formal assignment to a job.

In addition, legislative labor acts and collective bargaining influence the management criteria of a staffing program[10] (see Chapter 4).

Management efficiency

Management efficiency, in terms of human resource expenditures, is usually determined by a measured input used to produce a unit of output. In budgetary planning the cost factor is determined by the total number of nursing manhours required per patient each day in general and special services. For example, based on informational data the nursing service staffing program may state that in general patient units the staffing input will be limited to an average of 4.8 nursing hours per patient during each 24-hour period. In intensive care units the staffing input will be limited to 16.0 nursing manhours per patient during each 24-hour period. The preparation of a nursing service budget is discussed in Chapter 15.

The nurse-executive is ultimately responsible for achieving efficiency objectives and for significant deviations from defined objectives. However, professional nurse groups must share this accountability with their superiors. This "sharing" of responsibility is best accomplished through a collegial organizational communication process (see Chapter 12).

It should be mentioned that a high level of nursing service manhours allocated to nursing care does not necessarily result in a high quality of care. There are many difficult problems and hospital and nursing variables that nurses must cope with in planning and implementing an ongoing staffing program.

HOSPITAL CARE DELIVERY ENVIRONMENT

It is assumed that the daily patient census, admission policies, the architectural layout of units, and the input of supportive services influence the quantity and quality of nursing care.

Percentage occupancy rate and admission policy

For years the patient census or percentage occupancy has been an important factor in determining nursing care requirements. For example, administrators used the "average" occupancy rate on a particular service as the basis to determine the maximal nursing care input. Average determination creates problems for the nurse-executive when the unit census fluctuates or when the average occupancy rate increases by 15% for short periods of time.

Average nursing care inputs require a supportive contingency staffing plan. This plan may transfer regular staff members from their unit to another, use temporary personnel, or have the regular staff in a unit work additional hours each day. It is vital that professional nurse groups agree on the criteria of a contingency program. The plan should be reviewed with potential employees during their initial interview and again during their orientation period.

The admission, discharge, and transfer of patients can create difficulties or enhance the individualized care plan and workflow pattern of activities in the various units or areas.[23] Policies should encourage and support effective communication between de-

partments as well as between patient and physician.[25]

Studies indicate that when patient turnover is rapid, more personnel skills and time are spent in patient-orientation activities. Recent experiences of primary nurses in acute general hospitals state that planning the needs of patients on discharge must begin early in the patient's hospitalization. When a patient is hospitalized for 10 or more days and the occupancy rate is fairly stable, more nursing time is spent on teaching and rehabilitation activities.

The existence of an automated informational system enhances communications between the admitting office and the units.[18,25] The nurse receives advance information about the patient's arrival. The system, not nursing personnel, notifies the physician and the supportive services of the patient's arrival. By means of the automated system the nurse in the backup intensive care unit can inform the nurse in the general unit of a patient transfer and his or her clinical nursing care plan, prior to arrival on the unit. However, nursing care will be better only if that nursing service time is spent productively with patients.

An automated informational system and patients' shortened hospital stays require the continuation of needs after discharge. Most hospital-based continuing care programs lack effective communication within the hospital and between the hospital and the community. Thus, late referrals and last minute planning are necessary.[22] A health team approach to planning care for patients and their discharge is needed. Administrators should define objectives for patient discharge.

Unit layout

The physical layout of each unit should be designed around the care needs of patients on that unit. For example, in general adult units the one- and two-bed rooms with bathroom and shower and a storage alcove by the door for supplies and linens for use in the immediate future provide for smooth workflow patterns in rendering individualized care to each patient.

A quiet, efficient communication mechanism located at each patient's bed and connected to a console in the nursing station provides security to patients and saves the personnel's time. Architectural devices for the transfer of small materials such as requisitions from units to other departments decrease nursing service manhours.

A conference room located on a patient floor for the use of health care members and for in-service training purposes eliminates the need for staff to leave the unit. An office for the clinical nurse coordinator and the nurse specialist helps to provide closer relationships between superiors and subordinates.

Supportive services

Appropriate storage areas for sterile and unsterile supplies and equipment needed for immediate use that are controlled and serviced by the materials management staff decrease nursing service input. The hospital escort service enhances the workflow pattern of nursing personnel.

We know that modern hospital layouts, technological innovations, and the elimination of nonclinical tasks from nurses' duties can benefit patients and reduce the nursing service manhours allocated to units. However, research is needed to show that these improvements directly affect the quality of care. Results of projects on a patient-oriented system indicate that such a system can increase nurses' time in direct care activities and save costs in overtime pay for nurses, supplies, and pharmacy personnel. Such projects succeed when a participative approach and the problem-solving process are initiated by the hospital executive staff.

METHODOLOGY FOR DETERMINING NURSING CARE REQUIREMENTS

Several methods have been used to determine the amount of nursing hours required to meet the nursing care needs of patients.[24a]

Descriptive informational data such as percentage occupancy, medical diagnoses, and hospital variables are of little value in determining nursing care requirements. Industrial methodology may be used to identify various tasks and determine the time required to complete repetitive tasks in a controlled work environment. To determine direct nursing care requirements, data must present activities to meet the physical and psychosocial needs of each patient along his or her illness-health continuum.

The management engineering methodology applies systems analysis and operations research (see Chapter 6). Its elements include several strategies—stating performance objectives, analyzing components and functions, delegating functions to specific individuals for planning and directing activities, scheduling projects to meet desired outcomes, training individuals to initiate and evaluate the system, and quality control. The application of systems approach, based on the problem-solving process, requires gathering data, developing structures for solutions, testing the solutions, and selecting the best one for use.

Selecting a methodology

In selecting a methodology the nurse-executive and the staff must consider important existing variables. The objectives of the nursing practice statements of the nursing service organization must be considered. The interest and ability of the staff to conduct the study, the scope of the study, and the financial input required all influence the methodology used.[6]

When developing a staffing pattern for the effective distribution of professional or nonprofessional personnel for nursing care, several criteria must be established. Today the staff must consider a nursing practice act, patient safety, and differential abilities of nurses to perform legally acceptable activities.

In general, nurse administrators and staff are limited in their preparation of staffing methodologies or in the adoption of an experimental approach to nursing practice. The development of a methodology for staffing has been stymied by the concept that nurses must be infallible. This idea has impeded nurses from initiating scientific investigation. Moreover, many existing variables must be controlled to a degree for the effective practice of nursing in the care of patients. Alfano[2] and Georgopoulas[17] have done some valuable studies in areas of the nurses' role in meeting the needs of patients.

It should be mentioned that a successful staffing program to provide individualized care depends on five major factors: (1) A staff with the knowledge and ability to do their jobs in keeping with the care needs of the patients; (2) maximum contingency staffing plans; (3) qualified professional nurses for guidance in developing a plan of care for each patient in the performance of acceptable staff practices; (4) a built-in in-service training and continuing education program; and (5) a nonclinical staff to assume nonnursing supportive tasks.

Categorizing patients

To meet quantity and quality staffing standards for patients along their illness-health continuum, patient categorization methodology is used instead of the traditional method of counting the number of patients in beds and the number of personnel. The categorization method is not based on a patient's disease or medical diagnosis, but on each patient's nursing care requirements that must be performed by the nursing staff.[19,24a]

Patient classification systems. One method of patient classification is a scaling device in which the basic illness-health continuum of patients can be expressed in quantitative terms of each patient's requirements for nursing care and nursing services.

The range of patients' nursing care needs may vary from minimal requirements for those patients who have maximum self-help ability to continuous, complex requirements for those patients who have minimum or no self-help ability. A patient classification scale is not a perfect device to determine nursing care requirements. However, it can be an objective guide in helping nurses to make personnel staffing decisions to meet the ongoing daily needs of patients and to determine the basic manpower needs for groups of patients on a floor or unit area. It is a device whereby nursing service leaders can

determine the nature and general characteristics of the patients' requirements for planning future staffing standards; however, the supervisor will still be required to make some daily decisions. For example, the terminal cancer patient, who is classified at the lowest level of illness on the illness-health continuum, may require less professional nursing care than the healthy patient who is recovering from a hip-pinning surgical procedure and is classified at the moderate level of illness. Thus the type and frequency of nursing care activities are important aspects of a patient classification system for determination of nursing service manpower requirements.

The objective of a patient classification system is to make possible the matching of nursing service personnel manhour requirements with patient nursing care and service demands.

Patient category system. The literature describes three different categories:

I. Minimal (self)
II. Intermediate
III. Intensive

There seems to be no completely satisfactory system. Many nurses subdivide this system into five categories to describe more precisely the specific care needs of patients.

Wolfe and Young[39] conducted studies in 1965 using scientific methods to determine direct and indirect patient care requirements and to predict nursing loads. They listed a combination of factors for the categorization of patients grouped in category I (self care), category II (partial or intermediate care), and category III (intensive or total care).

The research findings of Wolfe and Young[40,41] conducted at the Johns Hopkins Hospital indicate that category I patients required 0.5 hour of direct care, category II patients required 1 hour of direct patient care, and category III patients required 2.5 hours of direct patient care. The study also indicated that activities other than direct care amounted to 20 hours of an 8-hour day on a general adult patient unit of 29 to 30 beds, regardless of the patient census or the number of nursing personnel on duty.

Thus the direct care index is computed

using the formula: $1 \times 0.5N_1 + 1N_2 + 2.5N_3$; 1 represents the direct care index in hours; N_1 represents the number of patients in category I; N_2 represents the number of patients in category II; and N_3 represents the number of patients in category III. In accordance with this patient classification formula, the amount of nursing hours required for 30 patients in a unit would be as follows:

4 patients in N_3 would be 4×2.5 hr. = 10 hr.
16 patients in N_2 would be 16×1 hr. = 16 hr.
10 patients in N_1 would be 10×0.5 hr. = 5 hr.
Total nursing care hours required
　　　　from 6 AM to 12 midnight = 31 hr.
Additional management activities
　　　　20 hr. $\times$ 2 shifts = 40 hr.
Total nursing service hours between
　　　　6 AM and 12 midnight = 71 hr.

During 18 hours the total nursing time for 30 patients would be 71 hours, plus coverage from 12 midnight to 6 AM. On the night shift if the nursing service input for the 30 patients on the floor included one registered graduate nurse, one licensed practical nurse and one nurse's aide each working 8 hours, total nursing service hours for a 24-hour period would be 95 hours. Thus the total nursing care and service requirements would be 95 nursing care and service hours for 30 beds. Based on this data, each patient would require an average of 3.16 nursing care hours each 24-hour period.

Some scientific methodologies focus on *the nursing care requirements of patients*, not on *what the patient is having done for him*. This requires the development of data collection forms, patient observations, the review of orders and chart recordings, conferences with nurses, the determination of categorization system, the establishment of the average number of minutes required to accomplish each nursing procedural activity, and assessment, planning, counseling, and evaluation.[24a,27]

This method requires knowledgeable nurses to collect data and make necessary judgments concerning patient care needs and the category of worker who should perform the activity. Based on the calcula-

tions for staffing patient care activities and human resource requirements for in-service training, nursing, and administration, the total nursing service staffing program is computed.

Scientific calculations of staffing require extensive hours of research to establish a data base for decision making. The determination of staffing needs is developed by reviewing existing and proposed operational systems.[24a]

Other methods described are based on the Standards for Nursing Practice in relation to the classification of patient care needs. Thomas[35] has classified clinical nurse positions according to their ability to meet specific Standards of Nursing Practice in relation to the acuity of nursing care needs of patients.[8]

Harman[18] describes an ongoing patient categorization instrument to provide a measure of nursing care requirements to meet patients' nursing care needs. The patient-categorization grouping and criteria are developed. The categories are given a weighted factor. Minimal care is given 4; partial, 6; full, 12; and constant care 24. Each category of personnel is given a weight factor. The registered staff nurse is assigned a weight factor of 10, and other workers are scaled using the registered nurse weighted factor of 10 as the reference point. This type of informational system, combined with quality of monitoring, is useful in identifying trends and in monitoring the appropriateness of resource allocation on a unit-to-unit basis and on a daily basis for each unit.

STAFFING SCHEDULE PATTERNS

In a hospital the nursing service's total human resources required for clinical care and nonclinical tasks are expressed in the master staffing program. The program is developed using the bottom-up approach by professional nurse groups in various units with the guidance and direction of the nurse-executive. The master staffing program is designed to meet defined objectives, assignment methodology, Standards of Nursing Practice, and the personnel policies of the organization.

Centralization and decentralization

The nurse-executive is ultimately responsible for the development and implementation of the master staffing program and for labor costs. Within a collegial organizational environment the nurse-executive shares the responsibility and authority for manhour inputs and costs required for the nursing care needs of patients in the various units.

The master staffing plan becomes an integral component of the nursing service budget. The determined human resource input for the different units is converted into positions. The position control for each unit becomes a measure of control for the approved budget (see Chapter 15).

The staffing program usually includes personnel who work consistently each week of the fiscal (full-time) year, those who work consistently several days each week (part-time); those who work several hours each week (complementary or float), and those who work occasionally when called (temporary). Difficulties arise in coordinating part-time workers' schedules and preferences with those of full-time workers of the same job classification. Part-time employees of the same job classification are grouped together to fill one full-time position during the fiscal year. The float group is used to meet heavy workloads, holidays, and staff vacations.

The professional nurse group should develop appropriate forms to record daily data on the census of patients in different nursing categories, the workload, and the staffing index.[18] The central nursing office should prepare weekly reports based on the daily data of each unit. This weekly report assists the staff members and administrators to identify trends and staffing problems and to monitor efficiency in the allocation of manhour input on a unit-to-unit and a day-to-day basis. Audit data feedback is often included in these reports (see Chapter 16).

In some hospitals maximum care needs are required 7 days a week. Frequently the available staffing input is inadequate, resulting in poor care.[29] In such situations, if the nurse group involved and the nurse-execu-

tive cannot provide safe care, the nurse-executive should request administration to restrict patient admissions for a specific period of time, even though this is a costly measure that creates dissatisfaction on the part of physicians and potential patients.

The professional nurse group in each unit should participate in the kind of scheduling pattern to be introduced to meet desired outcomes. Experimentation is needed to resolve ongoing staffing problems in accordance with nursing care objectives and available nursing resources.

Problems of traditional staffing patterns

In recent years the demands for quantity and quality care at a reasonable price and personnel requests for every other weekend off have forced nurses to consider new staffing patterns. In past years the nursing staff on the units worked 2 weekends out of every 3. Recently many hospitals have agreed to give all personnel every other weekend off. This step has been taken to reduce turnover and recruit qualified nursing personnel.

The traditional $7\frac{1}{2}$-hour day or 8-hour day and a 5-day week cannot meet patients' care needs 7 days a week without increasing labor costs or having periods of inadequate manhour input. The traditional staffing pattern tends to underutilize nursing resources on some days and overutilize them on weekends and holidays. Patients, nurses, and physicians become dissatisfied and frustrated when overutilization occurs.

Underutilization is further increased when nursing students and their instructor are on the units. Studies indicate that absenteeism results as much from underutilization as from overutilization. When manhour input fluctuates from day-to-day, a smooth workflow pattern is not possible. When overutilization exists, the staff uses the task-oriented functional assignment plan. Frequently the knowledge and expertise of the staff are not used efficiently in the care of patients.

Having most positions filled by full-time employees adds to the problem of underutilization of manhour input 1 or 2 days each week. Some departments use 1 day for in-service training and conferences. However, it is difficult to plan adequately for these activities.

To resolve the problem of providing a maximum level of care 7 days a week, some nursing services employ part-time personnel to relieve the regular staff members. However, it may be difficult to find part-time personnel who will work every other weekend. With personnel who are willing to work less than 8 hours, the full-time workers' shift requires adjustment.

To resolve some of the staffing problems, innovations have been introduced. A cyclic schedule plan, the use of two shifts pattern, or changing hours of shifts have been used.

The success of any schedule system depends on (1) the type of human resources available, (2) the staff members' willingness and motivation to accept their responsibility in making a plan work for the care of patients, (3) the staff members' creativity to test and evaluate ways to resolve their ongoing staffing problems, and (4) a collegial approach and an effective communication system between the *doers of care* and their superiors.[4]

Each nursing service must design its own staffing schedule pattern that will best meet its patients' care requirements, the need satisfactions of staff members, and the funds available for manhour inputs.

Purpose and criteria of staffing schedule plans

A staffing schedule plan is a means of allocating an appropriate amount of manhours produced by personnel in different job classifications for required care needs of each patient during each 24 hours, usually 7 days a week.[10,12]

The staffing schedule plan should enable the staff to meet the objectives, standards, and policies of the organization. It must stay within the limits set by the approved master staffing budget.[38]

The staffing schedule plan for each unit should inform all staff members of their work schedule for the coming consecutive 3 to 6 weeks including days off and shift of duty. At the completion of the planned sequence, the plan should be repeated with necessary adjustments.

The plan should provide for the satisfaction of staff members in their work and in planning their personal time. It should provide for some flexibility in meeting unexpected personnel changes such as terminations and sick leave, unanticipated care needs, and coverage for holidays and vacations. The staffing schedule plan must be in accord with the current Fair Labor Standard Act.

The plan should conserve nurses' time in preparing or changing work schedules. It should reduce interpersonal conflicts between staff and superiors created by changes made in scheduling.

Staffing coordinator responsibilities and duties

Experience has shown that a nonnurse who possesses the appropriate abilities can relieve professional nurses of preparing schedules and weekly time sheets.[37] In medium and large hospitals each department should have a staffing coordinator. However, in small hospitals the coordinator will work in the central nursing office under the supervision of the assistant director.

It is the professional nurses who develop the objectives and the schedule plan, but it is the coordinator who gives each employee a copy of the work schedule and posts the weekly time schedules in each unit a few days prior to the week it becomes effective.

The coordinator reviews the daily reports, makes the necessary adjustments to meet care needs, and may reassign the float individuals and call in temporary personnel if necessary. The coordinator keeps personnel records updated regarding absenteeism, overtime, and transfers. This data is used by the personnel and accounting departments for the personnel payroll.

Using daily unit reports, coordinators prepare the weekly staffing report for each unit. Coordinators work closely with clinical nurses and keep their superiors informed of major problems.

The staffing coordinator should take part in the orientation program for new nursing personnel. This gives new members an opportunity to know the role of the coordinator and emphasizes their responsibility to make the plan work successfully.

The coordinator should be a good typist, able to compute figures and percentages for the computerization of data, and should place a high value on effective communications.

Cyclical scheduling patterns

The cyclical schedules, produced for the workers of each patient unit, work best for everyone. Most cyclical patterns are based on 3-, 4-, and 6-week blocks. Cyclical scheduling of workhours and shifts removes the problems of personalities.[14,15,26] Once the cyclical pattern is established, all positions are assigned a number. New staff members are automatically assigned the number given the position before it becomes vacant. When an individual transfers to a different unit or shift, the person has to accept the schedule of that unit. Price,[26] Warstler,[37] and others provide detailed guidelines in developing cyclical schedules. A cyclical or block scheduling plan reduces nurses' time spent making out schedules.[15] The staff knows its days off in advance. Studies indicate that overtime is decreased, and personnel are treated fairly and equally.

Restructuring the work-week. Some nursing services have shortened the evening shift, and lengthened the day and night shifts. Fraser[13] describes a plan to meet the care needs and use the available part-time nurses as follows: The day shift, 7:00 AM to 5:00 PM; the night shift, 9:00 PM to 7:00 AM; and the evening shift, 5:00 PM to 10:00 PM. This schedule provides each employee with 2 consecutive days off in each week and a 3-day weekend every other week. The employees do not work more than 3 consecutive 10-hour workdays, and the evening (part-time) staff works a 4- to 5-hour shift.

This type of work cycle is based on a 2-week period. Each employee is scheduled on 1 week—Sunday through Thursday, and Monday through Saturday the other week.

This means 50% of the staff is scheduled for the first week, while the other half is scheduled for the second week of the cycle. In some institutions this plan has reduced turnover and labor cost with a better allocation of personnel input for patient care.

The 10-hour shift, 4-day work week. Some nursing services have found that this 6-week cyclical pattern has improved staffing as compared to the traditional 8-hour day, 5-day week. The part-time personnel cyclic pattern is interlocked with that of the schedule for the full-time personnel. According to Bauer,[7] the shifts developed for the 10-hour day were 7:00 AM to 5:30 PM, 1:00 PM to 11:30 PM, and 9:00 PM to 7:30 AM. Today nurses indicate that they appreciate the long weekends and the extra day off. This type of schedule seems effective in staffing intensive care units. Nurses are more satisfied because they can give comprehensive continuous care and because of the additional pay for overtime.

The 12-hour shift. In recent years some nursing service groups have introduced the 12-hour shift due to inadequate staffing input for nursing care of patients requiring intensive or modified intensive care.[36] The shift hours are usually 7:00 AM to 7:30 PM and 7:00 PM to 7:30 AM. When the 12-hour shift is used the personnel must have at least 2 days off prior to a change of shift.

Studies indicate that because few nurses are responsible for each patient, close relationships are established between the nurse, patient, and his family, and between the nurse and physician.[34] Time is saved in personnel shift changeover.

Ganong[16] and others studied the two-shift daily schedule of 12 hours each, with each employee working 7 days followed by 7 consecutive days off. The Ganong report indicates that there is a better use of nursing personnel; fewer nurses are required, and labor costs are decreased. The report also indicates that the level of productivity and the level of patient care were not really affected adversely. However, during some high work-load days, some nurses mentioned fatigue as a factor at the end of their shift and at the end of the week. Research studies indicate that biological rhythms are associated with temporal fluctuations in efficiency and performance.[11] However, this problem can be resolved by a predetermined staffing position for each position by means of a 6- to 8-hour week cyclical scheduling in advance, with a minimum of rotation to evening and night shifts and at least 16 to 24 hours between the change.

TRENDS IN SCHEDULING

In recent years, job enrichment (job expansion) of professional and technical nurses has required that they participate in planning and evaluating their work with less direct supervision and more self-evaluation. The literature indicates that job expansion produces lower absenteeism and reduces turnover costs. However, the job expansion of nurses and others must increase the quality of services. Some studies in nursing services indicate that the expansion of nurses' responsibility and accountability for patients' care and a systematic cyclical scheduling pattern result in a higher quality of services as compared to traditional approaches. In short, in terms of efficiency for the same input, patients can receive a higher quality of nursing care.

In the past 5 years nursing services have implemented several different scheduling workweek programs. This is in keeping with workweek programs used in industry. It is estimated that in 1974, over 4,000 companies in the United States had 4-day workweeks in operation. However, in hospitals patients require services during each of the 24 hours of a 7-day week.

Flex-time scheduling. Some researchers and nurse-executives have thought that the flex-time concept could be implemented for the services of highly trained clinical nurses and for nurses in in-service training or specialty programs.[28] Under flex-time, professional nurses agree to work a number of hours each week but are free to vary the hours of work within certain defined limits. For example, a professional nurse could be assigned to work from 7:30 AM to 3:30 PM (7½ hours) but would be allowed to work to 6:30 PM if patient care requirements demanded additional services. The nurse would be permitted to accumulate the additional hours of work for a free day each month.

Under flex-time the nurse assumes responsibility and accountability for the job. This plan is consistent with the view that individuals are paid for producing work while not being in their unit for a set period of hours. Several industrial firms who have implemented the flex-time plan report that it has resulted in increased employee productivity, a decrease in errors, improved employee morale, and reduced absenteeism. With increased functionalization and specialization in patient care services, the flex-time plan may become a useful technique that could be instituted for some professional nurse input at a relatively low cost.

Summary

Whatever cyclical staffing plan is used in the near future, most nursing services will be staffed by computer programming. By use of the computer, many variables can be fed into the staffing calculations that cannot be done by means of present cyclical scheduling forms. An effective staffing plan must provide the necessary quantity of nursing workers who have the proper qualifications and expertise to meet the nursing care requirements of patients as they pass through the various stages of acuity during each 24 hours of their hospitalization.[24a]

It seems evident that no one staffing scheduling workweek will eliminate all the staffing problems inherent in our present hospital structure. However, when all nurses work together, they can improve their staffing system to meet nursing service goals.

REFERENCES

1. Accreditation manual for hospitals, Chicago, 1976, Joint Commission on Accreditation of Hospitals.
2. Alfano, G.: The Loeb Center for nursing and rehabilitation: a professional approach to nursing practice, Nursing Clinics of North America 4:487, 1969.
3. American Nurses Association: Standards for organized nursing services, Kansas City, Mo., 1973, The Association.
4. Argyris, C.: Integrating the individual and the organization, New York, 1964. John Wiley & Sons, Inc.

5. Argyris, C.: The applicability of organizational sociology, London, 1972, Cambridge University Press.
6. Aydelotte, M. K.: Staffing for high-quality care, Hospitals 47(2):58, 60-65, 1973.
7. Bauer, J.: Clinical staffing with a 10-hour day, 4-day work week. In Journal of Nursing Administration staff, editors: Staffing, Wakefield, Mass., 1974, Contemporary Publishing, Inc., pp. 29-30.
8. Congress for Nursing Practice: A plan for implementation of the Standards of Nursing Practice, Kansas City, Mo., 1975, American Nurses Association.
9. Conover, W. J.: Practical nonparametric statistics, New York, 1971, John Wiley and Sons, Inc.
10. Coulton, M. R.: Labor disputes: a challenge to nurse staffing, Journal of Nursing Administration 6:15-20, May, 1976.
11. Felton G.: Body rhythm effects on rotating work shifts, Journal of Nursing Administration 5:16-19, March-April, 1975.
12. Fine, R. B.: Controlling nurses' workloads, American Journal of Nursing 74:2206-2207, Dec., 1974.
13. Fraser, L. P.: The reconstructed work week—one answer to the scheduling dilemma, Journal of Nursing Administration 2:12-16, Sept.-Oct., 1972.
14. Froebe, D.: Scheduling: by team or individually, Journal of Nursing Administration 4:34-36, May-June, 1974.
15. Gahan, K., and Talley, R.: A block scheduling system, Journal of Nursing Administration 5(9):39-41, 1975.
16. Ganong, W. L., et al.: The 12-hour shift: better quality, lower cost, Journal of Nursing Administration 6:17-29, Feb., 1976.
17. Georgopoulos, B., and Christman, L.: The clinical nurse specialist: a role model, American Journal of Nursing 75:1030, May, 1970.
18. Harman, R. J.: Nursing services information system, Journal of Nursing Administration 7:14-20, March, 1977.
19. Haussmann, R. K., and Dieter: A quality control programme for nursing services, Hospital Research and Educational Trust—Proceedings, March, 1975, The American Hospital Association.
20. Hegyvary, S. T., Haussmann, R. K. and Dieter.: Monitoring nursing care quality, Journal of Nursing Administration 5:17, May, 1975.
21. Herzberg, F., et al.: The motivation to work, ed. 2, New York, 1959, John Wiley & Sons, Inc.
22. La Montagne, M. E., and McKeehan, K. M.: Profile of a continuing care program emphasizing discharge planning, Journal of Nursing Administration 4(2):22-23, 1974.
23. Levine, H. D., and Phillips, P. J.: Factors affecting staffing levels and patterns of nursing personnel, pub. no. (HRA) 75-6, United States Department of Health, Education and Welfare, Washington, D.C., 1975, United States Government Printing Office.
24. Maslow, A. H.: Motivation and personality, New York, 1954, Harper & Row, Publishers, Inc.
24a. Norby, R. B., Freund, L. E., and Wagner, B.: A nurse staffing system based upon assignment difficulty, Journal of Nursing Administration 7:2-24, Nov., 1977.
25. Porter, A., Moschel, P., Liederman, B., and Pope, M.: Patient needs on admission, American Journal of Nursing 77:112-113, Jan., 1977.
26. Price, E. M.: Staffing for patient care (a guide for nursing service based on a research report). New York, 1970, Springer Publishing Co., Inc.
27. Ramey, I. G.: Staffing pattern. In Stone, S., Berger, M. S., Elhart, D., Firsich, S. C., and Jordan, S. B., editors: Management for nurses, St. Louis, 1976, The C. V. Mosby Co, chapter 12.
28. Robbins, P. S.: The administrative process—integrating theory and practice, Englewood Cliffs, N.J., 1976, Prentice-Hall, Inc., chapters 15 and 23.
29. Ryan, S. M.: The modified work week for nursing staff on two pediatric units, Journal of Nursing Administration 5:31-34, July-Aug., 1975. (Also in Nursing Digest, Winter issue, 1976, pp. 29-31.)
30. Ryan, T., et al.: A system for determining appropriate nursing staff, Journal of Nursing Administration 5:30-38, June, 1975.
31. Schneider, B.: Staffing organizations, Pacific Palisades, Calif., 1976, Goodyear Publishing Co., Inc.
32. Stinson, S. M., and Hazlett, C. B.: Nurse-physician opinion of a modified work week trial, Journal of Nursing Administration 5:21-26, Sept., 1975.
33. Tescher, B. E., and Colavecchio, R.: Definition of a standard for clinical nursing practice, Journal of Nursing Administration 7:32-44, March, 1977.
34. Thomas, L. A.: Predicting change in nursing values, Sloan Management Review 15:11-21, Fall 1973.
35. Thomas, L. A. Predicting changes in nursing values, focus on the work environment, Nursing Digest, Wakefield, Mass., 1975, Contemporary Publishing, Inc., pp. 126-134.
36. Underwood, A. B.: What a 12-hour shift offers, American Journal of Nursing 75:1176-1178, July, 1975.
37. Warstler, M. E.: Cyclic work schedules and a non-nurse coordinator of staffing, Journal of Nursing Administration 3:45-51, Nov.-Dec., 1973.
38. Warstler, M. E.: Some management techniques for nursing service administrators, Journal of Nursing Administration 2:25-34, Nov.-Dec., 1972.
39. Wolfe, H., and Young, J. P.: Staffing the nursing unit. I. Controlled variable staffing, Nursing Research 14(3):236-243, 1965.
40. Wolfe, H., and Young, J. P.: Staffing the nursing unit. II. The multiple assignment technique, Nursing Research 14(4):229-304, 1965.
41. Young, J. P.: A method for allocation of nursing personnel to meet inpatient care needs, Baltimore, 1962, Operations Research Division, The Johns Hopkins Hospital.

15 Budget planning and control

A constant concern of hospital executives and department heads is the budgeting of human, material, and financial expenses to meet objectives for a specific period of time; and how to use the controlling process effectively to measure actual results against determined objectives.

BUDGETING AND CONTRACTING AS MANAGEMENT PROCESSES

We would agree that the main goal of nursing is to provide adequate manpower to meet the care of each patient in a comprehensive, continuous fashion. Planning of resources for each unit or area is based on defined objectives (see Chapter 7). These objectives stem from the philosophy, goals, and standards agreed on by the nursing service and the institution (see Chapter 5). Professional nurse groups in the various services define subobjectives in keeping with the overall objectives of the organization.

In budgeting resources, quality factors must be expressed in quantitative terms to analyze and measure results against determined objectives. Subobjectives are translated into specific activities to attain the objectives. Thus, planning using problem-solving techniques is a prerequisite for budget planning (Fig. 8-1).

As discussed in Chapter 14, nursing service manhours are determined to meet the clinical care requirements of each patient in accordance with their acuity nursing care categories. The total manhour figures for the clinical care of patients and for nonclinical tasks are converted into positions in the job classification, and costs are determined.

Thus budget planning is setting objectives and cost limits. The plan describes anticipated activities in numerical terms to meet measurable objectives.[12] Nursing service budgets become an integral component of the total hospital budgeting system.[2,9]

Nursing service is responsible for preparing budget plans that cover manpower, operations, and capital expenditures. Most nursing services do not have an income estimate plan. If nursing students use the facilities several hours a week at periodic intervals during the hospital's fiscal year, a small portion of their input may be included in manpower input. Such input is not considered when calculating full- or part-time positions needed. The nursing student input, if it must be included in the budgeting plan, should appear under the "float" or "on-call" temporary resources.

Income from patients is usually calculated separately by the business office, even though the total patient costs may appear on the monthly accounting reports sent to nursing service departments. Thus nursing services are not considered a revenue source, although in reality they are.

Impact of budgets on human behavior

Argyris,[1] Newman,[12] and Likert,[6,7] in studying the effects of budgets and control on the supervisory staffs of organizations, conclude that the negative impact of budgets stems from their pressuring and needling effects. The pressures of budgets tend to create detrimental conflicts between workers and top management.[16]

Supervisors may be blamed for failure to

meet objectives, despite the fact that frequently they did not have an opportunity to participate in the planning.[11] This tends to encourage workers to join informal groups that may have objectives contrary to those of the institution.[4,18]

It is difficult for employees in lower and middle levels, who are not active participants in planning, to see the benefits of budgeting. When a top executive exercises control, the operational personnel often believe they lack an understanding of the practical ongoing problems and that it is an illegitimate source of pressure.[15,16]

Emerging trends in budgeting and control

In a collegial organizational behavior approach, budget planning and control are viewed as adaptive, dynamic, coordinated management processes. Newman,[12] Likert,[7] and others[14] indicate that the organizational character of the controlling process, as one variable, influences the effectiveness of budget planning and control.

The top management group of an organization should evaluate its existing operational approach in relation to participative concepts. In doing so, it may answer several questions. For example, are all individuals in supervisory positions at all levels of the hierarchy concerned about the performance of control functions, or do the major and primary concerns exist with the top administrators? Do the department heads and unit supervisors request complete and accurate data information to guide their own actions and the behavior of their workers? Do the executives of the organization exert strong pressure and provide procedural forms for the recording of specific information at appropriate intervals to assist them in decision making? Is the controlling process used for policing and interlocking reward with punishment?

It should be mentioned that corrective controlling analyzes the variances against the objectives after they occur. Preventive controlling anticipates the deviations by means of daily and weekly data and makes appropriate adjustments. An early diagnosis of variances and the adjustment of objectives tend

to decrease personnel problems as compared to changes made after the event has occurred.

Necessary management criteria

In a collegial, organizational, behavioral environment department heads and others need criteria as guidelines in budget planning and control. The criteria may include the following:

• The budget plan and controlling process of each division, department, and its units must be approved and supported by top management.

• The objectives, policies, and procedure related to budget planning and control are defined by top administration in consultation with department heads and usually by means of a budget committee.

• The managerial staff at all levels of each department must understand the budget planning and control processes. In nursing services all professional nurses should participate in the planning and controlling processes as part of their delegated responsibility and authority.

• Divisional directors and/or department heads of services must approve the budget plans for their units and the control system. For example, the nurse-executive is responsible for all budgets of nursing services and for the effectiveness of the control process.

• Each budget plan sets operating cost limits but should not be absolute. The plan must be broad enough to initiate alternate courses of action should unexpected conditions occur.

• A budget plan should identify what is to be done, how, by whom, and when. The organizational structure of each department should designate functional responsibilities and duties for budget planning and control and provide for effective communication feedback between superiors and subordinates.

• Administration must distribute predesigned budgetary forms with explicit instructions.

• Administration must also provide department heads with monthly expenses of each cost center indicating if below or above the anticipated objective (financial figure). The monthly report for the units also gives the year-to-date information for each accounting number such as salaries, supplies, and so forth, as well as the number of patient days and the direct cost per patient day.

- Monthly and summary reports must be used by the department heads and their assistants to analyze the actual activities against the objectives and initiate corrective action where necessary. Bauer,[3] in his article "Try a New Approach to Planning," describes a reporting system for communication accounting data. Long[9] and Baker[2] also discuss budgeting procedures for hospitals.

Predicting results

Department heads should not consider control only as the comparing of actual results with desired results. By the time actual results are known, it may be too late to do anything about them. Actually department heads and associates should predict the results. Effective managerial control should be based on predictions of results, not actual results.[12] For example, the medical and nursing staffs try to anticipate what is likely to happen to a patient suffering from a cardiovascular or diabetic condition, and on the basis of their diagnosis (predictions) take the corrective action that (they predict) will help bring actual results toward the patient's recovery. Thus, the controlling process is future oriented (Fig. 15-1).

INITIATION OF BUDGET PLANNING

Several months prior to a new fiscal year, top management initiates the planning and control phases of budgets with the department heads. This is done by forecasting and reexamining the planning premises of external conditions that will prevail in the coming year or 3 years hence (Fig. 15-1). Short-term plans must be linked to long-term premises (see Chapter 8 and Fig. 8-2).

Top administration provides department heads with information about the financial status of the organization and its anticipated revenue sources. Forecasting also includes projected activities and costs. This may involve closing a patient unit for 6 months for renovations, expansion of specific patient services such as unit management or materials management services, or installation of a hospital automated system. Many forecasting plans may require changing existing personnel inputs and reorganizing job activities.[5]

Forecasting is also based on external factors such as anticipated population changes in the surrounding community. For example, it may require a reduction in maternity services and an increase in geriatric rehabilitation services. State regulations of the adoption of Medicaid or national regulations for Medicare reimbursements will affect resources (see Fig. 6-9).

Changes in personnel policies, salaries, and wage schedules for various occupational classifications will be reviewed.

Each department is directed to consider the forecasting plans as they affect anticipated budgetary plans for the coming fiscal year and 3 years hence.[13] Departments are requested to submit preliminary budgets with interpretations for changes at a specific date.

Administration needs to clarify policies affecting budgeting techniques. Nurse-executives and associates need to understand the administrative policy for application to budget planning and control.

Personnel control policy

If position control in each job classification is used, it serves as the criterion for the employment of new personnel.[17] On the other hand, if the budget expense control is used, the nurse-executive is free to change the approved table of positions as long as the original approved manpower financial figure is not changed. Nursing service must follow the policy set by administration.

When nursing services want to increase or decrease the approved number of positions in each classification, the nurse-executive must make a formal request for changes to the top administrator delegated to supervise budget operations. The request must state the number of position changes, the results against the objectives, and reasons for the change.

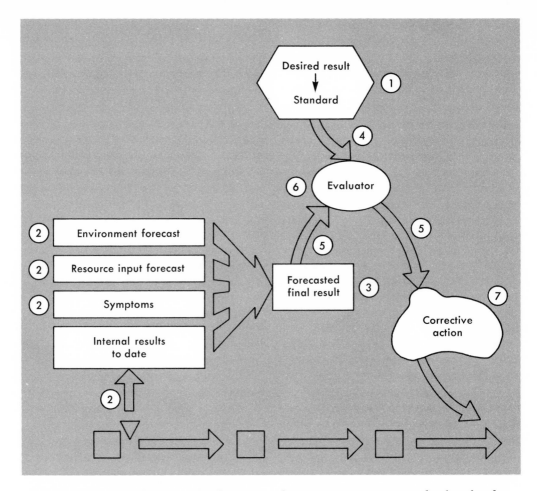

Fig. 15-1. Planning, directing, coordinating, and organizing activities are closely related to steering-control. (William H. Newman, Constructive control—design and use of control systems, © 1975, p. 13. Reprinted by permission of Prentice-Hall, Inc., Englewood Cliffs, New Jersey.)

The accounting cost center system

The accounting cost center system can be confusing and frustrating to managers of nursing services. A cost center is the smallest functional unit for which cost control and accountability can be assigned under the accounting system. Even with computers, setting up many cost centers increases input costs of the accounting department.

In nursing services, there is a clustering of similar activities in the cost centers; however, some cost centers create difficulties in measuring results against objectives. For example, the pediatric cost center may include expenses against collective subobjectives for children, toddlers, infants, and those patients in a six-bed intensive care unit. Also, a six-bed coronary care unit may be linked with expenses of a general medical patient unit. To examine ongoing manhour inputs to meet nursing care needs of patients in the intensive care unit requires nursing service to keep additional data apart from the monthly accounting report.

Cost centers should coincide with management centers; then the control responsibility becomes more meaningful to professional nurses who must control the plan.

Distribution of supply costs

Allocation of costs for supplies to units should be understood by all professional nurses. Many hospitals purchase supplies and other items in bulk. The cost of these supplies may be distributed to the various patient units in accordance with the patient occupancy percentage of each unit. This distribution of costs by formula does not indicate the actual use of supplies on each unit. When supply and equipment costs are based on actual use, the reports mean something to their users.

Cutoff figure for capital expenditures

In preparing the operational and capital budgets, department heads must know the hospital's cost-cut point for purchasing items. For example, the cutoff figure may be $100 or less. Any item above that figure is termed a capital instead of an operational expenditure. However, if the quantity of one item is above the cutoff point, the hospital may consider the request an operational expenditure. Administration must clarify their policy to be followed.

Allocation of manhours for personnel coverage

In preparation of the manpower budget, the nurse-executive develops a table of positions to provide the determined manhour needs for each patient, 24 hours a day, 7 days a week. Because personnel have days off, in accordance with personnel policies, the budget must include input to meet these policies. The nurse-executive reviews the historical data on the number of sick leave days taken by workers in the job classifications and the number of workers who will be entitled to 15 days vacation in the coming year. However, this analysis is not very reliable in predicting future inputs.

In budgeting it is more effective to use one figure in these calculations. For example, each worker may have 104 regular days off, 15 vacation days, 10 sick leave days, 8 holidays, 2 free days, and 3 days for continuing education, totaling 142 days off per year. Thus, each full-time employee works 223 days (365-142). If the full-time employee works an 8-hour day, the total manhours worked for 1 fiscal year would be 1784 hours.

Orientation manhours for new personnel

Most employees give advance notice of their resignation, thus permitting the hiring of other individuals. The nursing service may have an objective that states: allow the first 7 work days of each beginning employee to learn to do his or her job by means of an appropriate orientation program. In budget planning, historical data are reviewed and predictions are made for the coming year. To keep nursing care inputs at a safe determined level, additional manpower must be met by "float" input during the times that new personnel are in the program.

For example, if two registered staff nurses resign in each of three cost centers, totaling six nurses per month, then six nurses times 8 hours per day times 7 days totals 336 manhours for that month. If historical data indicate manhours for orientation of nurses equals 336 hours for 10 months of the year, then the budget plan should provide for sufficient input. In-service education input is discussed later in this chapter.

Nursing service must define objectives, translate them in clear dimensions that are measurable, and interpret policy in realistic terms.

MANPOWER BUDGET PLAN

There are two major phases to budget planning. The first phase is usually called preliminary planning based on the forecasting of plans. The second phase requires the translation of approved anticipated plans into realistic clear objectives and the input required to meet them.

Initial planning phase. The nurse-executive should present to the top professional nurse groups basic guidelines to meet realistic objectives. His or her forecasting is based on past performance results, predictions of top administrators, and initiation of hospital plans. Initial planning concerns what is to be done and how, by whom, and when during the coming year.

For example, if a patient unit is to be closed for 6 months for renovations, the manpower resources of that unit must be distributed to other units. During this period, nursing services may plan to develop a program for primary nursing to be introduced when the floor is opened. If so, in-service education resources may be used to train nurses for their roles. This requires new manhour inputs and costs that should be described in the budget. The architectural plan of the renovated unit and equipment needs will be described in the fiscal budget for that floor.

If an objective is to increase the percentage of nursing care to be given, the objective may use a ratio of 75% professional nursing staff to 25% technical nursing staff in some units, beginning with the last two quarters of the budget period. Quantitative inputs and costs must be reflected, and comparisons made with existing performance. Also, recruitment and in-service orientation inputs must be anticipated in terms of costs.

An objective may be to eliminate one shift, permitting nursing personnel to work 12-hour days in a unit. This requires the development of a cyclical schedule plan and the determination of the number of positions, costs, and the overtime pay policy (as discussed in Chapter 13).

The cost center of the in-service education program must define objectives for anticipated programs, resource inputs, and costs. As mentioned in Chapter 6, the staff may use the PERT technique in developing the programs. For example, they may participate in a recruitment program involving senior nursing students in the surrounding community. All resource inputs and costs must be determined to meet stated objectives.

The in-service staff will project the kind and number of in-service education programs for professional staff nurses to be given during the various quarters of the budget period. Human material and equipment resources must be anticipated to meet stated objectives.

The nurse-executive must prepare preliminary budgets with clearly stated interpretations of projected inputs against determined objectives. This initial budget plan with its modifications must be approved by top administration.

Final phase. The accounting office usually provides assistance in calculating figures for the budget. Each department head makes sure that personnel position sheets are in accordance with the existing budget cost centers. As mentioned in Chapter 14, several part-time workers in each job classification may fill one full-time position. The total manhours and costs for "float" input and "on-call" are also recorded.

Salaries and wages. Use of the predesigned budget forms, the total number of positions in each job classification, planned wages, and increases are reflected for each quarter of the budgetary year. Total projected wages and salary expenses in each cost center represent the planned expense for each quarter of the coming year.[9,10]

Other personnel costs. In some nursing services these anticipated costs are calculated in the cost centers of nursing services or centralized on a predesigned form. Manhour input and costs for overtime, sick leave, vacation, holidays, education, health insurance, and pension benefits must be anticipated in terms of expenditures.

OPERATIONAL BUDGET

The anticipated increases and decreases in each cost center are calculated and compared with past inputs. The administration and nursing service forecasting plans and the introduction of new technology and methods will influence the use of equipment and supplies.

In preparing operational budgets, the individuals responsible for the preparation of operational budgets must work closely with the medical staff, the materials management director, and others.

A hospital materials/equipment committee composed of physicians, nurses, and materials and management services including the central service supervisor can make an effective contribution in evaluating new products and equipment. This type of committee action can prevent the purchase of items that have not been tested and approved by administration. The operating room professional committee provides for decision making concerning surgical equipment and supplies. Thus, planning through committee action assists nurses in the preparation of operational and capital budgets.

The material management director can provide information on anticipated price increases, cost for repairs, and new equipment.

The indirect costs such as plant maintenance, heat, light, housekeeping, and general administration are part of the budget plan.

CAPITAL BUDGET

The capital budget plan describes the anticipated costs of major purchases of equipment or programs. Items appearing in the capital budget are usually those that are above the cutoff cost figure. These items have a reasonable expected life span of more than 3 years. For example, surgical appliances, patient beds, stretchers, emergency cardiac resuscitation equipment, visual aids equipment, and typewriters have a long life expectancy.

Documentation is required in preparing a capital expenditure budget. The use of a piece of equipment may pay for itself by decreasing manhours and use of other supplies. For example, the nursing staff and physicians may request the use of sterile spinal trays. The documentation of this request must include the amount of manhours saved by the sterile supply service over a specific period of time, and costs of items must be compared to the purchase price for the sterile trays.

EFFECTIVENESS OF BUDGET PLANNING AND CONTROL

When a hospital operates on a modern system of planning and control, considerable efficiency and cost saving can be realized. A collegial and organizational behavior environment is required so that all levels of management in each department are responsible within appropriate authority for setting anticipated resources and cost limits, for analyzing and measuring variances against objectives, and for initiating adjustments when necessary.

Budgeting and control become vital management processes. Budget planning and control can assist the nurse-executive and the professional nurse groups in introducing changes to improve nursing services.

The controls of nursing services should be integrated into a balanced subsystem of the hospital. The emerging control system of nursing services should be integrated with other managerial responsibilities of the staff for planning, organizing, and leading.

Good control design that is a part of the entire behavioral environment of nursing services has subtle benefits. When collegial, trusting relationships are operating, irritating and repressive influences disappear. The control activity of budgets is viewed as a positive force. Newman states that with the application of effective, modern controls we too can land on a moon.[12]

REFERENCES

1. Argyris, C.: The impact of budgets on people. In Litterer, J. A., editor: Organizations: structure and behavior, New York, 1969, John Wiley & Sons, Inc, pp. 282-295.
2. Baker, R. E.: Budgeting procedures for hospitals, Chicago, 1971, The American Hospital Association.
3. Bauer, R. W.: Try a new approach to planning. In Stone, S., Berger, M. S., Elhart, D., Firsich, S. C., and Jordan, S. B., editors: Management for nurses, St. Louis, 1976, The C. V. Mosby Co., pp. 199-210.
4. Hofstede, G. H.: The game of budget control, London, 1968, Tavistock Publications, Ltd.
5. Koontz, H., and O'Connell, C.: Essentials of management, New York, 1974, McGraw-Hill Book Co., chapter 24.
6. Likert, R.: The human organization: its management and value, New York, 1967, McGraw-Hill Book Co.
7. Likert, R., and Bowers, D. G.: Organizational theory and human resource accounting, American Psychologist 24(6):585-592, 1969.
8. Likert, R., and Likert, J. G.: New ways of managing conflict, New York, 1976. McGraw-Hill Book Co., chapters 2 and 18.
9. Longest, B., Jr.: Principles of hospital business office management, Chicago, 1975, Hospital Financial Management Association.
10. Marram, G., et al.: Cost-effectiveness of primary and team nursing, Wakefield, Mass., 1976, Contemporary Publishing, Inc.
11. Marrow, A. P., et al.: Management by participation: creating a climate for personal and organizational development, New York, 1967, Harper & Row, Publishers, Inc.
12. Newman, W. H.: Constructive control—design and use of control systems, Englewood Cliffs, N.J., 1975, Prentice-Hall, Inc.

13. Pluhacek, T. J.: If you've never prepared a budget before. In Stone, S., Berger, M. S., Elhart, D., Firsich, S. C., and Jordan, S. B., editors: Management for nurses, St. Louis, 1976, The C. V. Mosby Co., pp. 197-199.

14. Vatter, W. J.: Operating budgets, San Francisco, 1969. Wadsworth Publishing Co.

15. White, H. C.: Leadership: some behaviors and attitudes of hospital employees, Hospital Progress 52(1):46-50, 1971; 52(2):41-45, 1971.

16. White, H. C.: Some perceived behavior and attitudes of hospital employees under effective and ineffective supervisors, Journal of Nursing Administration 1:49-54, Jan., 1971.

17. Yoder, D.: Personnel management and industrial relations, ed. 6, Englewood Cliffs, N.J., 1970, Prentice-Hall Inc., chapter 25.

18. Zand, D. E.: Trust and managerial problem-solving, Administrative Science Quarterly 17(2):229-239, 1972.

16 | Quality control of nursing care

In the past decade across the country new demands for the accountability of health and sick care services by accreditating bodies, governmental agencies, and consumer groups have forced health providers to use and report the results of *quality assurance* (see Chapter 4).

Quality assurance refers to the mechanisms used for determining, effecting, and evaluating the quality of care. The quality, quantity, and costs of health and sick care services have become closely associated with social and professional issues (see Chapters 3 and 4). Quality assurance also refers to the results of estimation used to secure improvements and to assure the public of receiving effective services at a reasonable cost. Official and voluntary health agencies have become involved in current actions to monitor and control the components of quality assurance programs. Nurse practitioners and nurse administrators who are directly involved in the delivery of patient care are spending much time and energy to implement specific methods for evaluating the quality of nursing.[2,3,4,14,19]

RECENT OFFICIAL AND VOLUNTARY ACTIONS

The Social Security amendments of 1972 mandating the development of professional standards review organizations (PSROs)[28] and the active role of third parties in monitoring costs and the quality of care are forcing health care providers to become more involved in a single formal review system. The nationwide governmental system of PSROs is asking health care professionals to change their concept of private accountability to one of public accountability. During the past decade professionals continued to demonstrate their ability to monitor the activities and outcomes of health care services, thereby eliminating the need for government to take responsibility for quality assurance.

The American Hospital Association's Quality Assurance Program (QAP)[1] delegates the medical staff the requisite authority to perform quality assessment and evaluation activities. The AHA views the hospital as the agent who provides the sickness care services; therefore it should be responsible for quality monitoring and control and for implementing its own in-house quality assurance programs. In keeping with the option stated in Public Law 92-603, local PSROs may accept the results of a hospital in-house utilization review committee if the committee meets the PSRO standards and criteria.[6] The American Medical Association's Peer Review is another professional association sponsored program.

The Joint Commission on Accreditation of Hospitals (JCAH) states its medical and nursing audit requirements.[20] Its standard for the quality of professional services directs professionals to formulate criteria and implement a systematic evaluation system to assure optimal quality of care. The JCAH directs nonphysicians (nurses and others) to implement mechanisms to assure quality in those aspects of care that they provide. The JCAH Medical Care Evaluation and Utilization Review program is evidence of voluntary action.

The purpose of association-sponsored corporations such as the Wisconsin Health Care

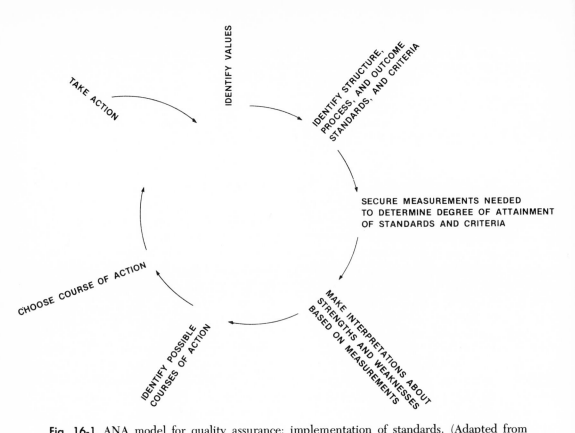

Fig. 16-1. ANA model for quality assurance: implementation of standards. (Adapted from Lang, N.: A model for quality assurance in nursing. In American Nurses' Association: a plan for implementation of the Standards of Nursing Practice, Kansas City, Mo., 1975, The Association, p. 15.)

Review, Incorporated (WHCRI), organized by state medical, dental, and hospital societies and associations, is to provide an external and statewide mechanism for the implementation of voluntary and mandatory requirements for quality assurance. The programs focus primarily on physician and institutional performance.

Hospital utilization review for medicare

Recent literature provides much information about hospital utilization programs. The criteria and mechanisms for accounting are described in the PSRO manual.[28] Davidson,[14] in the test PSRO—Utilization and Audit in Patient Care, presents the components and various systems used in monitoring and controlling the quality of patient care services. Snider,[34] Schueler,[31] and Davidson[14] give the reader a picture of the role

of the nurse-coordinator in hospital utilization review programs.

Donabedian[16] and others point out some inherent difficulties in the assessment and evaluation of care, activity, and other resource cost outcomes. Access to resources and their allocations are closely interrelated with who gets care, what kind, and how much. Moreover, care services in hospitals are highly organized, involving coordination of interdependent and intradependent responsibilities of professionals. Such managerial factors become important elements in the assessment and evaluation of quality care.

The ANA Technical Advisory Committee has made several recommendations for the utilization of PSRO programs. It has recommended that professional nurses assist the Bureau of Quality Assurance (BQA), the

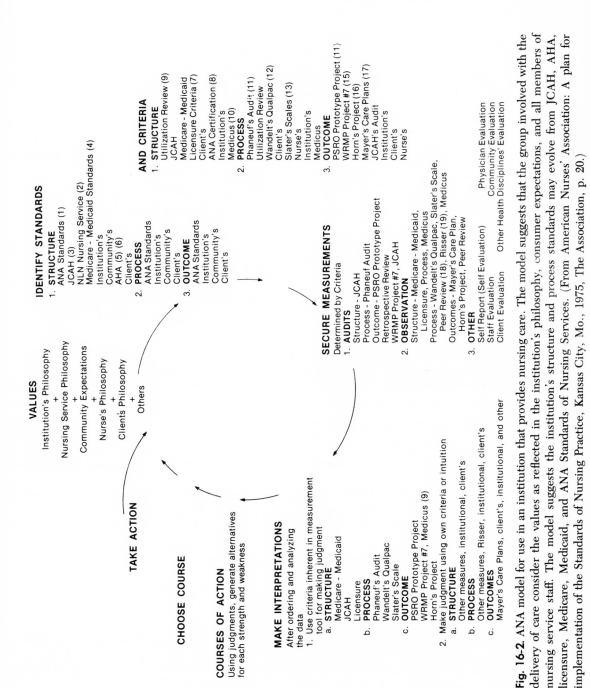

Fig. 16-2. ANA model for use in an institution that provides nursing care. The model suggests that the group involved with the delivery of care consider the values as reflected in the institution's philosophy, consumer expectations, and all members of nursing service staff. The model suggests the institution's structure and process standards may evolve from JCAH, AHA, licensure, Medicare, Medicaid, and ANA Standards of Nursing Services. (From American Nurses' Association: A plan for implementation of the Standards of Nursing Practice, Kansas City, Mo., 1975, The Association, p. 20.)

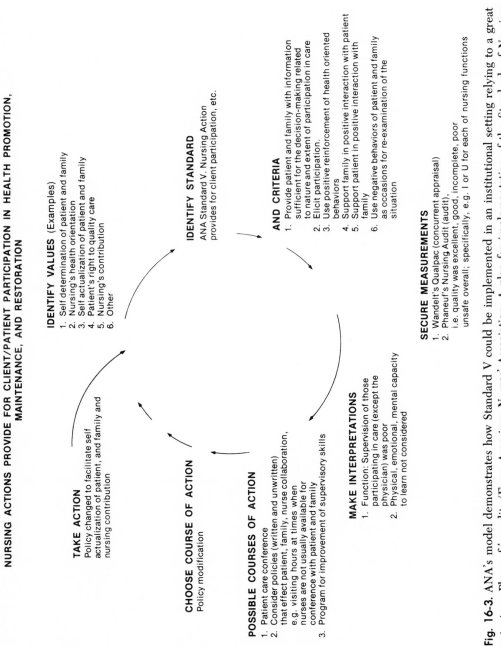

Fig. 16-3. ANA's model demonstrates how Standard V could be implemented in an institutional setting relying to a great extent on Phaneuf's audit. (From American Nurses' Association: A plan for implementation of the Standards of Nursing Practice, Kansas City, Mo., 1975, The Association, p. 24.)

The following text appears within the figure:

NURSING ACTIONS PROVIDE FOR CLIENT/PATIENT PARTICIPATION IN HEALTH PROMOTION, MAINTENANCE, AND RESTORATION

IDENTIFY VALUES (Examples)
1. Self determination of patient and family
2. Nursing's health orientation
3. Self actualization of patient and family
4. Patient's right to quality care
5. Nursing's contribution
6. Other

IDENTIFY STANDARD
ANA Standard V. Nursing Action provides for client participation, etc.

AND CRITERIA
1. Provide patient and family with information sufficient for the decision-making related to nature and extent of participation in care
2. Elicit participation.
3. Use positive reinforcement of health oriented behaviors
4. Support family in positive interaction with patient
5. Support patient in positive interaction with family
6. Use negative behaviors of patient and family as occasions for re-examination of the situation

SECURE MEASUREMENTS
1. Wandelt's Qualpac (concurrent appraisal)
2. Phaneuf's Nursing Audit (audit),
   i.e. quality was excellent, good, incomplete, poor unsafe overall; specifically, e.g. I or U for each of nursing functions

MAKE INTERPRETATIONS
1. Function: Supervision of those participating in care (except the physician) was poor
2. Physical, emotional, mental capacity to learn not considered

POSSIBLE COURSES OF ACTION
1. Patient care conference
2. Consider policies (written and unwritten) that effect patient, family, nurse collaboration, e.g. visiting hours at times when nurses are not usually available for conference with patient and family
3. Program for improvement of supervisory skills

CHOOSE COURSE OF ACTION
Policy modification

TAKE ACTION
Policy changed to facilitate self actualization of patient, and family and nursing contribution

Department of Health, Education, and Welfare, and the Office of Professional Standards and Review Organization (OPSRO) in ongoing modifications or supplementations of its policies and guidelines that influence local PSRO programs.[5]

The literature indicates that the nurse-coordinator in utilization review programs assists with the screening, using physician-developed criteria, as well as with the paper work. Some nurses are asking, What should be the responsibilities of nurses in such programs? Should not the paper work be done by clerical personnel trained in medical terminology?

In some hospitals, physicians are motivated to accept their responsibility to develop an acceptable quality assurance program. The nurses in these hospitals are attempting to gain professional status and to identify standards of nursing care. No doubt it will be some time before hospitals have a combined program of medical and nursing audit. Mutual understanding and awareness of each other's contribution to health care services is the first step toward a combined medical and nursing quality assurance program. Such a system would economize professional input.

American Nurses Associations' actions

Throughout the decades the actions of the ANA have been goal directed.[2,8,9] Its efforts have been to prepare nurses in institutions of higher education, to support continued education programs and new state nurse practice acts reflecting recognition of advancement of nursing practice, and to establish standards of nursing practice and of nursing services in keeping with current concepts innovations (see Chapters 4 and 5).

Certification of professional nurses, sponsored by the ANA Divisions on Practice, aims to provide tangible acknowledgment of nurses' achievement in a specific area of nursing practice to assure quality in nursing care (see Chapter 4).

The ANA's new Standards of Nursing Practice prepared by the ANA Congress of Nursing Practice[9] and the ANA Divisions of Practice aim to fulfill the profession's obligation to provide and improve nursing practice (see Chapter 5). The ANA believes that the new standards set forth by the Divisions on Practice can be applied to practice in any clinical situation. These goal-directed standards present desirable characteristics of the nursing process for the care of clients with certain health and illness problems.

ANA model for quality assurance. The implementation of standards is adapted from the Lang model (Figs. 16-1 to 16-3). The ANA provides a plan to implement the Standards of Nursing Practice by means of this model, which can be adapted for use in institutions providing nursing care for a specific client and in other settings. The ANA plan also demonstrates how Standard V could be implemented in an institutional setting.[9] The standards are guidelines for nurses as they formulate sets of criteria to measure the degree of excellence of care outcomes and make judgments on the weaknesses and strengths of the practice of nursing. Zimmer[41] indicates that the ANA standards sponsored by the Divisions on Practice are not tools for use in comparing actual results with desired outcomes to determine the degree of excellence.

FRAME OF REFERENCE FOR QUALITY ASSURANCE

One of the first steps in the development of a quality assurance nursing program is to clarify the values and attitudes of professional health groups and the public about nursing. Is the quality of nursing care to be viewed as minimal, optimal, moderate, or acceptable? What level of nursing care is the public willing to accept and pay for? Does the public accept the role of the nurse in accordance with the new state nurse acts?

Most professional nurses today recognize that the major sources of values are societal, professional, and scientific. As society and its values change, the nature of quality changes. The philosophy, objectives, and methodology of quality assurance for nursing care will be influenced by the values and attitudes of nurses toward their right and responsibility for the systematic quality appraisal of nursing practice and services.

In the development of a model for quality assurance in nursing, the components of quality assurance must be understood and agreed on by the planners and users of the methodology. A standard refers to an agreed on level of excellence in nursing care. In other words, it is an agreed on norm that is established for the assignment of a single score or value to a variable or criterion.[23,24] The ANA, in its Standards of Nursing Practice, provides Statements of Standards for adaptation of the ANA criteria.

Criterion refers to the characteristic of a variable that may be measured to provide scores by which subjects of the same classification can be compared in relation to the variable.

Donabedian[16] and Block[11,11a] have outlined and defined three major components of criteria for assessing the quality of care—structure, process, and outcome. Each of these criteria measures a different aspect of patient care.

Structure standards and criteria

Structure standards and criteria describe the purpose and objectives of the institution or program. Structure pertains to the status of the institution with regard to accreditation and certification, the physical facilities and equipment, the organizational design, and the management of human, material, and financial resources.

For example, the ANA Nursing Service Standards and the JCAH Accrediting Standards give direction in broad terms in the formulation of explicit, precise criteria to achieve desired outcomes. One nursing service may state a staffing criteria as follows: There shall be a minimum of one registered staff nurse on duty for every 10 patients during the day and evening shift, and one registered staff nurse on duty for every 20 patients during the night shift for 7 days a week, in x general medical patient unit.

A managerial criteria for individualized patient care may state that a professional nurse shall formulate a plan of nursing care for each patient within 2 hours after admission to the unit. Criteria are variables selected as relevant indications of the quality of nursing, or as the measures by which nursing care is judged as good.

Process standards and criteria

Process standards and criteria describe the nature and sequence of activities undertaken by nurses in the care of patients. Nursing activities aim to meet a plan of nursing care for each patient. In some situations, several different activities will be performed to achieve one desired outcome.

Process activity measures focus on what the nurse does for the patient, how it is done, and in what sequence it is done.

The Quality Patient Care Scale (QUAL-PACS), developed at Wayne State University, consists of a 68-item scale developed to evaluate the quality of care received by a patient.[39] The methodology involves persons directly observing patients as they receive care.

Hegyvary, Haussmann, and others[18,19] describe the development of criterion measures and methodology focusing on process. This methodology was developed in a joint effort of Rush-Presbyterian–St. Luke's Medical Center, The Medicus Systems Corporation, and the Division of Nursing, Department of Health, Education, and Welfare.

The operations of the nursing process model are shown in Exhibit A.

It should be mentioned that 6.3 and 6.4 were included in this model since they can influence the nursing process and since nurses frequently engage in those activities.

To identify specific indicators (criteria) of quality for each subobjective of the framework, the study group agreed that criteria must relate to nursing and provide for documentation and the predicted degree of reliability. In addition, criteria should be stated in specific, precise, measurable terms so that different observer-raters would interpret and apply them in the same manner.[3,18]

Each criterion is coded according to the type of patient categorization, such as self-care, partial, complete, or intensive. The criteria set, numbering 256, are grouped into homogeneous clusters to define a specific dimension of the nursing process. The patients are randomly selected for observation, and a subset of criteria appropriate to the patient's intensity of nursing care needs for assessment is used. The nursing process is evaluated on the basis of each sampled patient for a 1-month period. The researchers state that because not all criteria are applied to each patient, they do not measure the quality for each individual patient.

Outcome standards and criteria

Outcome standards and criteria pertain to the end results of nursing care. Patient outcome criteria are patients' behavior or clinical manifestations that represent desired patient responses to the nursing care process. Outcome measures focus on the consequences of care.

The outcome measures pertain to what the

EXHIBIT A*

Nursing process framework

1.0 *The plan of nursing care is formulated.*
1.1 The condition of the patient is assessed on admission.
1.2 Data relevant to hospital care are ascertained on admission.
1.3 The current condition of the patient is assessed.
1.4 The written plan of nursing care is formulated.
1.5 The plan of nursing care is coordinated with the medical plan of care.

2.0 *The physical needs of the patient are attended.*
2.1 The patient is protected from accident and injury.
2.2 The need for physical comfort and rest is attended.
2.3 The need for physical hygiene is attended.
2.4 The need for a supply of oxygen is attended.
2.5 The need for activity is attended.
2.6 The need for nutrition and fluid balance is attended.
2.7 The need for elimination is attended.
2.8 The need for skin care is attended.
2.9 The patient is protected from infection.

3.0 *The nonphysical (psychological, emotional, mental, social) needs of the patient are attended.*
3.1 The patient is oriented to hospital facilities on admission.

3.2 The patient is extended social courtesy by the nursing staff.
3.3 The patient's privacy and civil rights are honored.
3.4 The need for psychological-emotional well-being is attended.
3.5 The patient is taught measures of health maintenance and illness prevention.
3.6 The patient's family is included in the nursing care process.

4.0 *Achievement of nursing care objectives is evaluated.*
4.1 Records document the care provided for the patient.
4.2 The patient's response to therapy is evaluated.

5.0 *Unit procedures are followed for the protection of all patients.*
5.1 Isolation and decontamination procedures are followed.
5.2 The unit is prepared for emergency situations.

6.0 *The delivery of nursing care is facilitated by administrative and managerial services.*
6.1 Nursing reporting follows prescribed standards.
6.2 Nursing management is provided.
6.3 Clerical services are provided.
6.4 Environmental and support services are provided.

*From Hegyvary, S. T.: Development of criterion measures for quality of care: the Rush-Medicus experience, In Issues in evaluation research, an invitational conference, December 10-12, 1975, ANA pub. no. G-124 2M 9/76, pp. 108-109.

patient has learned, not to what the nurse has taught him. It also measures how the patient applies this knowledge and how it affects his personal goals and activities. Horn and Swain,[3] from the University of Michigan, describe methodology to measure the outcome of nursing care by classification of problems through considering the focus of nursing on the complete range of biopsychosocial functioning of individuals rather than on system problems or disease entities. Horn and Swain,[3] from a research point of view, recognize the need for a nursing classification system and for clinical research to determine reliable and valid measures of the outcomes of nursing care. Outcome criteria should focus on those dimensions on which nursing has an impact.

Zimmer[41] and her colleagues at the University of Wisconsin Hospital have formulated sets of outcome criteria and a quality review system. The methodology, referred to as Nursing Service Evaluation Program, consists of sets of criteria for defined patient populations in terms of medical diagnosis and other significant factors.

Bellinger[3] and his colleagues at Wayne State University have started a multiphase project to discover the relationships between nursing activities and patient outcomes. The system model of this project is concerned with all components of quality assurance. The researchers in this project view process and outcome as interdependent components, and therefore they should be approached as two interdependent dimensions in the evaluation of care quality.

RETROSPECTIVE AUDIT SYSTEM

As previously mentioned, concurrent appraisal evaluates care while it takes place and secures improvements if necessary. Retrospective evaluation is based on the documentation of that care recorded in the patient's chart.[32,40] This means the review of closed charts (those of patients who have been discharged).

Benedikter,[10] describing the rationale for retrospective evaluation of nursing care, states that it provides a determination of overall care, not the care of one patient given by one nurse in one unit. A nursing audit provides for more objectivity than a review of an active record while staff members are caring for a patient.

The nursing audit should not be viewed as a procedure to ensure completion of the medical record or as a punitive measure.

Basic organizational communication approach

The auditing program and its communication system should involve all professional nurses. In many nursing services, depending on the number and characteristics of the staff, the clinical practice committee is composed of representatives of staff nurse and clinical coordinator groups, clinical nurse-specialists, and educators and nurse-administrators. This committee is responsible for the final selection and definition of standards and criteria, methodology, and the evaluation of the program.

Zimmer[14] and Crawford[12] define the functions of the nurse-practitioner, clinical specialists, and the director of nursing. They and others emphasize that nursing practitioners in their specific areas of practice develop and write standards and criteria and actively participate in the review process. A collegial environment for peer action, effective communication feedback, appropriate material, and personnel resources are essential elements of an auditing program.

Selecting a tool

The Phaneuf[29] nursing audit is an instrument determining a source—a quantitative measurement of a quality of care using an audit of closed patients' medical record. The audit consists of 50 items. They are divided into seven functions in accordance with the legal functions of nursing. A nurse group can determine its own level of quality in nursing care using the Phaneuf profile of excellence in nursing care.

Selvaggi[32] and colleagues associated with the 1200-bed Jackson Memorial Hospital in Miami, Florida, have developed a retrospective audit system based on the JCAH's audit system. This system is used in conjunction with a process outcome methodology based on the Rush-Medicus process tool.

Ethridge and Packard[17] described a documentation system based on data gathered from set standard care plans. The basic objectives of this system were to simplify and replace the traditional charting procedures, use trained personnel, and medical record staff to assist in the scoring, and provide a quantification system that would be amenable to automation.

COMPETENCIES RATING SCALE

Both Slater and Tescher have developed competency rating scales. The Slater rating scale aims to provide an objective measure of nurse-practitioner performance. This scale is based on the concept that the patient will receive a higher quality of care from the nurse who possesses certain technical and interactional measured skills than from the nurse who has a low scale rating.[33] This evaluative tool, based on objective data, supports the concept of peer evaluation in a professional environment within the patient care setting.

It should be mentioned that a professional competencies rating of a nurse is not used in place of the institution's performance appraisal. Tescher[35] and others have developed a process by which job descriptions of nurses are based on a clinical ladder for nursing practice. The standards and criteria of each four clinical levels of practice are identified with the job descriptions.

QUESTIONNAIRE TO DETERMINE PATIENT SATISFACTION

The quality of nursing care that a patient received cannot be measured by a patient interview or a written questionnaire. However, this tool can assist the nursing staff to improve care and interactionary skills.[13,22]

Marram[27] describes the results of an open-ended questionnaire designed to determine patients' satisfactions with their care in hospitals practicing primary nursing. Kirchhoff[21] and colleagues designed a patient questionnaire to assist the supervisors and staff in

recognizing the value of patient input to secure improvements.

Research indicates that the concept of patient satisfaction should be investigated further.[25,26] Nursing has not defined the behavior necessary to achieve desired outcomes, even though specific nursing behaviors have been identified as important in providing individualized patient care.

A questionnaire sent by mail has some inherent limitations. It does not create a face-to-face feedback between the nurse and patient. In an interview-questionnaire the nurse should be most attentive to negative comments offered by the patient. In general, to minimize the possibility of subjectivity, the nurse who administers the interview questionnaire should not have been the one who gave a considerable amount of care to the patient.

It is important that data collected by means of questionnaires be shared and evaluated by the nurses of the unit. Patient input and nurse feedback should be an ongoing process at the patient's bedside.

The professional need for excellence in nursing has been closely associated with the public need for recognition of the capabilities and potential of the practice. Collaboration between nurses in health care settings, educators, and researchers is essential in the development of quality assurance objectives and methodology and its techniques.

It is evident that the components, structure, and process outcomes of the framework of quality assurance are interdependent and interrelated. There is a need for research groups to work together toward syntheses and the development of quality assurance systems. Phaneuf[29] recommends that quality assurance results be obtained by means of the fewest and simplest possible standards, criteria quantification measures, methods, and techniques needed. All these items are means to an end, not ends in themselves.

Recently Block[11a] emphasized the need to use the term *criterion* as the name of a variable; identify and name it, develop a method of measurement, and finally establish a standard for it. A standard is a desired and achievable range of performance.

SUMMARY

The development and implementation of quality assurance of patient care by members of the hospital staff and the evaluation of patients' satisfactions of care received can secure improvements in the quality of health and care services for future patients. There are many interrelated variables in the patient care system that influence the quality of the nursing process. Professional nurses and researchers will continue to find the most useful methodology to measure the health status of hospitalized patients as they pass through stages of acuity.

REFERENCES

1. American Hospital Association: Quality assurance program for medical care in the hospital, Chicago, 1972, The Association.
2. American Nurses Association: A plan for implementation of the standards of nursing practice (a report of the ANA Congress for Nursing Practice), Kansas City, Mo., 1975, The Association.
3. American Nurses Association: Report on issues in evaluation research, The ANA invitational conference Dec. 10-12, 1975. Kansas City, Mo., 1976, The Association.
4. American Nurses Association: Guidelines for peer review, Kansas City, Mo., 1973, The Association.
5. American Nurses Association: Guidelines for review of nursing care at the local level, contract HSA 105-74-207, November, 1975. (Submitted to the Office of Professional Standards Review and Bureau of Quality Assurance. Health Service Administrator Department of Health, Education, and Welfare.
6. American Nurses Association: Quality assurance of nursing care. (Proceedings of an institute jointly sponsored by the ANA and AHA, held Oct. 29-31, 1973.) Kansas City, Mo., 1975, The Association.
7. American Nurses Association: Standards of nursing practice, Kansas City, Mo., 1973, The Association.
8. American Nurses Association: Standards of organized nursing services, Kansas City, Mo., 1974, The Association.
9. American Nurses Association: Standards of nursing practice, Kansas City, Mo., 1975, The Association.
10. Benedikter, H.: Selecting appropriate assessment measures in the institutional setting. In Quality assessment and patient care (presentations at the fall 1974 forum for nursing service administration in the West). New York, 1975, The National League for Nursing.
11. Block, D.: Evaluation of nursing care in terms of process and outcome, Nursing Research **24:**256-263, July-Aug., 1975.
11a. Block, D.: Criteria, standards, norms, crucial terms in quality assurance, Journal of Nursing Administration **7**(7):20-30, 1977.
12. Crawford, J. E.: Hospital audit systems. In Davidson, S. V.: PSRO: utilization and audit in patient care, St. Louis, 1976, The C. V. Mosby Co., chapter 5.
13. Daeffler, R. J.: Patients' perception of care under team and primary nursing, Journal of Nursing Administration **5**(3):23, 1975.
14. Davidson, S. V.: PSRO: utilization and audit in patient care, St. Louis, 1976, The C. V. Mosby Co.
15. Dibbie, P.: Quality assurance—a general hospital meets a challenge, Journal of Nursing Administration **6**, July-Aug., 1976. Reprinted in Journal of Nursing Administration staff, editors: Quality control and performance appraisal, vol. 2, Wakefield, Mass., 1976, Contemporary Publishing, Inc., pp. 26-33.
16. Donabedian, A.: Evaluating the quality of medical care, Milbank Memorial Fund Quarterly **44**, July, 1966.
17. Ethridge, P., and Packard, R.: An innovative approach to measurement of quality through utilization of nursing care plans, Journal of Nursing Administration **6:**25-31, Jan., 1976.
18. Hegyvary, S., and Haussmann, R. K.: Monitoring nursing care quality, Journal of Nursing Administration **5**(5):17-26, 1975 and **6**(9):3-9, 1976.
19. Jekinek, R. C., et al.: A methodology for monitoring quality of nursing care, pub. no. HRA 74-25, United States Department of Health, Education, and Welfare, Washington, D.C., January, 1974, United States Government Printing Office.
20. Joint Commission on Accreditation of Hospitals: Accreditation manual for hospitals, Chicago, 1976, The Commission, pp. 27-28.
21. Kirchhoff, K. T.: Let's ask the patient: consumer input can improve patient care, Journal of Nursing Administration **6**(10):36-40, 1976.
22. Kramer, M.: The consumer's influence on health care, Nursing Outlook, **20**(9):576, 1972.
23. Lang, N. M.: A model for quality assurance in nursing. In Davidson, S. V.: PSRO: utilization and audit in patient care, St. Louis, 1976, The C. V. Mosby Co., chapter 3.
24. Lang, N.: Quality care—individual and collective responsibility, The American Nurse **9:**4-5, Sept., 1974.
25. Lindeman, C. A.: Measuring quality of nursing care. I. Journal of Nursing Administration **6:**7-9, June, 1975.
26. Lindeman, C. A.: Measuring quality of patient care, Part II, Journal of Nursing Administration **6**(7):16-19, 1976.
27. Marram, G., et al.: Cost-effectiveness of primary and team nursing, Wakefield, Mass., 1976, Contemporary Publishing, Inc., chapter 5.

28. Office of Professional Standards Review PSRO program manual, Rockville, Md., 1976, United States Department of Health, Education, and Welfare.
29. Phaneuf, M.: The nursing audit: profile for excellence, New York, 1972, Appleton-Century-Crofts, Inc.
30. Schlotfeldt, M.: Planning for progress, Nursing Outlook 21(12):766-769, 1973.
31. Schueler, A.: Utilization review for Medicare, American Journal of Nursing 77:110-111, Jan., 1977.
32. Selvaggi, L. M., et al.: Implementing a quality assurance program in nursing, Journal of Nursing Adminstration 7:37-43, Sept., 1976.
33. Slater, S., et al.: The Slater nursing competencies rating scale, Detroit, 1975, Wayne State University College of Nursing.
34. Snider, M. E.: Utilization review for Medicare, American Journal of Nursing 77:107-109, Jan., 1977.
35. Tescher, B. E., and Colavecchio, R.: Definition of a standard for clinical nursing practice, Journal of Nursing Administration 7:32-44, March-April, 1977.
36. U.S. Health Service Administration: Sample criteria for short stay hospital review: screening criteria to assist PSROs in quality assurance, contract no. NSA 105-74-206, Rockville, Md., June, 1976, The Administration.
37. U.S. Social Security Administration: Conditions of participation—hospitals and nursing facilities utilization review, Federal Register 39, no. 231, part 2, 41605 and 41606, Washington, D.C., Nov., 1974, The Administration.
38. U.S. Social Security Administration: Skilled nursing facilities manual; coverage of services, Washington, D.C. Feb., 1976, The Administration, pp. 6-15.
39. Wandelt, M., and Ager, L.: Quality patient care scales, New York, 1974, Appleton-Century-Crofts, Inc.
40. Watson, A., and Mayers, M.: Evaluating the quality of patient care through retrospective chart review, Journal of Nursing Administration 7:17-21, March-April, 1977.
41. Zimmer, M.: Quality assurance for outcomes, Nursing Clinics of North America 9:311-317, June, 1974.

17 Performance evaluation–a controlling process

It is through the efforts of people associated with a hospital that the organizational goals and objectives for the accomplishment of its primary mission are achieved—to provide an acceptable quality of health and sick-care services to people at a reasonable price.

Nursing services, as an integral part of the patient care system, are organized to accomplish the hospital's mission. The efforts of nurses and their assistants are important determinants of the success or failure in achieving desired outcomes in the care of patients.

DEFINITION AND PURPOSES

A well-designed performance evaluation program aims to secure a high standard of performance from all members of the organization. The program is composed of three major elements: (1) setting goals and objectives at key checkpoints in the controlling process, (2) evaluating progress or performance against determined standards, and (3) initiating preventive and corrective actions and making adjustments to improve workers' performance by means of ongoing coaching, orientation, and staff development programs.

A systematic evaluation and review of workers' performances should better integrate and coordinate interrelated activities so that the structured jobs fit together and become mutually supportive. The program provides an opportunity for subordinates and superiors to agree on corrective actions to improve performance and to use the capabilities of each worker as effectively as possible.

The communication of performance achievement in the form of evaluation feedback helps to satisfy the personal needs and goals of each worker. People have a natural desire to know how they are progressing in terms of the goals set for or by them. In addition, feedback is a necessary controlling device when results indicate that performance is substandard. The program encourages the subordinate, superior, and training instructor to initiate a specific plan that will help each worker attain the organization's desired outcomes and those of the worker.[12,36]

Promotion, demotion, and monetary rewards can be tied to the performance evaluation program. Personnel actions such as merit increases can be an effective way of rewarding good performance. However, such actions require setting standards, a consistency of rating by all superiors, and seeing that all workers understand how the program works for them.[18] The program should provide for the mutual protection of each individual. Each worker should be judged on the basis of individual performance. Performance evaluation is considered fair and productive by all who participate in it.

BASIC FOUNDATION

The total manpower planning, organizing staff development, and controlling processes should be viewed as one multiphase system.[4,5,19] Performance appraisal should not be viewed as an entity in itself.

Manpower control is a means of exacting a specific level of performance from all individuals in the organization. The controlling and motivating processes involve the monitoring and influencing of worker behavior to encourage effective quality of performance outputs.

When nursing service objectives are well defined (see Chapter 7), appropriate organizational structures are designed. This includes drawing together from, and for, a variety of roles to achieve objectives (see Chapters 9 and 10). Human material and financial resources are distributed (see Chapter 14), methods of performance plans and assignments are agreed on (see Chapters 12 and 13), and an effective communication system is used by staff members and others in the organization (see Chapter 11).

In such an organizational environment, administrators initiate periodic performance evaluation in relation to overall long term plans, so that ongoing operational activities can be monitored to determine if satisfactory progress is being made to achieve desired outcomes. Along with performance control, administrators establish other forms of control such as policies and regulations, to facilitate the attainment of desired performance. The external regulations and standards set by governmental and professional bodies influence the performance controlling processes (see Chapters 4 and 16).

NURSE-LEADER RESPONSIBILITIES

To design and implement an effective performance evaluation program, the first task of the nurse-executive and professional nursing staff includes the following steps:

1. Review the stated philosophy, purpose, and objectives of nursing services so that performance criteria and measurement tools can be designed to reflect them.

2. Make sure the general categories of the duties and responsibilities of each job description are stated in such a manner that standards of job performance can be identified for each job. For example, the job classification for nurse positions may be designed to achieve objectives and standards in clinical care, management, staff development (teaching), and research functions to achieve the goals and objectives of nursing services.

3. Consult with assistants and a quality control expert to develop an appraisal rating system for professional and nonprofessional employees. The

system must be appropriate to meet the purposes for which it will be used.

4. Develop and initiate a training program for all individuals who will use the appraisal tool.

5. Accept managerial and supervisory responsibilities to achieve organizational objectives and improve the performance of workers by means of effective communications.

6. Communicate with workers, informing them what is specifically expected of them, what is to be done, and how it is to be done for the attainment of both organizational and personal goals.

7. Assess workers' behavioral actions by close observation and provide guidance in setting their own objectives for effective behavioral changes over a period of time.

8. Assign appropriate authority to workers so they can act in an effective manner.

9. Interview, test, select, and train workers to perform the activities of their job to meet defined standards.

10. Initiate and support communication feedback among peers and between subordinates and their immediate superior.

11. Reduce and remove barriers and stumbling blocks to effective performance if possible.

12. Provide the necessary resources required for acceptable performance.

13. Use dimensions of a participative approach in performance appraisals to determine if the obligations and demands of the jobs are being met.

14. Implement the incentive compensation plan for commendable performance and penalties for substandard performance. The performance evaluation system must have the full support of top management.

15. Review periodically the effectiveness of the incentive plan and the total effectiveness of the performance evaluation program in consultation with staff members and top administrators.

PSYCHOLOGICAL CONSIDERATIONS OF WORK

When developing a sound, effective performance evaluation program, nurse-leaders should consider the psychological requirements as well as the technical content of each job. We might ask ourselves if we in practice accept the philosophy that each member of the organization has individual physical and psychological traits and an individual set of needs, drives, goals, and experiences?[36] Do the objectives and the organizational philosophy specifically support the psychological requirements of each job? Accepting Davis's concepts of each job,[4] one should recognize the following needs:

1. The job must be reasonably demanding of the worker in terms other than physical for it to provide for the full use of capacities in varied situations.
2. Each worker must know what the job is and how to perform in it.
3. Each worker must have the opportunity to learn on the job and to continue learning in a participative, trusting environment.
4. Each worker must have some area of decision making in order to exercise personal discretion.
5. Each worker must be able to relate the job to contributions to nursing, the hospital, and life in the community.
6. Each worker needs to feel that a standard performance of a job can lead to some kind of desirable future that may not necessarily involve promotion.

As we develop a controlling process as one element of a multiphase management system, we should consider the social system in our plans and actions. As the roles and environments of nursing services become more complex and jobs more flexible, nurse-leaders will need to vary their leadership behavior depending on the diagnosis of the problem and the individuals involved, such as a successful performance evaluation program, a trusting participative environment, and positive leadership roles.[8,13,34]

ESTABLISHMENT OF STANDARDS FOR PERFORMANCE

Most researchers agree that the validity of performance appraisals and their benefits for both the organization and employees in making decisions, determining who is best qualified for promotion, and determining needs depends on an established, planned program for evaluation. In addition, standards must be identified to compare and determine the level of a worker's performance. Appraisal results should never become a pseudo-objectivity of percentages and totals. MacKinnon and Eriksen[22] describe a flexible system for job descriptions, which also serves as an evaluation system by identifying the clinical or management components of positions as the standards for performance appraisal, using the checklist methodology.

Nelson and Arford[24] describe nurse positions in a progression of six steps from beginning staff nurse positions to top positions. The objectives and components of each job become the standard guidelines for performance appraisal and promotion. Marshall and Schau[23] describe a behaviorally oriented evaluation program for nursing assistants in which the staff identified and developed criteria for 18 categories of work performance such as emergency responsiveness, judgment, and skills. Harr and Kicks[11] point out the importance of identifying job duties and responsibilities of nurse jobs at the various levels of the hierarchy and the use of their general categories in preparing guidelines for performance appraisal.

Identifying a network of meaningful, desirable, and actionable standards for each job appears to be the best approach to performance appraisal for nursing service employees.

HISTORICAL DEVELOPMENT OF APPRAISAL METHODS

In the 1800s, Robert Owen introduced a formal rating system of appraisal in industry.[25] Using different colored blocks to indicate level of performance, Owen placed a colored block at each worker's bench to designate how well the worker had performed during the previous day. As mentioned in Chapter 6, Taylor[35] defined the basic measurement program for business enterprises. These early measurement systems were associated with various numerical efficiency factors involving work simplification and time and motion studies (see Chapter 9).

Between the 1920s and the 1940s, appraisal systems focused on rating the personality and behavioral traits of workers. In the 1950s the General Electric Company introduced the concept of management by objectives, measuring performance results against objectives. In 1970 a Supreme Court decision mandated that any type of testing procedure for a particular job must be directly related to the job duties to be performed, not to the person in the abstract. Reinforcing the Supreme Court's decision (Griggs vs. Duke Power Company), the guidelines of the Office of Federal Contract Compliance and the revised guidelines of the Equal Employment Opportunity Commission[7] in 1970 provided employee selection procedures. The EEOC guidelines define proper validation procedures and expectations for any test that is designed to facilitate personnel decisions for the purposes of selection, transfer, promotion, training, referral, or retention. In developing and implementing appraisal programs, it is vital that the evaluation criteria and rating methods should be constructed and validated in accordance with EEOC guidelines.

APPRAISAL METHODS

The traditional methods of performance appraisal include the forced-choice rating technique, the essay technique, the graphic rating scale, the checklist, field review methods, management by objectives, and the setting of standard techniques. Professional nurses and others should have a good understanding of the various techniques applied in rating a worker's performance, as well as the advantages and disadvantages of each technique when utilized for particular purposes.

Forced-choice rating technique

Forced-choice rating requires the rater to select from a group of statements those that best describe the individual being rated and that do not describe the performance. The statements are then weighted and scored, and workers with high scores are, by definition, better workers. The rater does not know the values assigned, and the worker's score is determined by someone other than the rater, reducing the possibility of bias on the part of the rater. However, this generally creates problems because raters feel they cannot be trusted to objectively evaluate their own workers. Forced-choice rating does not enhance trust between all employees, and furthermore, it is costly to develop the forms.[31]

Graphic rating scale

The graphic rating scale is commonly used. It requires the establishment of scales for each identified factor to be rated. Each individual who is rated is independently evaluated in relation to other individuals on graphic rating scale factors. The rater is required to assign a numerical value or letter grade to each dimension of performance, indicating judgments ranging from one (most unsatisfactory) to six (superior). Most raters accept this method, and it is easy to construct. The results, using the graphic rating scale, tend to be more consistent and fairly reliable.[33]

MacKinnon and Eriksen,[22] in developing a professional nurse classification and performance evaluation system, used the graphic scale technique. An individual nurse is evaluated only on those items that appear in the individualized job description. A rating scale from one (low) to seven (high) is used. For example, a nurse II task statement "initiates, implements, and modifies nursing care plans under the clinical practice components of the job description." The evaluation scale for this component provides several statements such as "interviews patients and families to obtain nursing history." The rater makes a judgment by circling the appropriate scale number from one to seven or opposite each statement.

The evaluations entered on a graphic rating scale represent evaluations in respect to job standards. Rating scale evaluations can be maintained over several years, and thus trends in a worker's specific behavior can be followed. Other worksheets are used to evaluate personal and professional attributes affecting job performance, such as attendance, communication, continuing education, and professional contributions. A final summary is made noting the major strengths and weaknesses of the worker's performance.

Marshall and Schau[23] also used the graphic scale technique to evaluate the performance of nursing assistants. Eighteen categories were involved. A weight of nine was given to the two highest categories, a weight of eight to the next two highest, and so on.

One of the problems with graphic scales is

that many ratings tend to be clustered toward the higher end, making it harder to differentiate performance levels of different people. Thus the graphic rating scale does not yield depth of information. The standards selected, based on the job description, must be comprehensive and chosen carefully. The rater must judge objectively. This scale is of little value in determining the training needs of the worker.

Checklist

The checklist was developed as an alternative to the graphic scales and is composed of a series of descriptive statements about the standard of performance of the job. The checklist requires the rater to make a "yes" or "no" judgment. In other words, it permits the rater to record whether behavior is present or absent or whether action was taken or not.

The items included in the checklist are weighted with preestablished values in order to secure a total rating. Thus, the relationships of each descriptive statement to the overall performance are determined before such a form can be used. A considerable amount of effort is required to develop a valid checklist form; however, it is easier to use than the graphic scale and tends to reduce bias.

Harr and Hicks[11] describe a periodic appraisal of workers' performance using the checklist technique. The rationale given for the use of the checklist included its efficiency and its use of specific behavioral language, thus permitting the evaluation of a large number of workers.

Critical incident technique

For some years, nurses have endeavored to use the critical incident technique to alert workers in particular areas of standard or substandard performance on a continuous basis. These critical incidents are recorded by the immediate superior and serve as the basis for the appraisal interview. The critical incidents method is directed primarily toward job performance without using predesignated standards. This method is useful in helping supervisors to do a better coaching

job and to communicate performance appraisal information to subordinates.

The critical incident technique does not provide an overall quantitative rating of each worker. However, it is helpful for identifying necessary areas of training or development. The disadvantage of this technique is that it requires the supervisor to record incidents daily or at least frequently. This can be time consuming and frequently difficult to accomplish.

Management by objectives

Management by objective depends on the superior's observations of the subordinate's performance, measured against specific predetermined goals that have been agreed on.[17] During the appraisal interview the superior discusses the evaluation results with the subordinate and they agree on new goals to be achieved in a specific period of time. This method encourages effective feedback in a participative, trusting climate. However, in some situations the worker's goals may not agree with those of management, and workers do not always want to participate in their own goal setting for the immediate future. Interview planning is discussed in Chapter 12.

Researchers emphasize that there is no one method of performance appraisal for use in every work setting with different individuals in different position classifications. However, the formulation of standards based on the duties of a job and the delegated responsibilities that use a checklist or graphic scale rating technique appear to be the best approaches for performance appraisal.

PERFORMING THE EVALUATION

The rater should review the previous appraisals and ongoing critical incidents of the subordinate who is to be evaluated. In many situations, individuals whose performances are subject to regular evaluation should have the opportunity for self-evaluation.[32] This means that performers should regularly be in a position to evaluate their own performances before being reviewed by the superior. When the coaching process is used effectively, workers do maintain an independent check on their work.

Traditionally, immediate superiors evaluate subordinates because of their delegated responsibility and accountability for the behavioral actions of workers on the unit. In addition to the authority-accountability factor, the immediate superior should be more knowledgeable than anyone, except the subordinates themselves, concerning the actions and efforts of the workers, because of ongoing close assessment and interactions that take place between subordinates and supervisors.

The rater uses the job description and the appraisal guidelines (standards) for each category of duties and responsibilities of the job when completing the predesigned evaluation forms, including remarks citing specific examples that relate to duties and responsibilities under each category.

One of the objectives of an evaluation performance program is to generate a fair and valid rating of each individual's performance and overcome all possible sources of bias. Frequently, when immediate su-

pervisors plan to evaluate nursing assistants, they will instruct staff nurses to fill out the rating forms on each nursing assistant. Then supervisors confer with staff nurses and compare scores to arrive at a consensus. This participative approach in decision making helps to reduce bias in rating a worker too high or too low on the form. However, the immediate supervisor of that unit is still responsible for the final decisions. Documentation of specific behavioral actions is most important.

As previously mentioned, professional nurses should be trained in rating workers and in counseling techniques so that a positive approach toward a good work performance becomes a reality.

The appraisal interview

Several goals of the performance evaluation program are to motivate workers to reach a higher level of performance, to set concrete goals, and to help the individual when performance should be improved.[42] The appraisal interview should provide for strengthening. It can serve to create better

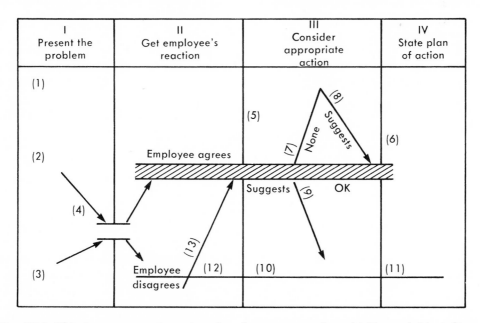

Fig. 17-1. This improvement interview chart has proven to be a highly workable indirect interview plan and should be helpful to nurses. The suggested "key phrases" are coded by numbers to correspond to the point where they would probably be used. (From Organizational communication, Chapter 3, p. 82 by Schneider, A. E. New York, 1975, McGraw-Hill Book Company. Used with permission of McGraw-Hill Book Company.)

understanding and trust between the supervisor and subordinate (see Fig. 17-1). The communication process, which is crucial in meeting the goals of both supervisor and worker, is discussed in detail in Chapter 12. The evaluator (source) should determine how much improvement can be expected of the worker and what approach will gain the performer's acceptance of goals.

Empathy is crucial in positive role leadership.[39] Kramer,[15] in a study of graduate nurses in their work environment, indicated that nurses in general do not rate particularly high on empathic ability related to cue sensitivity. Individuals with high empathic capacity can listen to feelings and nonverbal behavior as well as to words.

The worker being appraised should be encouraged to set work goals for the immediate future. The evaluation interview should focus on future performance instead of on the past. The primary functions of controls are prevention and adjustment as well as planning future actions.

An effective evaluation interview may fail if the supervisor does not follow-up on promises made during the interview. Coaching must be done to help the performer set goals. Checking progress with the worker periodically demonstrates the supervisor's sincerity in trying to make the evaluation an effective control process.

ACTING ON UNSATISFACTORY PERFORMANCE

When additional coaching, training, and disciplinary measures have failed to improve a worker's behavioral actions, the worker's immediate supervisor should initiate dismissal action.[9]

Prior to dismissal action, except in serious cases involving illegal acts or extreme subordination, the supervisor must follow proper disciplinary procedures that are formal written policies of the department and the hospital. If a worker's behavioral action presents dangers to patients and others, disciplinary procedures may be bypassed. However, explicit, specific documentation of the reasons for dismissal are necessary and must pertain to the duties of the job.

Disciplinary procedures usually include four steps:

1. Verbal warning documented by critical incident reports.[1] A copy of those reports should be filed in the worker's personal record, and the supervisor should retain the originals.

2. A documented written notice prepared by the supervisor, using the triplicate standard form which is signed by the supervisor and worker. The original copy is sent to the personnel department; one copy goes to the nurse-administrator, and the supervisor keeps the second copy.

3. Because of the legal, contractural, collective bargaining considerations involved in the dismissal of an employee, the supervisor must document the reasons for the action. The documentation must show that the employee received adequate training and appropriate coaching and assignments and that specific unsatisfactory behavioral actions did not improve after disciplinary action.[40,41]

4. The supervisor must review past and present appraisal ratings and written critical incident reports in preparing documentation. Administration does not want a losing case to go to grievance or arbitration, or to be placed in a position of rescinding a supervisor's dismissal action. Thus, documentation, coaching, and appraisal are important elements of the dismissal process.

ACTING ON GOOD PERFORMANCE

To reinforce and support workers who have given an exceptionally good performance, rewards should be given. Money is important to everyone but has a different significance depending on the content of variables of which it is a part.

For young people, money is a strong motivator because of its buying power. Money is a potential means of fulfillment for several of the higher needs of man. For example, increased monetary earnings that reward a good performance serve as a form of feedback to the worker. Money is a tangible gauge of achievement. Monetary and nonmonetary incentives can directly influence a worker's performance.[18]

When workers receive the expected reward for a good job, their motives are potentially fulfilled, and their trust and confidence in future motive-incentive situations are reinforced. Harris[12] presents a motivation model based on concepts of the Vroom[37] and

Porter and Lawler[27] models that describes a chain of events that must occur if action stimulated by incentives is to be attained and needs are to be fulfilled satisfactorily. On the other hand, if workers perform satisfactorily but do not receive the promised rewards, they will become distrustful of the incentive plan and disappointed at not earning the reward immediately.

Supervisors should know their workers' motives and how they evaluate rewards. A worker usually evaluates rewards on the basis of justice and fair treatment according to (1) the rewards first offered, (2) the personal input required to earn the rewards, and (3) the rewards that others have received for similar personal input. If workers perceive rewards as fair and equitable, the acceptance of them satisfies workers and gives them a feeling of accomplishment. This motivates them to reach for higher incentives for other rewards.

Thus, if wage or salary is related to performance, it is a motivator for efficient productivity. However, if it is unrelated to performance, it then serves as a maintenance factor or a dissatisfier. A merit raise recognizes an above average performance over a period of time. Studies indicate that merit increases above the promised yearly increment and other adjustments and benefits tend to attract and retain qualified professionals.

Compensation

The term *compensation* is generally preferred in describing organizational pay practices because the concept of compensation is broader in scope than other pay concepts.[33] Wage, salary, and remuneration pay concepts focus only on direct financial reimbursements, whereas the compensation pay design includes direct financial payments and indirect nonfinancial rewards. In general, some parties feel that a merit increase should be differentiated from other benefits and wage or salary adjustments such as the cost of living increase or yearly promised increments. There is a need to establish a logical, consistent, and systematic process. Factors or standards should be used to help

set pay rates and should be designed to measure pay adequacy, equity, need, and contribution. Different parties, in applying these criteria, frequently place more importance on some and less on others. Sikula[33] stresses that factors should not be considered separately, but should work together in determining pay rates.

PROBLEMS AND ISSUES OF WAGE AND SALARY ADMINISTRATION

In the United States, hospitals' wage and salary programs require careful planning and implementation. The criteria are prevailing pay, the ability to pay, union bargaining power, the cost of living, the average number of patient days and occupancy rates, and job requirements.[28]

The greatest difficulty in monetary motivation ties in with the expectancy part of the program. Organizations that use base pay supplemented by a merit-rating plan to determine periodic pay increases are less likely to create high expectancies than those that use individual incentive plans.[4]

How pay is actually administered is an important determinant of employees' perceptions concerning pay. The technical details of plans and the amount of distribution of monies cannot explain all the variances in individuals' perceptions because individuals often misperceive situations where wage or salary is involved.

Participation approach

Lawler[27] and Vroom,[38] based on research findings, indicate that the process, wage, and salary plans should be linked together as part of the elements of management to improve the effectiveness of the program. Some enterprises have found that employee participation has contributed to improving the total controlling manpower process. In a participative climate the employees gain more information about what is occurring and the problems of the organization to achieve desired outcomes.

Employees feel control over situations in their organization and possess a sense of commitment to decisions.[18] They also recognize more clearly the relationship between compensation and performance. The participative organizational approach between superiors and subordinates tends to create more pay satisfaction and to reduce absenteeism and turnover. On the other hand, underreward, overreward, and an inconsistent plan for rewards tend to create low satisfaction and encourage behavior that can prove dysfunctional to the attainment of organizational objectives.

A sound, consistent system of compensation helps to promote trust, equity, and satisfaction if the plan is understood and reasonably accepted by most of the employees.

Job evaluation

It should be mentioned that when new jobs are created or old ones revised they must be evaluated. As a first step in the pursuit of fairness, it is necessary to establish a consistent and systematic relationship among base compensation rates for all jobs in the hospital. This process is called "job evaluation."

In job evaluation, administrators endeavor to measure the inputs required of workers for minimum job performance and to translate such measures into specific monetary returns.[9] Thus, reasonably clear and accurate job descriptions and specifications must be available to provide data concerning the factors to be measured. In addition, a decision must be made concerning the groups of employees and jobs to be covered by a single evaluation plan.

Professional nurses and nurse-executives should be familiar with the job evaluation methods their institution uses. Alternative methods include simple ranking, job grading, the point system, and factor comparison. The grade description method may be used. General job classifications and grades are first established and then ranked in relation to one another (grade I, grade II, and so forth, to grade X). Specific positions are placed within and assigned to various grades. They are usually ranked in relationship to other positions within the same job classification, such as professional staff nurse I, II, and III. Thus wage and salary issues, prob-

lems, criteria, and systems are closely interrelated compensation matters. Sikula[33] views compensation and wage and salary administration as a multiphase interrelated system composed of three main elements: (1) principal wage and salary issues and problems, (2) wage and salary criteria, and (3) job evaluation.

MOTIVATIONAL, BEHAVIORAL, AND LEADERSHIP CONCEPTS

Motivation is concerned with the "why" of behavior and what makes us act as we do. We often hear, "How do I get my staff to do what I want them to do?" The leadership, regardless of the individual's position in an organization, is a relationship between one person and one or several others. Leadership is not a set of personality traits or characteristics of a particular individual, but a complexity of human and environmental interactions among individuals in a particular group. Vroom[38] emphasizes the fact that throughout the ages, no one has found the magical leadership trait, the one best management style, or the one single set of guidelines that, if followed, will ensure effective organizational performance.

Meaning of leadership

In management literature, one finds many definitions of leadership. However, researchers agree on several facts concerning effective leadership. They are as follows:

• Leadership is a process of influence in which one individual stimulates a positive response in other group members to achieve group goals. In work groups, formal leaders will engage in influential behavior more often than the group members. Also, most formal leaders receive much feedback from their subordinates, as well as from their supervisors.

• Effective leadership means effective and productive group performance. However, leaders who perform well in one group situation may not perform effectively in another. Thus, one can only say that a person performed well in one type of situation and poorly in another.

• Leadership may be viewed as a form of

dominance in which subordinates more or less willingly accept direction and control from their assigned leader toward goal setting and goal achievement. Thus, leadership is a relationship based on power and influence.

Likert[19] points out that effective supervision results when leaders pattern their behavior on the recognition of the values, drives, and interpersonal skills of those with whom they interact.

As organizational variables change, one determines to a degree if the present leader's personality and style will be effective in the leadership situation. When these variables change, the leader's style may not fit the leadership situation.

Various personnel strategies and organizational changes affect leadership control. When there are changes in superiors, control is temporarily decreased due to subordinates' uncertainty about their abilities to satisfy superiors' standards and goals. Likewise, a leader's control is temporarily decreased when there is a change in the work group or in the method of assignment, schedules, or job tasks.

Leadership attributes tend to be associated with judgment, facility, the desire to communicate with others, and the drive and confidence to achieve goals. A leader's intelligence should be close to that of the followers, for leaders who are too smart or not smart enough may lose their followers' respect.

BASIC MOTIVATIONAL CONCEPTS OF WORKERS

Human behavior must be understood before it can be effectively managed and controlled. This applies to the leader and the followers.

In management, Herzberg's[14] two-factor theory of satisfaction is that the primary determinants (satisfiers) of a job are the intrinsic factors such as the job content, responsibility, achievement, recognition, and advancement. These intrinsic factors become the motivators. It is perceived that individuals are motivated to obtain more of them through good work performance.

The environmental (hygienic) factors are termed the dissatisfiers of a job. They include schedules and other work conditions, salary, and supervisory practices and are the extrinsic factors that surround workers. Herzberg's[14] theory suggests that a job should produce positive work motivation and that workers should be satisfied because the job provides opportunities for recognition, growth, competence, and advancement.

In recent years researchers have found that satisfaction and dissatisfaction can be derived from both intrinsic and extrinsic job factors. Most modern motivation concepts are broader, including social, economic, and technological components and psychological, cultural, and ethical factors. For example, many external environmental actions that now affect the role of nursing have social, ethical, economic, and political implications. We also find that in designing the content of nurses' jobs for the clinical practice of nursing inpatient care one must consider the psychologic requirements of a job to achieve good performance results.

Motivational and environmental factors are somewhat interrelated and overlapping in nature. Sikula[33] and others classify all behavioral motivation theories into three categories—individual, group, and environmental factors within one interacting system (Fig. 17-2).

ORGANIZATIONAL CLIMATE, MORALE, AND LEADERSHIP

Organizational climate and morale are closely related and difficult to define. In general, an organization's climate consists of its unique culture, traditions, and methods of operation to achieve its goals. For example, the hospital climate consists of nurses' and physicians' ethical and cultural concepts about their respective professions, themselves in their jobs, and the hospital. Conflicts between nurses, physicians, and administrators stem from traditions and the traditional approaches toward patient care services. Morale is defined as the attitude of individuals and groups toward their work environment.

Data from researchers' findings show a

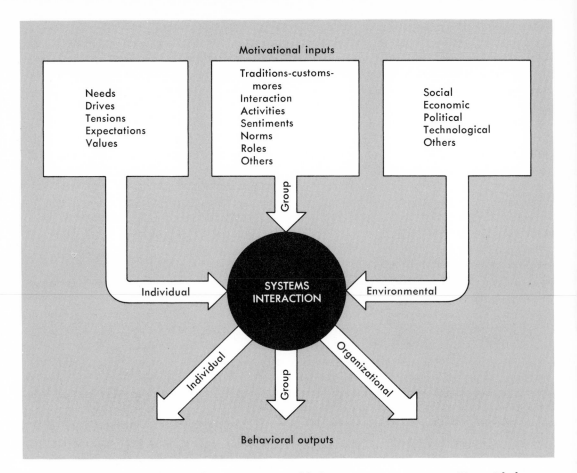

Fig. 17-2. A systems framework to motivation and behavior in an organization. (From Sikula, A. F.: Personnel administration and human resources management, New York, 1976, John Wiley & Sons, Inc., p. 89.)

lack of strong correlation between good organizational climate, high employee morale, and high quality of work performance. There are so many factors or variables that influence job satisfaction, morale, and climate that there are no definite conclusions.

Organizations attempt to assess the climate and workers' job satisfaction by studying such events as turnover, absenteeism, accidents, grievances, and interviews. Brief,[3] based on findings, states that the high rate of turnover exhibited by nurses is related to job content and salary dissatisfaction. The dissatisfaction factors were that the jobs lacked skill variety, task identity, autonomy, and feedback. A nurse who placed a high value on salary and did not derive satisfaction from the work became dissatisfied with the rewards and thus resigned.

The study by Kramer and Schmalenberg[16] on a staff nurse's first job indicates that the new graduate brings values and behaviors learned in the school subculture. Frequently these values and behaviors conflict with the subcultural values and behavior of the work, resulting in conflicts between the new staff member and established staff members. Here a leadership is needed that recognizes the value of empathy in interpersonal relations and coaching.

Gerstenfield's studies[10] indicate only one variable of the organization appeared to be related to employee absenteeism—the style of leadership. Frequently, the workers who felt that their superior was unfair had the poorest attendance records. He found that in these cases the leader was more important than the job itself.

Porter and others[27] state that the turnover organizations experience is controllable to a degree because it stems from individuals who are dissatisfied with how their careers are developing. The jobs they have taken do not give them the rewards and outcomes they expected, and they decide to try jobs in another organization that they perceive as more likely to satisfy their needs and goals. Thus the initial interview and testing of a candidate and ongoing evaluation and coaching by the superior or the staff development counselor could reduce turnover. Coaching is an effective tool to help individuals achieve present goals and prepare themselves to meet new needs and goals.

Leadership as a shared organizational process

Porter,[27] Likert,[19] and others emphasize that leadership requires power and influence. How much power and influence nurse-leaders get from their superiors, how their jobs and those of their followers are designed, and the degree of authority delegated and the support they obtain from group members and superiors are crucial factors in a leadership role.

When nurse-leaders know that subordinates will follow directions they feel more in control of the behavioral actions of the group. When nurse-leaders know all aspects, what, how, and when of their jobs and those of their followers, practice effective communication feedback, and have the opportunity and authority to do their jobs, they know they have control over their behavioral actions and those of others. Everyone knows that these leaders are good coaches and assessors who give rewards for good performance and take corrective action for poor performance.

On the other hand, if a leader is uncertain of the group's willingness to follow, if the jobs are unstructured or too rigid, and if authority is not clarified, this leader is unable to make decisions or control actions. Thus, the desired outcomes are unpredictable. The control of information and rewards can influence the attitudes and behavior of group members. A formal leader should be in a strong position to affect what followers do and how well they do it.

We hear it said that there is a critical need for effective clinical nurse-managers. Commonly cited is the Peter principle—that an individual is promoted to the level of incompetence that is beyond his capacity to effectively perform. All people have their level of incompetence, despite intense efforts to improve the technology and judgment in selection, and mistakes will continue to be made.

In recent years, nursing services have placed qualified professional nurses with patients to provide for quality nursing care. For years, fairly experienced leaders led the inexperienced in the most important elements of nursing service—the clinical care of patients and the management of that care. There is now evidence of more collaboration between superiors and subordinates; the multitiered hierarchy is being restructured to a minimum, and the climate of cooperation and trust is replacing uncertainty, tension, and conflict.

LEADERSHIP STYLES

Several approaches are used by those who serve in a formal leadership capacity. The three common styles are the autocratic, the participative, and the collegial, as discussed in Chapter 11.

Schien[29] emphasizes the value of McGregor's Theory in managing the behavioral actions of people in the organization (Fig. 17-2). Likert's[19] eight-fold leadership classification system and Davis's[4] four-fold classification leadership style (Fig. 17-3) depict managerial styles on the leadership continuum, according to their respective degrees of authoritarianism. Vroom and Yetton[38] have identified five behavioral styles.

The styles of leadership in decision making may be summarized as follows:

1. The leader solves the problem or makes the decision himself, using information available to him at that time.

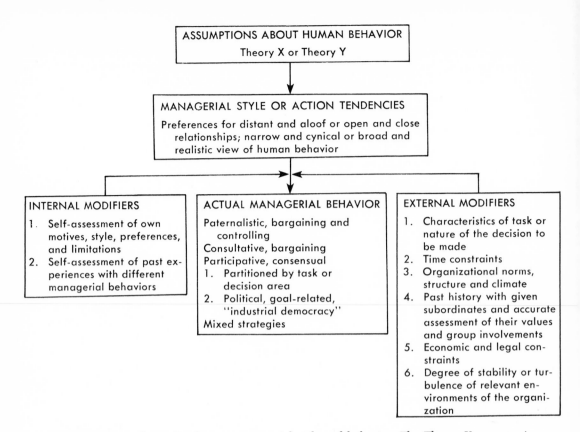

Fig. 17-3. How Theory Y relates to managerial style and behavior. The Theory Y manager is more likely to make an accurate internal and external diagnosis and consequently choose a behavior pattern that is appropriate to the realities of the situation. (From Man and work in society edited by Cass and Zimmer © 1975 Western Electric Company, Inc. Reprinted by permission of Van Nostrand Reinhold Company.)

2. The leader obtains necessary information from subordinates, and then decides on the solution to the problem himself. Subordinates are not involved in generating or evaluating alternative solutions.

3. The leader shares the problem with relevant subordinates individually, getting their ideas and suggestions without bringing them together as a group. Then the leader makes the decision—which may or may not reflect the influence of the subordinates.

4. The leader shares the problem with his subordinates as a group, collectively obtaining their ideas and suggestions. Then he makes the decision—which again may or may not reflect the influence of the subordinates.

5. The leader shares the problem with subordinates as a group. Together the leader and the subordinates generate and evaluate alternatives and attempt to reach agreement on a solution.

The nurse's position in the organization itself, specific problems to be resolved, characteristics of the individuals involved, and the nature of the communication process between superiors and subordinates all affect leadership behavior. The current emphasis is that managerial leadership should be flexible and adaptive in approach and that leaders should adjust their styles according to factors in the organization, within themselves, in subordinates, and in the task situation.

LEADERSHIP'S BEHAVIORAL FRAMEWORK

An individual who has leadership responsibilities concerning the management and control of human and financial resources performs different leadership functions at different times.

Dunnetter's[6] framework of effective

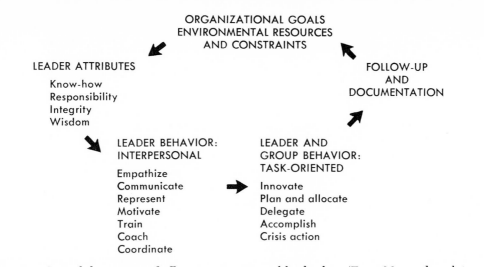

Fig. 17-4. Critical dimensions of effective organizational leadership. (From Man and work in society edited by Cass and Zimmer © 1975 Western Electric Company, Inc. Reprinted by permission of Van Nostrand Reinhold Company.)

leadership in organizations (Fig. 17-4) consists of 17 categories of what a manager must do to get his job done effectively and efficiently. Dunnetter's model emphasizes that the leader must depend on personal knowledge and capabilities to engage individuals and groups in social interaction toward decision making concerning resources and constraints to meet determined goals.

Leadership functions

If a group is to achieve its goals effectively over a period of time, two general types of leadership function must be fulfilled. They pertain to diagnoses and execution.

Porter[27] and others group administrative leadership functions and activities into two distinct yet interrelated functions: (1) diagnoses of internal and external functions by means of monitoring and forecasting and (2) execution of internal and external functions by taking action and creating conditions.

The challenge to each nurse-leader is to find the right approach for each situation and then to perform the role that is appropriate with that approach.

It seems evident that nursing, based on scientific and humanistic concepts, will be administered and coordinated by professional nurses who will be constantly intent on innovations and change and alert always

to the evaluation of change, according to how behavioral actions are affected and how they may be improved still further to provide quality nursing care to consumers in the years ahead.

REFERENCES

1. Baer, W. E.: Grievance handling, New York, 1970, The American Management Association.
2. Bailey, J. T., and Claus, K. E.: Decision making in nursing—tools for change, St. Louis, 1975, The C. V. Mosby Co., chapters 13 and 15.
3. Brief, A. P.: Turnover among hospital nurses: a suggested model, Journal of Nursing Administration **6**:55-57, Oct., 1976
4. Davis, K.: Human relations at work, New York, 1972, McGraw-Hill Book Co., chapter 24.
5. Donnelly, J. H., et al.: Fundamentals of management—functions, behavior, models, rev. ed., Dallas, 1975, Business Publications, Inc.
6. Dunnetter, M. D.: The Hawthorne effects: its societal meaning. In Cass, E., and Zimmer, F. G., editors: Man and work in society, New York, 1975, Van Nostrand Reinhold Co., pp. 237–245.
7. Equal Employment Opportunity Commission: Guidelines of employment and selection procedure, Federal Register **35**(149):12333-12336, 1970.
8. Fiedler, F. E., and Chemers, M. M.: Leadership and effective management, Glenview, Ill. 1974, Scott, Foresman & Company.
9. Flippo, E. B.: Principles of personnel management, ed. 4, New York, 1976, McGraw-Hill Book Co., chapters 12-15.
10. Gerstenfield, A.: Employee absenteeism—new insights, Business Horizons **12**(5):51-57, 1969.

11. Harr, L. P., and Hicks, J. H.: Performance appraisal: derivation of effective assessment tools, Journal of Nursing Administration **6:**20-29, Sept., 1976.

12. Harris, O. J., Jr.: Managing people at work, New York, 1976, John Wiley & Sons, Inc., chapters 7-13.

13. Harrison, R.: Understanding your organization's character, Harvard Business Review **50**(3):119-129, 1972.

14. Herzberg, F., et al.: The motivation to work, New York, 1959, John Wiley & Sons, Inc.

15. Kramer, M.: Reality shock: why nurses leave nursing, St. Louis, 1974, The C. V. Mosby Co.

16. Kramer, M., and Schmalenberg, C.: The first job: a proving ground—basis for empathy development, Journal of Nursing Administration **7:**13-20, Jan., 1977.

17. Levinson, H.: Management by whose objectives? Harvard Business Review, **48:**125-134, July-August, 1970.

18. Levinson, H.: The conceptual context for compensation. In Cass, E., and Zimmer, F. G., editors: Man and work in society, New York, 1976, Van Nostrand Reinhold Co., chapter 10.

19. Likert, R.: The human organization, New York, 1974, McGraw-Hill Book Co.

20. McGregor, D.: An uneasy look at performance. In Stone, S., Berger, M. S., Elhart, D., Firsich, S. C., and Jordan, S. B., editors: Management for nurses, St. Louis, 1976, The C. V. Mosby Co., chapter 9.

21. McGregor, D.: The professional manager, New York, 1967, McGraw-Hill Book Co.

22. MacKinnon, H. A., and Eriksen: C.A.R.E.—a four-track professional nurse classification performance evaluation system, Journal of Nursing Administration **7:**42-44, March-April, 1977.

23. Marshall, J. R., and Schau, E.: An evaluation process for nursing assistants. In Journal of Nursing Administration staff, editors: Quality control and performance appraisal, vol. 2, Wakefield, Mass., 1976, Contemporary Publishing, Inc., pp. 22-25.

24. Nelson, C. A., and Arford, P. H.: Strategy for clinical advancement, Journal of Nursing Administration **7**(4):46-51, 1977.

25. Owen, R.: The life of Robert Owen, New York, 1920, Alfred A. Knopf, pp. 111-112. (From the original published in 1857.)

26. Paul, W. J., et al.: Job enrichment pays off, Harvard Business Review **47:**61-78, 1969.

27. Porter, L. W., Lawler, E., and Hackman, J.: Behaviors in organizations, New York, 1975, McGraw-Hill Book Co.

28. Prasow, P., and Edwards, P.: Arbitration and collective bargaining, New York, 1970, McGraw-Hill Book Co.

29. Schein, E. H.: How theory Y relates to managerial style and behavior. In Cass, E., and Zimmer. F. G., editors: Man and work in society, New York, 1976, Van Nostrand Reinhold Co., chapter 6.

30. Schneider, A. E., et al.: Organizational communication, New York, 1975, McGraw-Hill Book Co., chapter 3.

31. Schneider, E. V.: The social relations of industry and the community, ed. 2, New York, 1969, McGraw-Hill Book Co., chapter 8.

32. Schranger, S., and Patterson, M. B.: Self-evaluation and the selection of dimensions for evaluating others, Journal of Personality **42**(4), 1974.

33. Sikula, A. F.: Personnel administration and human resources management, New York, 1976, John Wiley & Sons, Inc.

34. Tannenbaum, R., and Schmidt, W. H.: How to choose a leadership pattern. In Tannenbaum, R., editor: Leadership and organization, New York, 1961, McGraw-Hill Book Co., pp. 67-79.

35. Taylor, F. W.: The principles of scientific management, New York, 1911, Harper and Brothers.

36. Traux, C. B., et al.: Therapeutic relationships provided by various professionals, Journal of Community Psychiatry **2**(1):32-36, 1974.

37. Vroom, V. H.: Work and motivation, New York, 1964, John Wiley & Sons, Inc.

38. Vroom, V. H., and Yetton, P. W.: Leadership and decision-making, Pittsburgh, 1973, University of Pittsburgh Press.

39. Weinstein, E., Feldman, K. A., and Goodman N., et al.: Empathy and communication efficiency, Journal of Social Psychology **88:**247-254.

40. Woodworth, R. T., and Peterson, R. B.: Collective negotiations for public and professional employees, Glenview, Ill., 1969, Scott, Foresman & Co.

41. Yoder, D.: Personnel management and industrial relations, Englewood Cliffs, N.J., 1970, Prentice-Hall, Inc., pp. 229-231.

42. Zeitlin, L. R.: Planning for a successful performance review program, Personnel Journal Dec., 1969, p. 958.

INDEX